ESSENTIAL STATISTICAL METHODS
FOR MEDICAL STATISTICS

Essential Statistical Methods for Medical Statistics

A derivative of Handbook of Statistics: Epidemiology and Medical Statistics, Vol. 27

Edited by

C.R. Rao

Center for Multivariate Analysis
Department of Statistics, The Pennsylvania State University
University Park, PA, USA

J.P. Miller

Division of Biostatistics
School of Medicine, Washington University in St. Louis
St. Louis, MO, USA

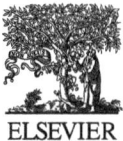

D.C. Rao

Division of Biostatistics
School of Medicine, Washington University in St. Louis
St. Louis, MO, USA

Amsterdam • Boston • Heidelberg • London • New York • Oxford
Paris • San Diego • San Francisco • Singapore • Sydney • Tokyo
North-Holland is an imprint of Elsevier

ELSEVIER

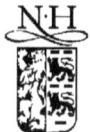

North Holland is an imprint of Elsevier
30 Corporate Drive, Suite 400, Burlington, MA 01803, USA
Linacre House, Jordan Hill, Oxford OX2 8DP, UK
Radarweg 29, PO Box 211, 1000 AE Amsterdam, The Netherlands

First edition 2011

British Library Cataloguing in Publication Data
A catalogue record for this book is available from the British Library

Library of Congress Cataloging-in-Publication Data
A catalog record for this book is available from the Library of Congress

ISBN: 978-0-444-53737-9

For information on all North Holland publications
visit our web site at books.elsevier.com

Transferred to Digital Printing in 2012

Table of Contents

Contributors

Bang, Heejung, *Division of Biostatistics and Epidemiology, Department of Public Health weill Medical college of Cornell University, New York, NY 10021; e-mail: heb2013@med.cornell.edu* (Ch. 9).

Bentler, Peter M., *University of California, Los Angeles, UCLA Psych-Measurement, Box 951563, 4627 FH, Los Angeles, CA 90095-1563; e-mail: bentler@ucla.edu* (Ch. 7).

Edwards, Lloyd J., *Department of Biostatistics, CB 7420, University of North Carolina, Chapel Hill, NC 27599-7420; e-mail: lloyd_edwards@une.edu* (Ch. 5).

Edwards, Michael C., *The Ohio State University, 1827 Neil Ave, Columbus, OH 43210; e-mail: edwards.134@osu.edu* (Ch. 6).

Glidden, David V., *Division of Biostatistics, Department of Epidemiology and Biostatistics, University of California, San Francisco, 185 Berry Street, 5700, San Francisco, CA 94143; e-mail: dave@biostat.ucsf.edu* (Ch. 3).

Greene, William H., *New York University, Henry Kaufman Mgmt Ctr, 44 West 4 Street, 7-78, New York City, NY 10012, NYU Mail Code: 0251; e-mail: wgreene@stern.nyu.edu* (Ch. 4).

Gurka, Matthew J., *Division of Biostatistics and Epidemiology, Department of Public Health Sciences, School of Medicine, University of Virginia, Charlottesville, VA 22908-0717; e-mail: mgurka@virginia.edu* (Ch. 5).

Hagan, Joseph L., *Biostatistics Program, School of Public Health, Louisiana State University Health Sciences Center, 2021 Lakeshore Dr., Suite 210, New Orleans, LA 70122; e-mail: jhagan@lsuhsc.edu* (Ch. 2).

Hayashi, Kentaro, *Department of Psychology, University of Hawaii at Manoa, 2430 Campus Drive, Honolulu, HI 96822; e-mail: hayashik@hawaii.edu* (Ch. 7).

Hernández, Bernardo, *Direccion de Salud Reproductiva Centro de Investigacion en Salud Poblacional, Instituto Nacional de Salud Publica, Cuernavaca, Morelos, Mexico 62508; e-mail: bhernand@insp.mx* (Ch. 10).

Hilbe, Joseph M., *School of Social and Family Dynamics, Arizona State University, Tempe, AZ 85232; e-mail: hilbe@asu.edu* (Ch. 4).

Horton, Nicholas J., *Department of Mathematics and Statistics, Smith College, Burton Hall 314, Northampton, MA 01063; e-mail: nhorton@email.smith.edu* (Ch. 10).

Laird, Nan M., *Department of Biostatistics, Harvard School of Public Health, Bldg 2, 4th FL, 655 Huntington Ave, Boston, MA 02115*; e-mail: *laird@biostat.harvard.edu* (Ch. 10).

Lecoutre, Bruno, *ERIS, Laboratoire de Mathématiques Raphael Salem, UMR 6085 C.N.R.S. and Université de Rouen, Avenue de l'Université, BP 12, 76801 Saint-Etienne-du-Rouvray (France)*; e-mail: *bruno.lecoutre@univ-rouen.fr* (Ch. 11).

Litman, Heather J., *New England Research Institutes, 9 Galen Street, Watertown, MA 02472*; e-mail: *litmanh@yahoo.com* (Ch. 10).

Looney, Stephen W., *Department of Biostatistics, Medical College of Georgia, 1120 15th Street, AE-3020, Augusta, GA 30912-4900*; e-mail: *slooney@mcg.edu* (Ch. 2).

Mazumdar, Madhu, *Division of Biostatistics and Epidemiology, Department of Public Health Weill Medical College of Cornell University, 411 East 69th Street, New York, NY 10021*; e-mail: *mam2073@med.cornell.edu* (Ch. 9).

McCulloch, Charles E., *Division of Biostatistics, Department of Epidemiology and Biostatistics, University of California, San Francisco, 185 Berry Street, 5700, San Francisco, CA 94143*; e-mail: *cmcculloch@epi-ucsf.org* (Ch. 3).

Prentice, Ross L., *Division of Public Health Sciences, Fred Hutchinson Cancer Research Center, 1100 Fairview Avenue North, Seattle, WA 98109-1024*; e-mail: *rprentic@fhcrc.org* (Ch. 1).

Shiboski, Stephen C., *Division of Biostatistics, Department of Epidemiology and Biostatistics, University of California, San Francisco, 185 Berry Street, 5700, San Francisco, CA 94143*; e-mail: *steve@biostat.ucsf.edu* (Ch. 3).

Vittinghoff, Eric, *Division of Biostatistics, Department of Epidemiology and Biostatistics, University of California, San Francisco, 185 Berry Street, 5700, San Francisco, CA 94143*; e-mail: *eric@biostat.ucsf.edu* (Ch. 3).

Woods, Carol M., *Psychology Department, Washington University in St. Louis, Campus Box 1125, St. Louis, MO 63130*; e-mail: *cwoods@artsci.wustl.edu* (Ch. 6).

Xiong, Chengjie, *Division of Biostatistics, Campus Box 8067, Washington University School of Medicine, 660 S. Euclid Ave, St. Louis, MO 63110-1093*; e-mail: *chengjie@wubios.wustl.edu* (Ch. 8).

Yu, Kai, *Biostatistics Branch, Division of Cancer Epidemiology and Genetics National Cancer Institute Executive Plaza South, Room 8050 Bethesda, MD 20892*; e-mail: *yuka@mail.nih.gov* (Ch. 8).

Yuan, Ke-Hai, *University of Notre Dame, 105 Haggar Hall, Notre Dame, IN 46556*; e-mail: *ke-hai.yuan.5@nd.edu* (Ch. 7).

Zhu, Kejun, *School of Management, China University of Geosciences, Wuhan, PRC 4330074*; e-mail: *zhubingl@public.wh.hb.cn* (Ch. 8).

Handbook of Statistics, Vol. 27
ISSN: 0169-7161
DOI: 10.1016/S0169-7161(07)27001-4

Statistical Methods and Challenges in Epidemiology and Biomedical Research

Ross L. Prentice

Abstract

This chapter provides an introduction to the role, and use, of statistics in epidemiology and in biomedical research. The presentation focuses on the assessment and understanding of health-related associations in a study cohort. The principal context considered is estimation of the risk of health events in relation to individual study subject characteristics, exposures, or treatments, generically referred to as 'covariates'. Descriptive models that focus on relative and absolute risks in relation to preceding covariate histories will be described, along with potential sources of bias in estimation and testing. The role, design, and conduct of randomized controlled trials will also be described in this prevention research context, as well as in therapeutic research. Some aspects of the sources and initial evaluation of ideas and concepts for preventive and therapeutic interventions will be discussed. This leads naturally to a discussion of the role and potential of biomarkers in biomedical research, for such purposes as exposure assessment, early disease diagnosis, or for the evaluation of preventive or therapeutic interventions. Recently available biomarkers, including high-dimensional genomic and proteomic markers, have potential to add much knowledge about disease processes and to add specificity to intervention development and evaluation. These data sources are attended by many interesting statistical design and analysis challenges. A brief discussion of ongoing analytic and explanatory analyses in the Women's Health Initiative concludes the presentation.

1. Introduction

The topic of this chapter is too broad to allow an in-depth coverage of its many important aspects. The goal, rather, will be to provide an introduction to some specific topics, many of which will be covered in later chapters, while attempting to provide a unifying framework to motivate statistical issues that arise in biomedical research, and to motivate some of the models and methods used to address these issues.

Much of epidemiology, and biomedical research more generally, involves following a set of study 'subjects', often referred to as the study cohort. Much valuable basic biological research involves the study of lower life forms. Such studies are often attended by substantial homogeneity among study subjects, and relatively short life spans. Here, instead, the presentation will focus on a cohort of humans, in spite of the attendant greater heterogeneity and statistical challenges. For research purposes the individuals in a cohort are of interest through their ability to yield health-related information pertinent to a larger population. Such a larger population may, for example, include persons residing in the geographic areas from which cohort members are drawn, who meet certain eligibility and exclusionary criteria. The ability to infer health-related information about the larger population involves assumptions about the representativeness of the cohort for the 'target' population. This typically requires a careful characterization of the cohort so that the generalizability of study findings can be defined. The target population is often somewhat conceptual, and is usually taken to be practically infinite in size. The major long-term goal of biomedical research is to decrease the burden of premature disease morbidity and mortality, and to extend the period of time that members of target populations live without major health-related restrictions.

The principal focus of epidemiologic research is understanding the determinants of disease risk among healthy persons, with a particular interest in modifiable risk factors, such as dietary or physical activity patterns, or environmental exposures. There is a long history of epidemiologic methods development, much of which is highly statistical, whose aim is to enhance the likelihood that associations between study subject characteristics or exposures and disease risk are causal, thereby providing reliable concepts for disease prevention.

The availability of disease screening programs or services, and the health care-seeking behavior of cohort members, have potential to affect the timing of disease diagnosis. Early disease detection may allow the disease course to be interrupted or altered in a manner that is beneficial to the individual. Disease screening research has its own set of methodologic challenges, and is currently the target of intensive efforts to discover and validate early detection 'biomarkers'.

Much biomedical research is directed to the study of cohorts of person having a defined disease diagnosis, with emphasis on the characterization of prognosis and, especially, on the development of treatments that can eradicate the disease or can facilitate disease management, while avoiding undue adverse effects.

The ultimate products of biomedical research are interventions, biomarkers, or treatments that can be used to prevent, diagnose, or treat disease. Additionally, the knowledge of the biology of various life forms and the methodologic knowledge that underlies the requisite research agenda, constitutes important and durable contributions from biomedical research. These developments are necessarily highly interdisciplinary, and involve a wide spectrum of disciplines. Participating scientists may include, for example, molecular geneticists studying biological processes in yeast; technologists developing ways to assess a person's genome or proteome in a rapid and reliable fashion; population scientists studying disease-occurrence patterns in large human cohorts; and expert panels and government regulators synthesizing research developments and providing recommendations and regulations for consumption by the general population.

Statisticians and other quantitative scientists have important roles to fulfill throughout this research spectrum. Issues of study design, quality control, data analysis, and reporting are important in each biomedical research sector, and resolving methodologic challenges is crucial to progress in some areas. The biomedical research enterprise includes natural tensions, for example, basic versus applied research; in-depth mechanistic research versus testing of current concepts; and independent versus collaborative research. Statisticians can have a unifying role across related cultural research norms, through the opportunity to bring ideas and motivations from one component of this research community to another in a non-threatening manner, while simultaneously applying critical statistical thinking and methods to the research at hand.

2. Characterizing the study cohort

A general regression notation can be used to represent a set of exposures and characteristics to be ascertained in a cohort under study. Let $z(u)' = \{z_1(u), z_2(u), \ldots\}$ be a set of numerically coded variables that describe an individual's exposures and characteristics at 'time' u, where, to be specific, u can be defined as time from selection into the cohort, and a prime ($'$) denotes vector transpose. Let $Z(t) = \{z(u), u < t\}$ denote the history of each covariate at times less than t. The 'baseline' covariate history $Z(0)$ may include information that pertains to time periods prior to selection into the cohort.

Denote by $\lambda\{t, Z(t)\}$ the occurrence rate for a health event of interest in the targeted population at cohort follow-up time t, among persons having a preceding covariate history $Z(t)$. A typical cohort study goal is to assess the relationship between aspects of $Z(t)$ and the corresponding disease rate $\lambda\{t; Z(t)\}$. Doing so involves recording over time the pertinent covariate histories and health event histories for cohort members, whether the cohort is comprised of healthy individuals as in an epidemiologic cohort study or disease prevention trial, or persons having a defined disease in a therapeutic context. The notation $Z(t)$ is intended to encompass evolving, time-varying covariates, but also to include more restrictive specifications in which, for example, only baseline covariate information is included.

A cohort available for study will typically have features that distinguish it from the target population to which study results may be applied. For example, an epidemiologic cohort study may enroll persons who are expected to continue living in the same geographic area for some years, or who are expected to be able and willing to participate in research project activities. A therapeutic cohort may have characteristics that depend on institutional referral patterns and clinical investigator experience and expertise. Hence, absolute health event (hereafter 'disease') occurrence rates may be less pertinent and transferable to the target population, than are relative rates that contrast disease rates among persons receiving different treatments or having different exposures.

The hazard ratio regression model of Cox (1972) captures this relative risk notion, without imposing further restrictions on corresponding absolute rates. It can be written

$$\lambda\{t; Z(t)\} = \lambda_0(t) \exp\{x(t)'\beta\}, \tag{1}$$

where $x(t)' = \{x_1(t), \ldots, x_p(t)\}$ is a modeled regression p-vector formed from $Z(t)$ and product (interaction) terms with t, $\beta' = (\beta_1, \ldots, \beta_p)$ is a corresponding hazard ratio, or relative risk, parameter to be estimated, and $\lambda_0(\cdot)$ is an unrestricted 'baseline' hazard function corresponding to $x(t) \equiv 0$. For example, $x(t) \equiv x_1$ may be an indicator variable for active versus placebo treatment in a prevention trial, or an indicator for test versus the standard treatment in a therapeutic trial, in which case e^{β_1} is the ratio of hazard rates for the test versus the control group, and there may be special interest in testing $\beta_1 = 0$ ($e^{\beta_1} = 1$). Such a constant hazard ratio model can be relaxed, for example, to $x(t) = \{x_1, x_1 \log t\}$ in which case the 'treatment' hazard ratio function becomes $e^{\beta_1} t^{\beta_2}$, which varies in a smooth manner with 'follow-up time' t. Alternatively, one may define $x(t)$ to include a quantitative summary of a study subject's prior exposure to an environmental or lifestyle factor in an epidemiologic context.

Let T be the time to occurrence of a disease under study in a cohort. Typically some, and perhaps most, of cohort members will not have experienced the disease at the time of data analysis. Such a cohort member yields a 'censored disease event time' that is known to exceed the follow-up time for the individual. Let Y be a process that takes value $Y(t) = 1$ if a subject is 'at risk' (i.e., without prior censoring or disease occurrence) for a disease event at follow-up time t, and $Y(t) = 0$ otherwise. Then a basic independent censoring assumption requires

$$\lambda\{t; Z(t), Y(u) = 1, u < t\} = \lambda\{t; Z(t)\},$$

so that the set of individuals under active follow-up is assumed to have a disease rate that is representative for the cohort given $Z(t)$, at each follow-up time t. The hazard ratio parameter β in (1) is readily estimated by maximizing the so-called partial likelihood function (Cox, 1975)

$$L(\beta) = \prod_{i=1}^{k} \left[\frac{\exp\{x_i(t_i)'\beta\}}{\sum_{l \in R(t_i)} \exp\{x_l(t_i)'\beta\}} \right], \tag{2}$$

where $t_1, \ldots, t_k$ are the distinct disease occurrence times in the cohort and $R(t)$ denotes the set of cohort members at risk (having $Y(t) = 1$) at follow-up time t. Standard likelihood procedures apply to (2) for testing and estimation on β, and convenient semiparametric estimators of the cumulative baseline hazard function $\Omega_0(t) = \int_0^t \lambda_0(u)\, du$ are also available (e.g., Andersen and Gill, 1982) thereby also providing absolute disease rate estimators.

The score test $\partial \log L(\beta)/\partial \beta$ for $\beta = 0$ is referred to as the logrank test in the special case in which $x(t) \equiv x$ is comprised of indicator variables for p of $p+1$

groups, for which disease rates are to be compared. A simple, but practically useful refinement of (1) replaces the baseline hazard rate $\lambda_0(t)$ by $\lambda_{0s}(t)$ thereby allowing the baseline rates to differ arbitrarily among strata $s = 1, 2, \ldots$ that may be time-dependent. This refinement allows a more flexible modeling of disease rates on stratification factors, formed from $\{Z(t), t\}$, than would conveniently be possible through hazard ratio regression modeling. The partial likelihood function under a stratified Cox model is simply the product of terms (2) formed from the stratum-specific disease occurrence and covariate data. Other modifications are needed to accommodate tied disease occurrence times, and for more complex disease occurrence time data as may arise with specialized censoring schemes or with recurrent or correlated disease occurrence times. The Cox regression method has been arguably the major statistical advance relative to epidemiology and biomedical research of the past 50 years. Detailed accounts of its characteristics and extensions have been given various places (e.g., Andersen et al., 1993; Kalbfleisch and Prentice, 2002).

The Cox model provides a powerful and convenient descriptive tool for assessing relative associations with disease incidence. There are other descriptive models, such as accelerated failure time models

$$\lambda\{t, Z(t)\} = \lambda_0 \left(\int_0^t e^{x(u)'\beta} du \right) e^{x(t)'\beta},$$

for which the regression parameter may have a more useful interpretation in some contexts. This model tends to be rather difficult to apply, however, though workable implementations have been developed, with efficiency properties dependent on the choice of model for $\lambda_0(\cdot)$ that is used to generate estimating functions (e.g., Jin et al., 2003).

In some settings mechanistic or biologically-based disease occurrence rate models are available (e.g., Moolgavkar and Knudson, 1981). The parameters in such models may characterize aspects of the disease process, or provide specific targets for treatments or interventions that allow them to valuably complement descriptive modeling approaches. Biologically based models with this type of potential also tend to be more challenging to apply, but the payoff may sometimes justify the effort. Of course, it is useful to be able to examine a cohort dataset from more than a single modeling framework, to assure robustness of principal findings, and to garner maximal information.

The statistical issues in study design, conduct, and analysis differ somewhat between the epidemiologic, early detection, and therapeutic contexts, according to differences in disease outcome rates and outcome ascertainment issues, and according to covariate definition and measurement issues. However, there are also some important commonalities; for example, issues of multiple hypothesis testing, especially in relation to high-dimensional covariate data and study monitoring procedures, arise in each context. We will proceed by describing some of the context-specific statistical issues first, and subsequently include a discussion of shared statistical issues.

3. Observational study methods and challenges

3.1. Epidemiologic risk factor identification

3.1.1. Sampling strategies
Cohort studies provide a mainstay epidemiologic approach to the identification of disease risk factors. A single cohort study has potential to examine the associations between multiple exposures, behaviors or characteristics and the risk of various diseases, and has potential to examine both short- and long-term associations. A distinguishing feature of the epidemiologic cohort study is the typical low incidence rates for the diseases under study. Even such prominent chronic diseases as coronary heart disease or lung cancer typically occur at a rate of 1% or less per year among ostensibly healthy persons. It follows that epidemiologic cohorts may need to be quite large, often in the range of tens of thousands to more than 100,000, depending on the age distribution and on the frequencies of 'exposures' of interest in the cohort, to provide precise estimates on association parameters of interest in a practical time frame. Well-characterized cohorts tend to be followed for substantial periods of time, as their value typically increases as more disease events accrue, and marginal costs for additional years of follow-up tend to diminish.

The rare disease aspect of epidemiologic cohort studies opens the way to various design and analysis simplifications. For example, the partial likelihood-based estimating function for β from (2) can be written

$$\partial \log L(\beta)/\partial \beta' = \sum_{i=1}^{k} \left\{ x_i(t_i) - \frac{\sum\limits_{l \in R(t_i)} x_l(t_i) W_{il}(\beta)}{\sum\limits_{l \in R(t_i)} W_{il}(\beta)} \right\}, \tag{3}$$

where $W_{il}(\beta) = \exp\{x_l(t_i)'\beta\}$, which contrasts the modeled regression vector for the individual developing disease at time t_i (the case), to a suitably weighted average of the regression vectors, $x_l(t_i)$, for cohort members at risk at t_i (the controls). Most of the variance in this comparison derives from the 'case' regression vector, and the summations over the 'risk set' at t_i can be replaced by a summation over a few randomly selected controls from this risk set with little loss of estimating efficiency. This 'nested case–control' (Liddell et al., 1977; Prentice and Breslow, 1978) approach to estimation is attractive if the determination of some components of $x(t)$ is expensive. Often only one, or possibly two or three, controls will be 'time-matched' to the corresponding case. Depending somewhat on the covariate distribution and hazard ratio magnitude, the efficiency reduction for a nested case–control versus a full-cohort analysis is typically modest if, say, five or more controls are selected per case. With large cohorts, it is often possible to additionally match on other factors (e.g., baseline, age, cohort enrollment date, gender) to further standardize the case versus control comparison. Another within-cohort sampling strategy selects a random subcohort, or a stratified random subcohort, for use as the comparison group for the case at each t_i, instead of the entire risk set $R(t_i)$ in (3). If some care is taken to ensure that the subcohort is well aligned with the case group, there will be little to choose between this case–cohort (e.g., Prentice, 1986) estimation approach and the nested case–control approach, and there may be value in having covariate data determination on a random subcohort. Within-cohort sampling strategies of this type are widely used in epidemiology when the focus is on blood or urine biomarkers for which determinations on the entire cohort may be prohibitively expensive, and has application also to the analysis and extraction of information from stored records, for example, nutrient consumption estimates from food records, or occupational exposure estimates from employer records.

In a large cohort with only a small fraction experiencing disease one can, with little concern about bias, select a distinct comparison group to replace $R(t_i)$ in (3) for the case occurring at t_i, for each $i = 1, 2, \ldots$. The estimating equation (3) is then formally that for a conditional logistic regression of case versus control status at t_i on the corresponding regression vectors $x(t)$. In fact, since most association information for baseline risk factors derives from whether or not disease occurs during cohort follow-up, rather than from the timing of case occurrence, it is often convenient to pool the case and the control data and analyze using unconditional logistic regression, perhaps including follow-up duration and other matching characteristics as control variable in the regression model. The estimates and interpretation of odds ratios from such a logistic regression analysis will typically differ little from that for hazard ratios defined above. Breslow and Day (1987) provide a detailed account of the design and analysis of these types of case–control studies.

Note that the case–control analyses just described do not require a cohort roster to be available. Rather, one needs to be able to ascertain representative cases and controls from the underlying cohort, and ascertain their covariate histories in a reliable fashion. In fact, the classic case–control study in the context of a population-based disease register proceeds by randomly sampling cases occurring during a defined accrual period along with suitably matched controls, and subsequently ascertains their covariate histories. The challenges with this study design include avoiding selection bias as may arise if the cases and controls enrolled are not representative of cases and controls in the cohort, and especially, avoiding 'recall bias', as persons who have recently experienced a disease may recall exposures and other characteristics differently than do continuing healthy persons. The classic case–control study may be the only practical study design for rare diseases, but in recent years, as several large cohort studies have matured, this design has been somewhat overtaken by cohort studies having a defined roster of members and prospective assessment of covariate histories and health events.

3.1.2. Confounding
The identification of associations that are causal for the study disease represents a major challenge for cohort studies and other observational study (OS) designs. The association of a disease incidence rate at time t with a covariate history $Z_1(t)$ may well depend on the histories $Z_2(t)$ of other factors. One can then model the hazard rate $\lambda\{t; Z(t)\}$, where $Z(t) = \{Z_1(t), Z_2(t)\}$ and examine the association between λ and $Z_1(t)$ in this model, that has now 'controlled' for factors $Z_2(t)$ that may otherwise 'confound' the association. Unfortunately, there is no objective means of knowing when the efforts to control confounding are sufficient, so that

one can only argue toward causation in an OS context. An argument of causation requires a substantial knowledge of the disease processes and disease determinants. The choices of confounding factors to control through regression modeling or through stratification can be far from straightforward. For example, factors that are time-dependent may offer greater confounding control (e.g., Robins, 1987), but if such 'factors are on a causal pathway' between Z, and disease risk, they may 'overcontrol'. Some factors may both confound and mediate, and specialized modeling techniques have been proposed to address this complex issue (e.g., Hernan et al., 2001). Randomized controlled trials provide the ability to substantially address this confounding issue. However, randomized prevention trials having disease outcomes tend to be very expensive and logistically difficult, so that for many important prevention topics one must rely strongly on observational associations. OS findings that are consistent across multiple populations may provide some reassurance concerning confounding, but it may be unclear whether the same sources of confounding could be operative across populations or whether other biases, such as may arise if common measurement instruments are used across studies, are present.

3.1.3. Covariate measurement error

The issue of measurement error in covariate data is one of the most important and least developed statistical topics in observational epidemiology. Suppose that some elements of $Z(t)$, and hence of the modeled regression vector $x(t)$ in (2) are not precisely measured. How might tests and estimation on β be affected? Some of the statistical literature on covariate measurement error assumes that $x(t)$ is precisely measured in a subset of the cohort, a so-called validation subsample, while some estimate, say $w(t)$ of $x(t)$ is available on the remainder of the cohort. The hazard rate at time t induced from (1) in the non-validation part of the cohort is then

$$\lambda_0(t)E\{\exp\{x(t)'\beta\}|w(t),\ Y(t) = 1\}. \tag{4}$$

The expectation in (4) can be estimated using the validation sample data on $\{x(t),\ w(t)\}$ and consistent non-parametric estimates of β are available (Pepe and Fleming, 1991; Carroll and Wand, 1991) with the measurement error simply reducing estimating efficiency.

Frequently in epidemiologic contexts, however, the 'true' covariate history is unascertainable for any study subjects, and only one or more estimates thereof will be available. Important examples arise in nutritional and physical activity epidemiology where $Z(t)$ may include the history of consumption of certain nutrients over preceding years, or aspects of lifetime physical activity patterns. A classical measurement model, ubiquitous in the statistical measurement error literature, assumes that available measurements $w_1(t)$, $w_2(t)$, ... of $x(t)$ are the sum of $x(t)$ plus error that is independent across replicates for an individual, and that is independent of $x(t)$ and of other study subject characteristics. A variety of hazard ratio estimators are available from this type of reliability data including regression calibration (Carroll et al., 1995), risk set regression calibration (Xie et al., 2001), conditional score (Tsiatis and Davidian, 2001), and non-parametric corrected score procedures (Huang and Wang, 2000; Song and Huang, 2005). These modeling assumptions and estimation procedures may be sufficient for objectively assessed covariates (e.g., certain exposure biomarkers), but the classical measurement model may be inadequate for many self-reported exposures. For example, the relationship between the consumption of fat, carbohydrate, and total energy (calories) to the risk of chronic disease has been the subject of continuing cohort and case–control study research for some decades. Almost all of this work has involved asking cohort members to self-report their dietary patterns, most often in the form of the frequency and portion size of consumption of each element of a list of foods and drinks. For certain nutrients, including short-term total energy and protein energy, there are objective consumption markers that plausibly adhere to a classical measurement model. Though published data on the relationship of such markers to corresponding self-reported consumption remains fairly sparse, it is already evident, for example for total energy, that the measurement error properties may depend on such individual characteristics as body mass (e.g., Heitmann and Lissner, 1995), age, and certain behavioral characteristics, and that replicate measurements have measurement errors that tend to be positively correlated (e.g., Kipnis et al., 2003). This work underscores the need for more flexible and realistic models (e.g., Carroll et al., 1998; Prentice et al., 2002) for certain exposure assessments in epidemiologic cohort settings, and for the development of additional objective (biomarker) measures of exposure in nutritional and physical activity epidemiology. Typically, it will not be practical to obtain such objective measures for the entire epidemiologic cohort, nor can some key biomarkers be obtained from stored specimens. Hence, the practical way forward appears to be to use the biomarker data on a random subsample to calibrate (correct) the self-report data for the entire cohort prior to hazard ratio estimation or odds ratio estimation (e.g., Sugar et al., 2006). This is a fertile area for further data gathering and methods development, and one where statisticians have a central role to fulfill.

3.1.4. Outcome data ascertainment

A cohort study needs to include a system for regularly updating disease event information. This may involve asking study subjects to periodically self-report any of a list of diagnoses and to report all hospitalizations. Hospital discharge summaries may then be examined for diagnoses of interest with confirmation by other medical and laboratory records. Sometimes outcomes are actively ascertained as a part of the study protocol; for example, electrocardiographic tracings for coronary heart disease or mammograms for breast cancer. Diagnoses that require considerable judgment may be adjudicated by a committee of experts, toward standardizing the accuracy and timing of disease event diagnoses. Disease incidence or mortality registers can sometimes provide efficient outcome ascertainment, or can supplement other ascertainment approaches.

Unbiased ascertainment of the fact and timing of disease events relative to the elements of $Z(t)$ under study is needed for valid hazard ratio estimation. Valid absolute risk estimation has the more stringent requirement of comprehensive disease event ascertainment. For example, a recent NIH workshop assessed the state-of-the science in the topic of multivitamin and multimineral (MVM)

supplements and chronic disease risk. MVM users tend to have many characteristics (e.g., highly educated, infrequent smoking, regular exercise, low-fat and
high-fruit and vegetable dietary habits) that could confound a disease association, but also MVM user engage more frequently in such disease-screening
activities as mammography or prostate-specific antigen testing (e.g., White et al.,
2004). Hence, for example, a benefit of MVMs for breast or prostate cancer could
be masked by earlier or more complete outcome ascertainment among users.
Careful standardization for disease screening and diagnosis practices, at the
design or analysis stages, may be an important element of cohort study conduct.
Similarly, differential lags in the reporting or adjudication of disease events can
be a source of bias, particularly toward the upper end of the distribution of
follow-up time for the cohort.

3.2. Observational studies in treatment research

Observational approaches are not used commonly for the evaluation of a treatment for a disease. Instead, the evaluation of treatments aimed at managing
disease, or reducing disease recurrence or death rates, rely primarily on randomized controlled trials, typically comparing a new treatment or regimen to a
current standard of care. Because of the typical higher rate of the outcome events
under study, compared to studies of disease occurrence among healthy persons,
therapeutic studies can often be carried out with adequate precision with at most
a few hundred patients. Also, the process for deciding a treatment course for a
patient is frequently complex, often involving information and assumption
related to patient prognosis. Hence, the therapeutic context is one where it may
be difficult or impossible to adequately control for selection factors, confounding
and other biases using an OS design.

Observational studies do, however, fulfill other useful roles in disease-
treatment research. These include the use of data on cohorts of persons having a
defined diagnosis to classify patients into prognostic categories within which
tailored treatments may be appropriate, and supportive care measures may need
to be standardized. For example, classification and regression trees (e.g., LeBlanc
and Tibshirani, 1996), as well as other explanatory and graphical procedures, are
used by cooperative oncology and other research groups. Also, observational
studies in patient cohorts, often under the label 'correlationals studies' are frequently used as a part of the treatment development enterprise. For example,
observational comparisons, between persons with or without recurrent disease, of
gene expression patterns in pre-treatment tissue specimens may provide important insights into the 'environment' that allows a disease to progress, and may
suggest therapeutic targets to interrupt disease progression and improve prognosis.

3.3. Observational studies in disease-screening research

Disease-screening research aims to identify sensitive and specific means of
diagnosing disease prior to its clinical surfacing. In conjunction with effective
means of disease treatment, such screening programs can reduce disease-related
mortality, and can reduce morbidity that accompanies advanced stage disease.

For similar reasons to the therapeutic area, observational studies to evaluate screening programs are most challenging, and randomized controlled trials offer important advantages.

At present, substantial efforts are underway to discover biomarkers for the early detection of various cancers. These research efforts can be expected to identify a number of novel early detection markers in upcoming years. The cost and duration of disease-screening trials encourage additional research to enhance the reliability of observational evaluations in this setting, including the possibility of joint analyses of observational and randomized trial data.

Observational studies play a crucial role in the identification of disease-screening biomarkers and modalities. For example, a current concept in the early detection of cancer is that, early in their disease course, malignant tumors may shed minute amounts of novel proteins into the blood stream, whence the presence of, or an elevated concentration of, the protein could trigger biopsy or other diagnostic work-up. For such a protein to yield a test of sufficient sensitivity and specificity to be useful as a screening tool, corresponding hazard ratios need to be considerably larger than is the case for typical epidemiologic risk factors. Hence, stored blood specimens from rather modest numbers of cases and controls (e.g., 100 of each) from an epidemiologic cohort may be sufficient to allow identification of a biomarker that would satisfy demanding diagnostic test criteria.

In terms of the notation of Section 2, the principal covariate in the diagnostic test setting is a binary variable that specifies whether or not the test is positive (e.g., prostate-specific antigen concentration, or change in concentration, above a certain value), so that the issue of converting a quantitative variable (e.g., PSA concentration) to a binary variate is important in this context.

This leads to a focus on receiver-operator characteristic (ROC) curves from case–control data, with test evaluation based in part on 'area under' the ROC 'curve' (AUC), or partial AUC if one chooses to focus on a range of acceptable specificities. A focus on the predictiveness of a diagnostic marker, typically using a logistic regression version of (3), is also important in this context and requires a linkage of the case–control data to absolute risks in the target population. This too is an active and important statistical research area. See Pepe (2003) and Baker et al. (2006) for accounts of the key concepts and approaches in evaluating diagnostic tests. Issues requiring further development include study design and analysis methods with high-dimensional markers, and methods for the effective combination of several screening tests (e.g., McIntosh and Pepe, 2002).

3.4. Family-based cohort studies in genetic epidemiology

There is a long history of using follow-up studies among family members to study genetic aspects of disease risk. For example, one could compare the dependence patterns among times to disease occurrence in a follow-up study of monozygotic and dizygotic twins having shared environments to assess whether there is a genetic component to disease risk. The so-called frailty models that allow family members to share a random multiplicative hazard rate factor are often used for this type of analysis (e.g., Hougaard, 2000). Such models have also been adapted to case–control family studies in which one compares the disease-occurrence patterns of family members of persons affected by a disease under study to corresponding patterns for unaffected persons (e.g., Hsu et al., 1999).

Often the ascertainment schemes in family-based studies are complex, as families having a strong history of the study disease are selected to increase the probability of harboring putative disease genes. Linkage analysis has been a major approach to the mapping of genes that may be related to disease risk. Such analyses proceed by determining the genotype of family members for a panel of genetic markers, and assessing whether one or more such markers co-segregate with disease among family members. This approach makes use of the fact that segments of the chromosome are inherited intact so that markers over some distance on a chromosome from a disease gene can be expected to associate with disease risk. There are many possible variations in ascertainment schemes and analysis procedures that may differ in efficiency and robustness properties (e.g., Ott, 1991; Thomas, 2004). Following the identification of a linkage signal, some form of finer mapping is needed to close in on disease-related loci.

Markers that are sufficiently close on the genome tend to be correlated, depending somewhat on a person's evolutionary history (e.g., Felsenstein, 1992). Hence, if a dense set of genetic markers is available across the genome, linkage analysis may give way to linkage-disequilibrium (LD) analyses. Genome-wide association studies with several hundred thousand single-nucleotide polymorphism (SNP) markers have only recently become possible due to efficient high-throughput SNP genotyping. High-dimensional SNP panels can be applied in family study contexts, or can be applied to unrelated cases and controls. There are many interesting statistical questions that attend these study designs (Risch and Merikangas, 1996; Schork et al., 2001), including the choice of SNPs for a given study population, and the avoidance of the so-called population stratification wherein correlations with disease may be confounded by ethnicity or other aspects of evolutionary history. Some further aspects of high-dimensional SNP studies will be discussed below.

4. Randomized controlled trials

4.1. General considerations

Compared to purely observational approaches, the randomized controlled trial (RCT) has the crucial advantage of ensuring that the intervention or treatment assignment is statistically independent of all pre-randomization confounding factors, regardless of whether or not such factors can be accurately measured and modeled, or are even recognized. The randomization assignment is also independent of the pre-randomization disease-screening patterns of enrollees. Hence, if outcomes of interest during trial follow-up are equally ascertained, tests to compare outcome rates among randomized groups represent fair comparisons, and a causal interpretation can be ascribed to observed differences. Such tests are often referred to as 'intention-to-treat (ITT)' tests, since the comparisons is among the entire randomized groups, without regard to the extent to which the assigned intervention or treatment was adhered to by trial enrollees. Note that the validity of comparisons in RCTs depends on the equality of outcome ascertainment (e.g., disease-occurrence times) between randomization groups. This implies an important role for an outcome ascertainment process that is blinded to randomization group, and implies the need for a protocol that standardizes all aspects of the outcome identification and adjudication. The RCT often provides a clinical context, which makes such unbiased outcome data ascertainment practical.

4.2. Prevention trials

For the reasons just noted, RCTs have some major advantages compared to observational studies for the evaluation of preventive interventions. The major limitations of the RCT design in this context are the typical large sample sizes, challenging logistics, and very substantial costs. For example, a simple sample size formula based on the approximate normality of the logarithm of the odds ratio indicates that a trial cohort sample size must be at least

$$n = \{p_2(1 - p_2)\}^{-1}(\log \lambda)^{-2}Q, \tag{5}$$

for a trial having active and control groups, assigned with probabilities γ and $1 - \gamma$ that have corresponding outcome event probabilities of p_1 and p_2 over trial follow-up. In this expression $\lambda = p_1(1 - p_2)/\{p_2(1 - p_1)\}$ is the active versus control group odds ratio, and

$$Q = \{\gamma(1 - \gamma)\}^{-1}[W_{\alpha/2} - W_{1-\eta}\{\gamma + \lambda^{-1}(1 - p_2 + \lambda p_2)^2(1 - \gamma)\}^{1/2}]^2,$$

is a rather slowly varying function of λ and p_2 at specified test size (type I error rate) α and power η, while $W_{\alpha/2}$ and $W_{1-\eta}$ are the upper $\alpha/2$ and $1-\eta$ percentiles of the standard normal distribution. The above formula also allows calculation of study power at a specified trial sample size. For example, that a trial of size 10,000 study subjects with randomization fraction $\gamma = 0.50$, control group incidence rate of 0.30% per year, and an odds ratio of 0.67, would have power of about 61% over an average 6-year follow-up period, and of 79% over an average 9-year follow-up period. Although more sophisticated power and sample size formulas are available (e.g., Self et al., 1992), the simple formula (5) illustrates the sensitivity to the magnitude of the intervention effect, and secondarily to the control group incidence rate. Primarily because of cost, it is common to design prevention trials with power that is just adequate under design assumptions, for the overall ITT comparison. It follows that trial power may be less than desirable if the intervention effect is somewhat less than designed. Often there will not be firm preliminary information on the magnitude, or especially the time course, of intervention effects and less than designed adherence to the assigned interventions or treatments can reduce the trial odds ratio. Less than expected control group outcome rates (p_2) also reduces trial power, as may occur if extensive eligibility or exclusionary criteria are applied in trial recruitment, or because volunteers for a prevention trial, that may be time consuming and of long duration, have distinctive biobehavioral characteristics that are related to the

outcome of interest. Also, there may be substantive questions of intervention
benefits and risks in relation to important subsets of trial enrollees, but power
may be marginal for such subset intervention comparisons and for related
interaction tests. In summary, sample size and power is an important topic for
RCTs in the prevention area, particularly since such full-scale trials typically
have little chance of being repeated. Additional statistical work on design procedures to ensure sufficient robustness of study power would be desirable.

On the topic of intervention effects within subsets, the typical low hazard rates
in prevention trials implies a role for 'case–only' analyses (e.g., Vittinghoff and
Bauer, 2006). Let $s = 1, 2, \ldots$ denote strata formed by baseline characteristics in a
prevention trial, and let $x(t) \equiv x$ take values 1 and 0 in the active and control
groups. A simple calculation under a stratified Cox model

$$\lambda_s(t; x) = \lambda_{0s}(t) \exp(x\beta_s)$$

gives

$$p(x = 1|s, T = t) = \frac{\exp \beta_s p(s, t)/\{1 - p(s, t)\}}{1 + \exp \beta_s p(s, t)/\{1 - p(s, t)\}}, \tag{6}$$

where $p(s,t) = p(x = 1|s, T \geq t)$. If outcome and censoring rates are low during
trial follow-up, then $p(s,t)$ is very close to γ, the active group randomization
fraction, and (6) is approximately

$$\frac{\{\gamma/(1 - \gamma)\}e^{\beta s}}{1 + \{\gamma/(1 - \gamma)\}e^{\beta s}}.$$

Hence, logistic regression methods can be applied for estimation and testing on
$\beta_1, \beta_2, \ldots$. This type of analysis evidently has efficiency very similar to a 'full-
cohort' analysis under this stratified Cox model, and hence may be more efficient
than case–control or case–cohort estimation for this specific purpose. The case–
only analyses may provide valuable cost saving if the baseline factors to be
examined in relation to the hazard ratio involve expensive extraction of information from stored materials.

Ensuring adequate adherence to intervention goals can be a substantial challenge in prevention trials, as such trials are typically conducted in free living,
ostensibly healthy, persons who have many other priorities, and may have other
major life events occur during a possible lengthy trial intervention period. Various types of communications, incentives, and adherence initiatives may help
maintain adherence to intervention goals, for either pill taking or behavioral
interventions. If the adherence to intervention goals is less than desirable, there is
a natural desire to try to estimate the intervention effects that may have arisen
had there been full adherence to intervention goals. An interesting approach to
such estimation (Robins and Finkelstein, 2000) involves censoring the follow-up
times for study subjects when they are no longer adherent to their assigned
intervention and weighting the contributions of each individual in the risk set
$R(t)$ by the inverse of the estimated adherence probability at time t. Following
the development of a model for time to non-adherence, perhaps using another

Cox model, these weights can be estimated, thereby allowing the continuing adherent study subjects, in a sense, to 'represent' those with the same risk factors for non-adherence in the overall trial cohort. This approach has considerable appeal, but it is important to remember that the validity of the 'full adherence' comparison among randomization groups is dependent on the development of an adequate adherence rate model, and that one never knows whether or not residual confounding attends any such adherence model specification.

Most chronic disease-prevention trials to date have involved pill-taking interventions, with tamoxifen for breast cancer prevention (Fisher et al., 1998), statins for heart disease prevention (Shepherd et al., 1995), and alendronate for fracture prevention (Cummings et al., 1998) providing examples of important advances. Behavioral and lifestyle interventions arguably provide the desirable long-term targets for chronic prevention and for public health recommendation. There have been fewer such trials, with the Diabetes Prevention Program trial of a combination of a dietary pattern change and physical activity increase standing out as providing impressive findings (Diabetes Prevention Program Research Group, 2002). An analytic challenge in this type of 'lifestyle' trial is the estimation of the contributions of the various components of a multi-faceted intervention to the overall trial result. Usually, it will not be practical to blind study participants to a behavioral intervention assignment, so that unintended, as well as intended, differences in behaviors between intervention groups may need to be considered in evaluating and interpreting trial results. These are complex modeling issues where further statistical methodology research is needed.

4.3. Therapeutic trials

As noted above, RCTs provide the central research design for the evaluation and comparison of treatment regimens for a defined population of patients. Compared to prevention trials, therapeutic trials are typically smaller in size and of shorter duration though, depending on the disease being treated and the interventions being compared may require a few hundred, or even a few thousand, patients followed for some years.

For some diseases, such as coronary disease or osteoporosis, there is an underlying disease process that may be underway for some years or decades and intervention concepts arising, for example, in risk factor epidemiology might logically apply to either primary prevention or recurrence prevention. Because of sample size and cost issues, it may often be reasonable to study the intervention first in a therapeutic setting, perhaps using trial results to help decide whether a subsequent primary prevention trial is justified. The above examples of tamoxifen, statins, and alendronate each followed this pattern, as is also the case for ongoing trials of estrogen deprivation agents (aromatase inhibitors) for breast cancer treatment and prevention.

Therapeutic interventions may particularly target diseased tissue or organs. Surgical interventions to remove cancerous or damaged tissue, or to arrest the progression of an infectious disease, provide a classic example. Other therapeutic interventions for cancer may, for example, restrict the blood supply to tumor tissue (angiogenesis inhibitors), induce cancerous cells to self-destruct (apoptosis inducers), or interfere with signal transduction or other biological processes relevant to tumor progression. Some such interventions have potential for adverse effects during an early intensive treatment phase followed by longer-term benefit. Statistical tools of the type already described are useful for trial evaluation. Further developments would be useful in relation to hazard ratio models that reflect time-dependent treatment effects, and in relation to summary measures that can bring together such time-to-response outcomes as time to disease response to treatment, disease-free survival time, and overall survival toward a comparative summary of treatment benefits and risks. The development and evaluation of a therapeutic intervention is typically a multiphase process, and important statistical issues attend study design and analyses at each phase, including methods for deciding which treatments move on for testing in subsequent phases.

4.4. Disease-screening trials

There have been rather few RCTs of interventions for the early detection of disease, with mortality outcomes. As an exception there have been several trials of mammography, or of mammography in conjunction with other breast-screening modalities, for the reduction in breast cancer mortality, including the classic New York Health Insurance Plan breast-screening trial (Shapiro, 1977), which is often credited with establishing the value of mammography screening among older women, the Canadian National Breast Screening Study (Miller et al., 1992a, 1992b), and several group randomized trials in Europe. The latter pose some interesting analytic challenges as persons randomized in the same group to active screening or control tend to have correlated mortality times that give rise to inflation in the variance of test statistics, like the logrank test from (3), that need to be acknowledged. Such acknowledgement can take place by allowing a robust variance estimator (Wei et al., 1989) for the logrank test from (3), or by adopting a permutation approach to testing with the randomized group as the unit of analysis (Gail et al., 1996; Feng et al., 1999).

Another special feature of a screening trial with disease outcomes is the presence of a strong correlate of the primary outcome, disease-specific mortality. Specifically one observes the occurrence of the targeted disease during the course of the trial, and disease occurrence is a strong risk factor for the corresponding mortality. A statistical challenge is to use the disease incidence data in a manner that strengthens mortality comparisons relative to analyses based on the mortality data alone. To do so without making additional modeling assumptions requires a nonparametric estimator of the bivariate survivor function that can improve upon the efficiency of the Kaplan–Meier estimator, for separate application in each randomization group. Such estimation is known to be possible asymptotically (Van der Laan, 1996), but estimation procedures that can make practical improvements to the KM estimator with a moderate number (e.g., a few hundred) of disease events have yet to be developed. This 'auxiliary data' problem is one of a range of statistical challenges related to the use of intermediate outcomes and biomarkers.

5. Intermediate, surrogate, and auxiliary outcomes

The cost and duration of RCTs in the treatment area, and especially in the disease prevention and screening areas, naturally raises questions about whether some more frequently occurring or proximate outcome can suffice for the evaluation of an intervention. Alternatively, there may be a battery of intermediate outcomes that together convey most information concerning intervention benefits and risks.

On the contrary, it is clear that there are often readily available intermediate outcomes that are highly relevant to intervention effects. The effects of statin family drugs on blood lipids and lipoproteins, is undoubtedly a major aspect of the associated heart disease risk reduction, and the effects of the bone-preserving agent alendronate on bone mass and bone mineral density is likely an important determinant of fracture risk reduction. But one is typically not in a position to know whether or not such intermediate outcomes are comprehensive in respect to pathways relevant to the targeted disease, or are comprehensive in relation to unrecognized adverse effects. Recent controversy surrounding the use of the Cox-2 inhibitor VIOXX for colorectal adenoma recurrence prevention and an unexpected increase in cardiovascular disease risk illustrate the latter point (Bresalier et al., 2005). See Lagakos (2006) for a discussion of related interpretational issues. On the data analysis side, we often lack indices that bring together data on several pertinent intermediate outcomes for a meaningful projection of benefits versus risks for a disease outcome of interest, so that intermediate outcome trials typically play the roles of refinement and initial testing of an intervention, rather than of definitive testing in relation to a subsequent 'hard' endpoint.

In some circumstances, however, one may ask whether there is an intermediate outcome that so completely captures the effect of an intervention of interest on a 'true' outcome, that treatment decisions can be based on the intermediate outcome alone – the so-called surrogate outcome problem. Unfortunately, such circumstances are likely to be quite rare unless one defines a surrogate that is so proximate as to be tantamount to the true outcome. Specifically, the conditions for a test of the null hypothesis of no relationship between an intervention and intermediate outcome to be a valid test for the null hypothesis concerning the treatment and a true outcome require the surrogate to fully mediate the intervention effect on the time outcome (Prentice, 1989). This assumption is very restrictive, and one can never establish full mediation empirically. Nevertheless, the lack of evidence against such mediation in sizeable data sets is sometimes used to argue the practical surrogacy of certain intermediate outcomes, as in recent analysis of prostate-specific antigen 'velocity' as a surrogate for prostate cancer recurrence for the evaluation of certain types of treatments (D'Amico et al., 2003).

A rather different 'meta-analytic' approach to this issue of replacing a true outcome by a suitable intermediate outcome arises by modeling joint treatment effect parameters for the intermediate and true outcome in trials of similar interventions to that under study, and assuming some aspects of this joint distribution to apply to a subsequent trial in which only the intermediate ('surrogate') is observed (e.g., Burzykowski et al., 2005). It is not clear how often one would be in a position to have sufficient prior trial data available to apply this concept, and the issues of how one decides which treatments or interventions are close enough to the test treatment to support this type of approach also appears to be challenging.

The approaches described thus far in this section may not often allow a definitive evaluation of a treatment effect on a clinical outcome, such as disease incidence or mortality. The auxiliary data idea mentioned in Section 4.4 may have potential to streamline a definitive intervention evaluation, without making additional strong assumptions, if short-term and frequent outcomes exist that correlate strongly with the clinical outcome of interest. Essentially, the short-term outcome data provide dependent censorship information for the true clinical outcome, which may be able to add precision to comparative analysis of the clinical outcome data. High-dimensional short-term outcome data (e.g., changes in the proteome following treatment initiation) may offer particular opportunities, but, as noted previously, the requisite statistical methodology has yet to be developed.

In some circumstances, available data sources will have established an adverse effect of an exposure on disease risk. Cigarette smoking in relation to lung cancer or heart disease, occupational asbestos exposure and mesothelioma and lung cancer, human papilloma virus exposure and cervical cancer, provide important examples. RCTs in such contexts may be aimed at finding effective ways of reducing the exposures in question, for example, through smoking cessation or prevention educational approaches, through protective strategies in the workplace, or through safe-sex practices. Related dissemination research projects fulfill an important role in the overall epidemiology and biomedical research enterprise.

6. Multiple testing issues and high-dimensional biomarkers

6.1. Study monitoring and reporting

It is well recognized that Type I error rates may be inflated if trial data are analyzed periodically with analytic results having potential to alter trial conduct or to trigger trial reporting. Monitoring methods that preserve the size of tests to compare randomized group disease rates (e.g., Jennison and Turnbull, 2000) are widely used in RCT settings. These methods tend to depend strongly on proportional hazards assumptions. Settings in which the intervention may plausibly affect multiple clinical outcomes, either beneficially or adversely, present participation challenges in trial monitoring. For example, Freedman et al. (1996) propose a global index that is defined as the time to the earliest of a set of outcomes that may be affected by an intervention, and propose a monitoring process that first examines designated primary outcomes for the trial, but also examines at the global index to determine whether early trial stopping should be considered. Special efforts are required to estimate treatment effect parameters in the presence of sequential monitoring (Jennison and Turnbull, 2000). Conditional power calculations that make use of the data in hand in projecting study power also have value for trial monitoring.

It is interesting that most attention to the specification of testing procedures that acknowledge multiplicity of tests occurs in the RCT setting; where this is typically a well-defined treatment or intervention, a specified primary outcome, a specified test statistic for intervention group comparisons, and a trial monitoring plan. In contrast multiple testing issues are often not formally addressed in OS settings where there may be multiple covariate and covariate modeling specifications, multiple possible outcome definitions, multiple association test statistics, and where associations may be repeatedly examined in an ad hoc fashion. See Ioannidis (2005) for an assertion that 'most published findings are false', as a result of these types of multiple testing issues, and other sources of bias. The development of testing procedures that can avoid error rate inflation as a result of this array of multiplicities could add substantial strength to observational epidemiologic studies.

6.2. High-dimensional biomarker data

The development of high-dimensional biologic data of various types has greatly stimulated the biomedical research enterprise in recent years. One example is the identification of several million SNPs across the human genome (e.g., Hinds et al., 2005) and the identification of tag SNP subsets that convey most genotype information as a result of linkage disequilibrium among neighboring SNPs. Tag SNP sets in the 100,000 to 500,000 range, developed in part using the publicly funded HapMap project (The International HapMap Consortium, 2003), have recently become commercially available for use in a sufficiently high-throughput fashion that hundreds, or even thousands, of cases and controls can be tested in a research project. The photolithographic assessment methods used for high-dimensional SNP studies can also be used to generate comparative gene expression (transcript) assessments for cases versus controls, or for treated versus untreated study subjects, for thousands of genes simultaneously, also in a high-throughput fashion. There are also intensive technology developments underway to assess the concentrations of the several thousands of proteins that may be expressed in specific tissues, or may be circulating in blood serum or plasma. The genomic and transcriptomic methods rely on the chemical coupling of DNA or RNA in target tissue with labeled probes having a specified sequence. This same approach is not available for studying the proteome, and current technologies mainly rely on separation techniques followed by tandem mass spectrometry in subfractions for comparative proteomic assessments (e.g., Wang et al., 2005a). Antibody arrays involving a substantial number of proteins are also beginning to emerge as a useful proteomic platform (e.g., Wang et al., 2005b). Technologies for interrogating the metabolome (small molecules) are also under intensive investigation (e.g., Shurubor et al., 2005). High-dimensional data sources also include various other types of scans and images that may be of interest as risk factors, as early detection markers, or as outcomes (e.g., PET scans for neurologic disease progression) in RCTs.

High-dimensional genomic, transcriptomic, or proteomic data, or combinations thereof, even on a modest number of persons, may provide valuable insights into biological processes and networks, or intervention mechanisms that can lead to the development of novel treatments or interventions. Evaluation of the relationship of high-dimensional data to disease rates, however, can be expected to require large sample sizes to identify associations of moderate strength and to control for various sources of heterogeneity and bias. In fact, these studies may require sample sizes much larger than the corresponding low-dimensional problems, or a multistage design, to eliminate most false positive findings. For example, 1000 cases and 1000 controls from a study cohort may yield an association test of acceptable power for a 0.01 level test of association for a candidate SNP. Testing at this significance level for 500,000 SNPs would be expected to yield 5000 false positives under the global null hypothesis. A test at the 0.00001 (10 in a million) level would reduce this expected false positive number to 5, but corresponding study power would be greatly reduced.

A multistage design in which only markers satisfying statistical criteria for association with disease move on to a subsequent stage can yield important cost savings, as less promising markers are eliminated early. In the case of SNP association tests, pooled DNA provides the opportunity for much additional cost saving, but there are important trade-offs to consider (Downes et al., 2004; Prentice and Qi, 2006).

Proteomic markers in blood may have particular potential as early detection biomarkers. Special efforts may be needed to ensure equivalent handling of serum or plasma specimens between cases of the study disease and matched controls. Specimens that are stored prior to diagnosis are much to be preferred in this context, even for biomarker discovery. For cancer early detection markers, controls having benign versions of the disease under study may be needed to identify markers having acceptable specificity. Multistage designs again may be needed if a large number of proteins are being investigated (e.g., Feng et al., 2004).

Proteomic approaches also provide an opportunity for more targeted preventive intervention development, which heretofore has relied mainly on leads from observational epidemiology, or from therapeutic trials. For example, there is potential to examine the effects of an intervention on the plasma proteome, in conjunction with knowledge of proteomic changes in relation to disease risk, as a means for the development and initial testing of biobehavioral interventions.

Much additional research is needed to identify study designs that make good use of these types of emerging high-dimensional data. The high-dimensionality also opens the way to some novel empirical testing procedures (Efron, 2004), that may provide valuable robustness compared to standard tests that assume a theoretical null distribution. Also, false discovery rate procedures (Benjamini and Hochberg, 1995) provide a useful alternative to controlling experiment-wise Type I error rates in these contexts. Additional statistical research is needed on parameter estimation, and simultaneous confidence interval specification, in the context of multistage designs in which the biomarkers of interest satisfy a series of selection criteria (e.g., Benjamini and Yekutieli, 2005).

7. Further discussion and the Women's Health Initiative example

The Women's Health Initiative (WHI) clinical trial (CT) and OS in which the author has been engaged since its inception in 1992, provides a context for illustrating a number of the points raised above. The WHI is conducted among postmenopausal women, in the age range 50–79 when enrolled during 1993–1998 at one of 40 clinical centers in the United States. The CT is conducted among 68,132 such women and evaluates four interventions in a randomized, controlled fashion in a partial factorial design (WHI Study Group, 1998). Two CT components involve postmenopausal hormone therapy, either conjugated equine estrogen alone (E-alone) among women who were post-hysterectomy at enrollment, or the same estrogen plus medroxyprogesterone acetate (E + P) among women with a uterus. The E + P trial among 16,608 women ended early in 2002 (Writing Group for the WHI, 2002) when an elevated risk of breast cancer was observed, and the 'global index' was also elevated, in part because of an unexpected increase in the designated primary outcome, coronary heart disease, as well as increases in stroke and venous thromboembolism. The E-alone trial among 10,739 women also ended early in 2004 (WHI Steering Committee, 2004) largely because of a stroke elevation, along with little potential for showing a heart disease benefit by the planned completion date in 2005.

The WHI OS includes 93,676 women recruited from the same populations, over the same time period, with much common covariate data collection, and with similar outcome ascertainment procedures. Comparison of study findings between the CT and OS provides a particular opportunity to identify sources of bias and to improve study design and analysis procedures. In the case of hormone therapy and cardiovascular disease joint analyses of the two cohorts using Cox models that stratify on cohort and baseline age reveal that careful control for confounding and for time from hormone therapy initiation provide an explanation for substantially different hazard ratio functions in the two cohorts (Prentice et al., 2005a; Prentice et al., 2006b). Corresponding unpublished breast cancer analyses draw attention to the need to carefully control for mammography patterns in outcome ascertainment, and also raise thorny issues of assessment when the intervention has potential to affect outcome ascertainment.

A series of case–control studies are underway using candidate biomarkers to elucidate hormone therapy effects on cardiovascular disease, breast cancer, and fractures. For example, the cardiovascular disease studies focus on blood-based markers of inflammation, coagulation, lipids, and candidate gene polymorphisms. A genome-wide association study involving 360,000 tag SNPs is also underway in collaboration with Perlegen Sciences to identify genetic risk factors for coronary heart disease, stroke, and breast cancer, and to elucidate hormone therapy effects in these three diseases (e.g., Prentice and Qi, 2006).

The WHI specimen repository also serves as a resource for a wide range of biomarker studies by the scientific community. A novel ongoing example aims to identify colon cancer early detection markers by studying prediagnostic stored plasma from 100 colon cancer cases and matched controls. A total of 10 labs across the United States are applying various proteomic platforms for shared discovery analyses, under the auspices of the NCI's Early Detection Research Network and WHI.

The other two CT components involve a low-fat dietary pattern for cancer prevention (48,835 women) and calcium and vitamin D supplementation for fracture prevention (36,282 women). Initial reports from these trials have recently been presented (Prentice et al., 2006a, 2006b; Beresford et al., 2006; Howard et al.,

2006, for the low-fat trial; Jackson et al., 2006; Wactawski-Wende et al., 2006, for the calcium and vitamin D trial), with much further analytic work, and explanatory analyses underway. Biomarker studies are underway in both the dietary modification trial cohort and the OS to examine the measurement properties of frequencies, records, and recalls for self-reporting both dietary consumption and physical activity patterns. These same biomarkers will be used to calibrate the self-report data for a variety of disease association studies in WHI cohorts. See Prentice et al. (2005b) for a detailed discussion of statistical issues arising in the WHI, and for commentary by several knowledgeable epidemiologists and biostatisticians.

In summary, epidemiology and biomedical research settings are replete with important statistical issues. The population science and prevention areas have attracted the energies of relatively few statistically trained persons, even though the public health implications are great, and methodologic topics often stand as barriers to progress. These and other biomedical research areas can be recommended as stimulating settings for statistical scientists at any career stage.

Acknowledgement

This work was supported by grants CA 53996, CA86368, and CA106320.

References

Andersen, P.K., Borgan, D., Gill, R.D., Keiding, N. (1993). *Statistical Models Based on Counting Processes.* Springer, New York.

Andersen, P.K., Gill, R.D. (1982). Cox's regression model for counting processes: A large sample study. *The Annals of Statistics* **10**, 1100–1120.

Baker, S.G., Kramer, B.S., McIntosh, M., Patterson, B.H., Shyr, Y., Skates, S. (2006). Evaluating markers for the early detection of cancer: Overview of study designs and methods. *Clinical Trials* **3**, 43–56.

Benjamini, Y., Hochberg, Y. (1995). Controlling false discovery rate: A practical and powerful approach to multiple testing. *Journal of the Royal Statistical Society. Series B* **57**, 289–300.

Benjamini, Y., Yekutieli, D. (2005). False discovery rate-adjusted multiple confidence intervals for selected parameters (with discussion). *Journal of the American Statistical Association* **100**, 71–93.

Beresford, S.A., Johnson, K.C., Ritenbaugh, C., Lasser, N.L., Snetselaar, L.G., Black, H.R., Anderson, G.L., Assaf, A.R., Bassford, T., Bowen, D., Brunner, R.L., Brzyski, R.G., Caan, B., Chlebowski, R.T., Gass, M., Harrigan, R.C., Hays, J., Heber, D., Heiss, G., Hendrix, S.L., Howard, B.V., Hsia, J., Hubbell, F.A., Jackson, R.D., Kotchen, J.M., Kuller, L.H., LaCroix, A.Z., Lane, D.S., Langer, R.D., Lewis, C.E., Manson, J.E., Margolis, K.L., Mossavar-Rahmani, Y., Ockene, J.K., Parker, L.M., Perri, M.G., Phillips, L., Prentice, R.L., Robbins, J., Rossouw, J.E., Sarto, G.E., Stefanick, M.L., Van Horn, L., Vitolins, M.Z., Wactawski-Wende, J., Wallace, R.B., Whitlock, E. (2006). Low-fat dietary pattern and risk of colorectal cancer: The Women's Health Initiative randomized controlled dietary modification trial. *The Journal of the American Medical Association* **295**, 643–654.

Bresalier, R.S., Sandler, R.S., Quan, H., Bolognese, J.A., Oxenius, B., Horgan, K., Lines, C., Riddell, R., Morton, D., Lanas, A., Konstam, M.A., Baron, J.A., Adenomatous Polyp Prevention on Vioxx (APPROVe) Trial Investigators. (2005). Cardiovascular events associated with rofecoxib in a colorectal cancer chemoprevention trial. *The New England Journal of Medicine* **352**, 1092–1102.

Breslow, N.E., Day, N.E. (1987). Statistical methods in cancer research, Vol. 2. The Design and Analysis of Cohort Studies. IARC Scientific Publications No. 82, International Agency for Research on Cancer, Lyon, France.

Burzykowski, T., Molenberghs, G., Buyse, M. (2005). *The Evaluation of Surrogate Endpoints.* Springer, New York.

Carroll, R.J., Freedman, L., Kipnis, V., Li, L. (1998). A new class of measurement error models, with application to dietary data. *Canadian Journal of Statistics* **26**, 467–477.

Carroll, R.J., Ruppert, D., Stefanski, L.A. (1995). *Measurement Error in Nonlinear Models.* Chapman & Hall, London.

Carroll, R.J., Wand, M.P. (1991). Semiparametric estimation in logistic measurement error models. *Journal of Royal Statistical Society. Series B* **53**, 573–585.

Cox, D.R. (1972). Regression models and life tables (with discussion). *Journal of Royal Statistical Society. Series B* **34**, 187–220.

Cox, D.R. (1975). Partial likelihood. *Biometrika* **62**, 269–276.

Cummings, S.R., Black, D.M., Thompson, D.E., Applegate, W.B., Barrett-Connor, E., Musliner, T.A., Palermo, L., Prineas, R., Rubin, S.M., Scott, J.C., Vogt, T., Wallace, R., Yates, A.J., LaCroix, A.Z. (1998). Effect of alendronate on risk of fracture in women with low bone density but without vertebral fractures. *The Journal of the American Medical Association* **280**, 2077–2082.

D'Amico, A.V., Moul, J.W., Carroll, P.R., Sun, L., Lubeck, D., Chen, M.H. (2003). Surrogate endpoint for prostate cancer-specific mortality after radical prostatectomy or radiation therapy. *Journal of the National Cancer Institute* **95**, 1376–1383.

Diabetes Prevention Program Research Group (2002). Reduction in the incidence of Type 2 diabetes with lifestyle intervention or metformin. *The New England Journal of Medicine* **346**, 393–403.

Downes, K., Barratt, B.J., Akan, P., Bumpstead, S.J., Taylor, S.D., Clayton, D.G., Deloukas, P. (2004). SNP allele frequency estimation in DNA pools and variance component analysis. *BioTechniques* **36**, 840–845.

Efron, B. (2004). Large-scale simultaneous hypothesis testing: The choice of a null hypothesis. *Journal of the American Statistical Association* **99**, 96–104.

Felsenstein, J. (1992). *Theoretical Evolutionary Genetics.* University of Washington/ASUW Publishing, Seattle, WA.

Feng, Z., Diehr, P., Yasui, Y., Evans, B., Beresford, S., Koepsell, T. (1999). Explaining community-level variance in group randomized trials. *Statistics in Medicine* **18**, 539–556.

Feng, Z., Prentice, R.L., Srivastava, S. (2004). Research issues and strategies for genomic and proteomic biomarker discovery and validation: A statistical perspective. *Pharmacogenomics* **5**, 709–719.

Fisher, B., Costantino, F.P., Wickerham, J.L., Redmond, C.K., Kavanah, M., Cronin, W.M., Vogel, V., Robidoux, A., Dimitrov, N., Atkins, J., Daly, M., Wieand, S., Tan-Chiu, E., Ford, L., Wolmark, N. (1998). Tamoxifen for prevention of breast cancer: Report of the National Surgical Adjuvant Breast and Bowel Project P-1 study. *Journal of the National Cancer Institute* **90**, 1371–1388.

Freedman, L., Anderson, G., Kipnis, V., Prentice, R., Wang, C.Y., Rossouw, J., Wittes, J., DeMets, D. (1996). Approaches to monitoring the results of long-term disease prevention trials: Examples from the Women's Health Initiative. *Controlled Clinical Trials* **17**, 509–525.

Gail, M.H., Mark, S.D., Carroll, R.J., Green, S.B., Pee, D. (1996). On design considerations and randomization-based inference for community intervention trials. *Statistics in Medicine* **15**, 1069–1092.

Heitmann, B.L., Lissner, L. (1995). Dietary underreporting by obese individuals – is it specific or non-specific? *British Medical Journal* **311**, 986–989.

Hernan, M.A., Brumback, B., Robins, J.M. (2001). Marginal structural models to estimate the joint causal effect of nonrandomized treatments. *Journal of the American Statistical Association* **96**, 440–448.

Hinds, D.A., Stuve, L.L., Nilsen, G.B., Halperin, E., Eskin, E., Ballinger, D.G., Frazer, K.A., Cox, D.R. (2005). Whole-genome patterns of common DNA variation in three human populations. *Science* **307**, 1072–1079.

Hougaard, P. (2000). *Analysis of Multivariate Survival Data.* Springer, New York.

Howard, B.V., Van Horn, L., Hsia, J., Manson, J.E., Stefanick, M.L., Wassertheil-Smoller, S., Kuller, L.H., LaCroix, A.Z., Langer, R.D., Lasser, N.L., Lewis, C.E., Limacher, M.C., Margolis, K.L., Mysiw, W.J., Ockene, J.K., Parker, L.M., Perri, M.G., Phillips, L., Prentice, R.L., Robbins, J., Rossouw, J.E., Sarto, G.E., Schatz, I.J., Snetselaar, L.G., Stevens, V.J., Tinker, L.F., Trevisan, M., Vitolins, M.Z., Anderson, G.L., Assaf, A.R., Bassford, T., Beresford, S.A., Black, H.R., Brunner, R.L., Brzyski, R.G., Caan, B., Chlebowski, R.T., Gass, M., Granek, I., Greenland, P., Hays, J., Heber, D., Heiss, G., Hendrix, S.L., Hubbell, F.A., Johnson, K.C., Kotchen, J.M. (2006). Low-fat dietary pattern and risk of cardiovascular disease: The Women's Health Initiative randomized controlled dietary modification trial. *The Journal of the American Medical Association* **295**, 655–666.

Hsu, L., Prentice, R.L., Zhao, L.P., Fan, J.J. (1999). On dependence estimation using correlated failure time data from case–control family studies. *Biometrika* **86**, 743–753.

Huang, Y., Wang, C.Y. (2000). Cox regression with accurate covariate unascertainable: A nonparametric correction approach. *Journal of the American Statistical Association* **45**, 1209–1219.

Ioannidis, J.P.A. (2005). Why most published findings are false. *PLoS Medicine* **2**(8), e124.

Jackson, R.D., LaCroix, A.Z., Gass, M., Wallace, R.B., Robbins, J., Lewis, C.E., Bassford, T., Beresford, S.A., Black, H.R., Blanchette, P., Bonds, D.E., Brunner, R.L., Brzyski, R.G., Caan, B., Cauley, J.A., Chlebowski, R.T., Cummings, S.R., Granek, I., Hays, J., Heiss, G., Hendrix, S.L., Howard, B.V., Hsia, J., Hubbell, F.A., Johnson, K.C., Judd, H., Kotchen, J.M., Kuller, L.H., Langer, R.D., Lasser, N.L., Limacher, M.C., Ludlam, S., Manson, J.E., Margolis, K.L., McGowan, J., Ockene, J.K., O'Sullivan, M.J., Phillips, L., Prentice, R.L., Sarto, G.E., Stefanick, M.L., Van Horn, L., Wactawski-Wende, J., Whitlock, E., Anderson, G.L., Assaf, A.R., Barad, D., Women's Health Initiative Investigators. (2006). Calcium plus vitamin D supplementation and the risk of fractures. *The New England Journal of Medicine* **354**, 669–683.

Jennison, C., Turnbull, B.W. (2000). *Group Sequential Methods with Application to Clinical Trials*. Chapman & Hall/CRC, Boca Raton, LA.

Jin, Z., Lin, D.Y., Wei, L.J., Ying, Z. (2003). Risk-based inference for the accelerated failure time model. *Biometrika* **90**, 341–353.

Kalbfleisch, J.D., Prentice, R.L. (2002). *The Statistical Analysis of Failure Time Data*, 2nd ed. Wiley, New York.

Kipnis, V., Subar, A.F., Midthune, D., Freedman, L.S., Ballard-Barbash, R., Troiano, R.P., Bingham, S., Schoeller, D.A., Schatzkin, A., Carroll, R.J. (2003). Structure of dietary measurement error: Results of the OPEN biomarker study. *American Journal of Epidemiology* **158**, 14–21.

Lagakos, S. (2006). Time-to-event analyses for long-term treatments in the APPROVE trial. *The New England Journal of Medicine* **355**, 113–117.

LeBlanc, M., Tibshirani, R. (1996). Combining estimates in regression and classification. *Journal of the American Statistical Association* **91**, 1641–1650.

Liddell, F.D.K., McDonald, J.C., Thomas, D.C. (1977). Methods for cohort analysis: Appraisal by application to asbestos mining. *Journal of Royal Statistical Society Series A* **140**, 469–490.

McIntosh, M., Pepe, M.S. (2002). Combining several screening tools: Optionality of the risk score. *Biometrics* **58**, 657–664.

Miller, A.B., Baines, C.J., To, T., Wall, C. (1992a). Canadian National Breast Screening Study. I. Breast cancer detection and death rates among women aged 40–49 years. *Canadian Medical Association Journal* **147**, 1459–1476.

Miller, A.B., Baines, C.J., To, T., Wall, C. (1992b). Canadian National Breast Screening Study. 2. Breast cancer detection and death rates among women aged 50–59 years. *Canadian Medical Association Journal* **147**, 1477–1488.

Moolgavkar, S.H., Knudson Jr., A.G. (1981). Mutation and cancer: A model for human carcinogenesis. *Journal of the National Cancer Institute* **66**, 1037–1052.

Ott, J. (1991). *Analysis of Human Genetic Linkage*. Johns Hopkins University Press, Baltimore, MD.

Pepe, M.S. (2003). *The Statistical Evaluation of Medical Tests for Classification and Production*. Oxford University Press, London.

Pepe, M., Fleming, T.R. (1991). A nonparametric method for dealing with mis-measured covariate data. *Journal of the American Statistical Association* **86**, 108–113.

Prentice, R.L. (1986). A case–cohort design for epidemiologic cohort studies and disease prevention trials. *Biometrika* **73**, 1–11.

Prentice, R.L. (1989). Surrogate endpoints in clinical trials: Discussion, definition and operational criteria. *Statistics in Medicine* **8**, 431–440.

Prentice, R.L., Breslow, N.E. (1978). Retrospective studies and failure time models. *Biometrika* **65**, 153–158.

Prentice, R.L., Caan, B., Chlebowski, R.T., Patterson, R., Kuller, L.H., Ockene, J.K., Margolis, K.L., Limacher, M.C., Manson, J.E., Parker, L.M., Paskett, E., Phillips, L., Robbins, J., Rossouw, J.E., Sarto, G.E., Shikany, J.M., Stefanick, M.L., Thomson, C.A., Van Horn, L., Vitolins, M.Z., Wactawski-Wende, J., Wallace, R.B., Wassertheil-Smoller, S., Whitlock, E., Yano, K., Adams-Campbell, L., Anderson, G.L., Assaf, A.R., Beresford, S.A., Black, H.R., Brunner, R.L., Brzyski, R.G., Ford, L., Gass, M., Hays, J., Heber, D., Heiss, G., Hendrix, S.L., Hsia, J., Hubbell, F.A., Jackson, R.D., Johnson, K.C., Kotchen, J.M., LaCroix, A.Z., Lane, D.S., Langer, R.D., Lasser, N.L., Henderson, M.M. (2006a). Low-fat dietary pattern and risk of invasive breast cancer: The Women's Health Initiative randomized controlled dietary modification trial. *The Journal of the American Medical Association* **295**, 629–642.

Prentice, R.L., Langer, R., Stefanick, M.L., Howard, B.V., Pettinger, M., Anderson, G., Barad, D., Curb, J.D., Kotchen, J., Kuller, L., Limacher, M., Wactawski-Wende, J., for the Women's Health Initiative Investigators. (2005a). Combined postmenopausal hormone therapy and cardiovascular disease: Toward resolving the discrepancy between Women's Health Initiative clinical trial and observational study results. *American Journal of Epidemiology* **162**, 404–414.

Prentice, R.L., Langer, R.D., Stefanick, M.L., Howard, B.V., Pettinger, M., Anderson, G.L., Barad, D., Curb, J.D., Kotchen, J., Kuller, L., Limacher, M., Wactawski-Wende, J., for the Women's Health Initiative Investigators. (2006b). Combined analysis of Women's Health Initiative observational and clinical trial data on postmenopausal hormone treatment and cardiovascular disease. *American Journal of Epidemiology* **163**, 589–599.

Prentice, R.L., Pettinger, M., Anderson, G.L. (2005a). Statistical issues arising in the Women's Health Initiative (with discussion). *Biometrics* **61**, 899–941.

Prentice, R.L., Qi, L. (2006). Aspects of the design and analysis of high-dimensional SNP studies for disease risk estimation. *Biostatistics* **7**, 339–354.

Prentice, R.L., Sugar, E., Wang, C.Y., Neuhouser, M., Peterson, R. (2002). Research strategies and the use of nutrient biomarkers in studies of diet and chronic disease. *Public Health Nutrition* **5**, 977–984.

Risch, N., Merikangas, K. (1996). The future of genetic studies of complex human diseases. *Science* **273**, 1516–1517.

Robins, J. (1987). A graphical approach to the identification and estimation of causal parameters in mortality studies with sustained exposure periods. *Journal of Chronic Diseases* **2**, 139–161.

Robins, J.M., Finkelstein, D.M. (2000). Correcting for noncompliance and dependent censoring in an AIDS clinical trial with inverse probability of censoring weighted (IPCW) log-rank tests. *Biometrics* **56**, 779–781.

Schork, N.J., Fallin, D., Thiel, B., Xu, X., Broeckel, U., Jacob, H.J., Cohen, D. (2001). The future of genetic case–control studies. *Advances in Genetics* **42**, 191–212.

Self, S.G., Mauritsen, R.H., Ohara, J. (1992). Power calculations for likelihood ratio tests in generalized linear models. *Biometrics* **48**, 31–39.

Shapiro, S. (1977). Evidence of screening for breast cancer from a randomized trial. *Cancer* **39**, 2772–2782.

Shepherd, J., Cobbe, S.M., Ford, I., Isles, C.G., Lorimer, A.R., MacFarlane, P.W., McKillop, J.H., Packard, C.J. (1995). Prevention of coronary heart disease with pravastatin in men with hypercholesterolemia. West of Scotland Coronary Prevention Study Group. *The New England Journal of Medicine* **333**, 1301–1307.

Shurubor, Y.I., Matson, W.R., Martin, R.J., Kristal, B.S. (2005). Relative contribution of specific sources of systematic errors and analytic imprecision to metabolite analysis by HPLC-ECD. *Metabolomics: Official Journal of the Metabolomic Society* **1**, 159–168.

Song, X., Huang, Y. (2005). On corrected score approach to proportional hazards model with covariate measurement error. *Biometrics* **61**, 702–714.

Sugar, E.A., Wang, C.Y., Prentice, R.L. (2007). Logistic regression with exposure biomarkers and flexible measurement error. *Biometrics* **63**, 143–151.

The International HapMap Consortium (2003). The International HapMap Project. *Nature* **426**, 789–796.

Thomas, D.C. (2004). *Statistical Methods in Genetic Epidemiology*. Oxford University Press, London.

Tsiatis, A.A., Davidian, M. (2001). A semiparametric estimator for the proportional hazards model with longitudinal covariates measured with error. *Biometrika* **88**, 447–458.

Van der Laan, M.J. (1996). Efficient estimation in the bivariate censoring model and repaired NPMLE. *The Annals of Statistics* **24**, 596–627.

Vittinghoff, E., Bauer, D. (2006). Case–only analysis of treatment-covariate interactions in clinical trials. *Biometrics* **62**, 769–776.

Wactawski-Wende, J., Kotchen, J.M., Anderson, G.L., Assaf, A.R., Brunner, R.L., O'Sullivan, M.J., Margolis, K.L., Ockene, J.K., Phillips, L., Pottern, L., Prentice, R.L., Robbins, J., Rohan, T.E., Sarto, G.E., Sharma, S., Stefanick, M.L., Van Horn, L., Wallace, R.B., Whitlock, E., Bassford, T., Beresford, S.A., Black, H.R., Bonds, D.E., Brzyski, R.G., Caan, B., Chlebowski, R.T., Cochrane, B., Garland, C., Gass, M., Hays, J., Heiss, G., Hendrix, S.L., Howard, B.V., Hsia, J., Hubbell, F.A., Jackson, R.D., Johnson, K.C., Judd, H., Kooperberg, C.L., Kuller, L.H., LaCroix, A.Z., Lane, D.S., Langer, R.D., Lasser, N.L., Lewis, C.E., Limacher, M.C., Manson, J.E., Women's Health Initiative Investigators. (2006). Calcium plus vitamin D supplementation and the risk of colorectal cancer. *The New England Journal of Medicine* **354**, 684–696.

Wang, H., Clouthier, S.G., Galchev, V., Misek, D.E., Duffner, U., Min, C.K., Zhao, R., Tra, J., Omenn, G.S., Ferrara, J.L., Hanash, S.M. (2005a). Intact-protein-based high-resolution three-dimensional quantitative analysis system for proteome profiling of biological fluids. *Molecular and Cellular Proteomics* **4**, 618–625.

Wang, X., Yu, J., Sreekumar, A., Varambally, S., Shen, R., Giacherio, D., Mehra, R., Montie, J.E., Pienta, K.J., Sanda, M.G., Kantoff, P.W., Rubin, M.A., Wei, J.T., Ghosh, D., Chinnaiyan, A.M. (2005b). Autoantibody signatures in prostate cancer. *The New England Journal of Medicine* **353**, 1224–1235.

Wei, L.J., Lin, D.Y., Weissfeld, L. (1989). Regression analysis of multivariate incomplete failure time data by modeling marginal distributions. *Journal of the American Statistical Association* **84**, 1065–1073.

White, E., Patterson, R.E., Kristal, A.R., Thornquist, M., King, I., Shattuck, A.L., Evans, I., Satia-Abouta, J., Littman, A.J., Potter, J.D. (2004). Vitamins and lifestyle cohort study: Study design and characteristics of supplement users. *American Journal of Epidemiology* **159**, 83–93.

Women's Health Initiative (WHI) Steering Committee (2004). Effects of conjugated equine estrogen in postmenopausal women with hysterectomy. *The Journal of the American Medical Association* **291**, 1701–1712.

Women's Health Initiative Study Group (1998). Design of the Women's Health Initiative clinical trial and observational study. *Controlled Clinical Trials* **19**, 61–109.

Writing Group for the Women's Health Initiative (WHI) Investigators (2002). Risks and benefits of estrogen plus progestin in healthy postmenopausal women: Principal results from the Women's Health Initiative randomized controlled trial. *The Journal of the American Medical Association* **288**, 321–333.

Xie, S., Wang, C.Y., Prentice, R.L. (2001). A risk set calibration method for failure time regression by using a covariate reliability sample. *Journal of Royal Statistical Society. Series B* **63**, 855–870.

Handbook of Statistics, Vol. 27
ISSN: 0169-7161
© 2007 Elsevier B.V. All rights reserved
DOI: 10.1016/S0169-7161(07)27004-X

2

Statistical Methods for Assessing Biomarkers and Analyzing Biomarker Data

Stephen W. Looney and Joseph L. Hagan

Abstract

The analysis of biomarker data often requires the proper application of statistical methods that are typically not covered in introductory statistics textbooks. In this chapter, we use examples from the biomarker literature to illustrate some of the challenges faced in handling data from biomarker studies and describe methods for the appropriate analysis and interpretation of these data.

1. Introduction

According to the *Dictionary of Epidemiology*, a *biomarker* is "a cellular or molecular indicator of exposure, health effects, or susceptibility" (Last, 1995, p. 17). Our primary focus here will be on markers of exposure, although the techniques we describe can be applied to any type of biomarker.

In this chapter, we provide descriptions and illustrations of many of the statistical methods that we have found useful in the analysis of biomarker data. It is often the case that data collected in studies involving biomarkers require "non-standard" analyses because of the presence of such characteristics as non-normality, heterogeneity, dependence, censoring, etc. In addition, sample sizes in biomarker studies can be rather small, so that large-sample approximations to the null distributions of test statistics are no longer valid. For these reasons, we have emphasized using exact methods whenever possible, and have recommended distribution-free and robust methods in many situations. In some instances, we have illustrated improper applications of "standard" statistical analyses by citing articles from the biomarker literature. It is not our intention to be overly critical of the authors of these articles, but rather to demonstrate that many of the published accounts of biomarker data analyses have not made proper use of the methods included in this chapter. It is often the case that the statistical analyses that appear in print represent the best that could be done at the time of publication due to unavoidable limitations on time, personnel, or resources, and that more thorough analyses could have been performed under different circumstances. It is hoped, however, that those who read this chapter will be better able to assess the quality of a biomarker and to conduct proper analyses of biomarker data in their future research endeavors.

It should also be noted that our discussion of the statistical analysis of biomarker data is not intended to be comprehensive. We have attempted instead to offer practical advice on the appropriate methods to use when analyzing biomarker data and we hope that our recommendations will be helpful to those who perform statistical analyses of these data on a regular basis. To the greatest extent possible, we have based our recommendations on the published advice of recognized authorities in the field. Our emphasis is on statistical methods and procedures that can be implemented using widely available statistical software, and we have indicated how commonly used statistical packages (primarily StatXact (Cytel Inc., Cambridge, MA) and SAS (SAS Institute Inc., Cary, NC)) can be used to carry out the recommended analyses. However, since statistics is a dynamic field, many of the recommendations contained in this chapter may soon prove to be obsolete because of new developments in the discipline and/or new advances in statistical software.

2. Statistical methods for assessing biomarkers

2.1. Validation of biomarkers

The proper statistical analysis of biomarker data cannot proceed unless it has been established that the biomarker has been *validated*; i.e., that it is known to be both valid and reliable. *Reliability* refers to "the degree to which the results obtained by a measurement procedure can be replicated" (Last, 1995). The reliability of a measurement process is most often described in terms of intra-rater and inter-rater reliability. *Intra-rater reliability* refers to the agreement between two different determinations made by the same individual and *inter-rater reliability* refers to the agreement between the determinations made by two different individuals. A reliable biomarker must exhibit adequate levels of both types of reliability. *The reliability of a biomarker must be established before validity can be examined*; if the biomarker cannot be assumed to provide an equivalent result upon repeated determinations on the same biological material, it will not be useful for practical application.

The *validity* of a biomarker is defined to be the extent to which it measures what it is intended to measure. For example, Qiao et al. (1997) proposed that the expression of a tumor-associated antigen by exfoliated sputum epithelial cells could be used as a biomarker in the detection of preclinical, localized lung cancer. For their biomarker to be valid, there must be close agreement between the classification of a patient (cancer/no cancer) using the biomarker and the diagnosis of lung cancer using the gold standard (in this case, consensus diagnosis using "best information"). As another example, body-fluid levels of cotinine have been proposed for use as biomarkers of environmental tobacco smoke exposure (Benowitz, 1999). For cotinine level to be a valid biomarker of tobacco exposure, it must be the case that high levels of cotinine consistently correspond to high levels of tobacco exposure and low levels of cotinine consistently correspond to low levels of exposure.

The appropriate statistical methods for assessing the reliability and validity of a biomarker are discussed in detail in Looney (2001) and therefore will not be treated fully in this chapter. However, there are two types of statistical analyses involving biomarker comparisons that are typically part of the validation process for a biomarker that we feel are worthy of consideration here. These analyses are discussed in Sections 2.2 and 2.3.

2.2. Comparing biomarkers with other diagnostic tests in terms of accuracy

It is often of interest to compare the accuracies of two or more biomarkers or to compare the accuracy of a biomarker with those of other diagnostic tests. One may wish to determine which of several newly proposed biomarkers is the most accurate, or to compare one or more newly proposed biomarkers to an existing measure of exposure or disease. For example, Qiao et al. (1997) used the "paired χ^2 test" to compare the accuracy of a new biomarker they were proposing with two "routine clinical detection methods" for lung cancer (sputum cytology and chest X-ray). When analyzing paired data of this type, the appropriate method for comparing two biomarkers in terms of accuracy is McNemar's test (Conover, 1999, pp. 166–170). There is no statistical method that is commonly known as the "paired χ^2 test." Although a χ^2 approximation is available for McNemar's test, it is preferable to use the exact version of the test (Siegel and Castellan, 1988, pp. 78–79; Suissa and Shuster, 1991). When comparing the accuracies of three or more biomarkers (as in the Qiao et al. study), the preferred method to use is the Cochran Q test (Lehmann, 1975, pp. 267–270).

2.2.1. McNemar test
Qiao et al. (1997) did not present sufficient data in their article for us to be able to perform the exact version of McNemar's test. A hypothetical 2×2 table for the comparison of their biomarker with chest X-ray based on the assumption that their biomarker agreed with the result of the chest X-ray on all true cases of the disease is given in Table 1.

To perform McNemar's test, let $n_{ij} = $ # of subjects in the (i,j) cell of Table 1. Let $\pi_{ij} = $ true probability that a subject falls into cell (i,j) in Table 1. Then the

Table 1
Hypothetical 2×2 table for comparison of accuracy of a new biomarker for lung cancer vs. chest X-ray

Biomarker	Chest X-Ray		
	Positive	Negative	Total
Positive	24	41	65
Negative	7	61	68
Total	31	102	133

true probabilities of accurate lung cancer diagnoses by the two methods are given by π_{1+} and π_{+1}, respectively. When $\pi_{1+} = \pi_{+1}$, we say that *marginal homogeneity* is present. Since $\pi_{1+} - \pi_{+1} = \pi_{12} - \pi_{21}$, marginal homogeneity in a 2×2 table is equivalent to equality of the "off-diagonal" probabilities, i.e., $\pi_{12} = \pi_{21}$. Let $n^* = n_{12} + n_{21}$ denote the total count in the two off-diagonal cells. Conditional on the value of n^*, the allocation of the n^* observations to one of the two off-diagonal cells is a binomial random variable (RV) with n^* trials and probability of "success" π. Under the null hypothesis H_0: $\pi_{12} = \pi_{21}$, each of the n^* observations has probability $1/2$ of being in cell $(1,2)$ and probability $1/2$ of being in cell $(2,1)$. So, n_{12} and n_{21} are the number of "successes" and "failures" for a binomial RV having n^* trials and probability of success $1/2$. Thus, a conditional test of H_0: $\pi_{12} = \pi_{21}$ can be performed using the binomial distribution to calculate the exact p-value. First, consider the one-sided alternative hypothesis H_a: $\pi_{1+} > \pi_{+1}$ or, equivalently, H_a: $\pi_{12} > \pi_{21}$. From Table 1, $n_{12} = 41$, $n_{21} = 7$, and $n^* = 48$. The reference distribution (conditional on the value of n^*) is a binomial with $n^* = 48$ and $\pi = 0.5$. The p-value for the one-sided alternative above is then $\Pr(n_{12} \geqslant 41 | n^* = 48, \pi = 0.5) = 0.0000003$. For the two-sided alternative H_a: $\pi_{1+} \neq \pi_{+1}$, the two-tailed p-value would be twice the upper-tailed p-value, or 0.0000006. Thus, there is very strong evidence of a difference in diagnostic accuracy between the new biomarker and chest X-ray.

2.2.2. Cochran Q test

Let n denote the number of biological specimens under study, and let k denote the number of biomarkers being compared. Let y_{ij} denote the determination (usually "positive" or "negative") based on the jth biomarker for the ith specimen, where $y_{ij} = 1$ for "positive" and $y_{ij} = 0$ for "negative," and let

$$y_{i.} = \sum_{j=1}^{k} y_{ij}$$

denote the total number of positive findings for the ith specimen. Similarly, let

$$y_{.j} = \sum_{i=1}^{n} y_{ij}$$

denote the total number of specimens that are classified as positive by the jth biomarker.

The test statistic for Cochran's Q test is

$$Q = \frac{k(k-1) \sum_{j=1}^{k} (y_{.j} - (y_{..}/k))^2}{ky_{..} - \sum_{i=1}^{n} y_{i.}^2}, \tag{1}$$

where $y_{..}$ denotes the total number of specimens that are classified as positive by any biomarker. The test statistic Q is asymptotically distributed as χ^2_{k-1}, so an approximate two-sided p-value is given by $p = \Pr(Q \geq Q_{cal})$, where Q_{cal} is the

Table 2
Data layout for hypothetical agreement among three diagnostic tests for lung cancer

Pattern of Agreement[a]	Frequency
Cases	
1 1 1	12
1 0 1	12
0 0 1	18
0 0 0	15
Controls	
1 1 1	0
1 0 0	7
0 0 1	16
0 0 0	53

[a] The first value in each pattern indicates the result for sputum cytology, the second value indicates the result for chest X-ray, and the third value indicates the result of the new biomarker. The pattern 1 0 1, for example, indicates that sputum cytology classified the specimen as positive, the chest X-ray classified the specimen as negative, and the new biomarker classified the specimen as positive.

observed value of the test statistic given by (1) above. The exact two-sided p-value for Cochran's Q test can be obtained using the permutation approach, as described by Mehta and Patel (2005, p. 227).

Qiao et al. (1997) did not present sufficient data in their article for us to perform Cochran's test. A hypothetical data set for the comparison of their biomarker with sputum cytology and chest X-ray was generated based on the assumption that their biomarker agreed with the sputum cytology and X-ray results on all true cases of the disease. This hypothetical data set is given in Table 2.

The value of Cochran's Q for the data in Table 2 is 122.43 and with df $= 2$, the χ^2 asymptotic p-value is <0.001. The exact p-value, approximated by StatXact using simulation, is also <0.001. Thus, there is strong evidence to indicate that there is a difference in the accuracies of the three classifiers.

2.3. Measuring agreement among biomarkers

2.3.1. Dichotomous biomarkers

Tockman et al. (1988) examined the use of murine monoclonal antibodies to a glycolipid antigen of human lung cancer as a biomarker in the detection of early lung cancer. As part of their assessment of the inter-rater reliability of scoring stained specimens, they compared the results obtained on 123 slides read by both a pathologist and a cytotechnologist (Table 3). The authors stated that they used McNemar's test to test for "significant agreement ($P = 1.000$)" between the readers. However, what they really did was to test for a significant difference in classification accuracy between the two readers. While such a test is often informative, one should also measure the degree of agreement between the readers (Kraemer, 1980). The generally accepted method for assessing agreement between two dichotomous biomarkers, neither of which can be assumed to be the gold standard, is Cohen's kappa, although alternative measures are also

Table 3
2 × 2 Table showing agreement between a pathologist and a cytotechnologist when scoring the same stained specimen

Pathologist's Reading	Cytotechnologist's Reading	
	Positive	Negative
Positive	31	1
Negative	0	91

Source: Reprinted from Table 4 of Tockman et al. (1988) with permission from the American Society of Clinical Oncology.

Table 4
2 × 2 Table showing agreement between two dichotomous variables

Variable A	Variable B		
	Positive	Negative	Total
Positive	n_{11}	n_{12}	$n_{1.}$
Negative	n_{21}	n_{22}	$n_{2.}$
Total	$n_{.1}$	$n_{.2}$	n

available (see Section 2.3.1.1). When measuring agreement among three or more dichotomous biomarkers, we recommend the method of Fleiss (1971), which is described in Section 2.3.1.2.

2.3.1.1. Cohen's kappa and alternatives (two dichotomous biomarkers). Consider the general 2 × 2 table showing agreement between two dichotomous variables A and B given in Table 4. The two most commonly used measures of agreement between two dichotomous variables are the *Index of Crude Agreement*, given by

$$p_0 = \frac{n_{11} + n_{22}}{n}, \tag{2}$$

and *Cohen's kappa*, given by

$$\hat{\kappa} = \frac{p_0 - \hat{p}_e}{1 - \hat{p}_e},$$

where p_e is the percentage agreement between the two variables that "can be attributed to chance" (Cohen, 1960). This degree of agreement is estimated by

$$\hat{p}_e = p_1 p_{.1} + p_2 p_{.2},$$

where $p_{1.} = n_{1.}/n$, $p_{.1} = n_{.1}/n$, $p_{2.} = 1 - p_{1.}$, and $p_{.2} = 1 - p_{.1}$. The formula for Cohen's kappa now becomes

$$\hat{\kappa} = \frac{2(n_{11}n_{22} - n_{12}n_{21})}{n^2(p_{1.}p_{.2} + p_{.1}p_{2.})}. \tag{3}$$

The approximate variance of $\hat{\kappa}$ is given by

$$\widehat{\text{Var}}(\hat{\kappa}) = \frac{1}{n(1-\hat{p}_e)^2} \times \left(\sum_{i=1}^{2} p_{ii} \left\{ 1 - (p_{i.} + p_{.i})(1-\hat{\kappa}) \right\}^2 \right.$$

$$\left. + (1-\hat{\kappa})^2 \sum_{i \neq j} p_{ij}(p_{i.} + p_{.j})^2 - \left\{ \hat{\kappa} - \hat{p}_e(1-\hat{\kappa}) \right\}^2 \right), \qquad (4)$$

where n is the number of subjects being rated by the two raters, and $p_{ij} = n_{ij}/n$, $i = 1, 2$; $j = 1, 2$.

Approximate $100(1-\alpha)\%$ confidence limits for κ are given by $\hat{\kappa} \pm z_{\alpha/2}\sqrt{\widehat{\text{Var}}(\hat{\kappa})}$. For the data given in Table 3, we obtain $\hat{\kappa} = 0.98$ using Eq. (3) and $\widehat{\text{Var}}(\hat{\kappa}) = 0.0004494$ using (4).

This yields an approximate 95% confidence interval (CI) for κ of (0.94, 1.00). These results indicate excellent inter-rater reliability for the biomarker proposed by Tockman et al. (1988).

Cohen's kappa is the generally accepted method for assessing agreement between two dichotomous variables, neither of which can be assumed to be the gold standard (Bartko, 1991), but several deficiencies have been noted (Feinstein and Cicchetti, 1990, p. 545; Byrt et al., 1993, p. 425). These deficiencies include: (i) If either method classifies no subjects into one of the two categories, $\hat{\kappa} = 0$. (ii) If there are no agreements for one of the two categories, $\hat{\kappa} < 0$. (iii) The value of $\hat{\kappa}$ is affected by the difference in the relative frequency of "disease" and "no disease" in the sample. The higher the discrepancy, the larger the value of $\hat{p}_e$ and the smaller the value of $\hat{\kappa}$. (iv) The value of $\hat{\kappa}$ is affected by any discrepancy between the relative frequency of "disease" for Method A and the relative frequency of "disease" for Method B. The greater the discrepancy, the smaller the expected agreement, and the larger the value of $\hat{\kappa}$.

To adjust for these deficiencies, Byrt et al. (1993) propose that, in addition to $\hat{\kappa}$, one also reports the prevalence-adjusted and bias-adjusted kappa (*PABAK*),

$$\text{PABAK} = \frac{(n_{11} + n_{22}) - (n_{12} + n_{21})}{n} = 2p_0 - 1,$$

where p_0 is the index of crude agreement given in Eq. (2). (Note that *PABAK* is equivalent to the proportion of "agreements" between the variables minus the proportion of "disagreements.") The approximate variance of PABAK is given by $\text{Var}(\text{PABAK}) = 4p_0(1-p_0)/n$ and approximate $100(1-\alpha)\%$ confidence limits for the true value of PABAK are given by

$$\text{PABAK} \pm z_{\alpha/2}\sqrt{\widehat{\text{Var}}(\text{PABAK})}.$$

As an illustration of some of the deficiencies of $\hat{\kappa}$, consider the hypothetical data on the agreement between two dichotomous biomarkers given in Table 5. Even though the two biomarkers agree on 80% of the specimens, the value of

Table 5
Hypothetical 2×2 table showing agreement between two dichotomous biomarkers

| | Biomarker B | | |
Biomarker A	Positive	Negative	Total
Positive	80	15	95
Negative	5	0	5
Total	85	15	100

$\hat{\kappa}$ is -0.08, indicating poor agreement (Landis and Koch, 1977, p. 165). Two of the previously mentioned deficiencies are at work here. First, since the two bio-markers did not agree on any of the subjects who were classified as "negative," $\hat{\kappa} < 0$. Second, the value of $\hat{\kappa}$ is adversely affected by the difference in the relative frequencies of "disease" (90%) and "no disease" (10%) in the sample. The *PABAK* coefficient, which adjusts for both of these shortcomings, has the value $2p_0 - 1 = 2(0.80) - 1 = 0.60$, with an approximate 95% CI for the true value of PABAK of $(0.44, 0.76)$. We contend that the PABAK coefficient is a much more accurate measure than $\hat{\kappa}$ of the agreement between the two biomarkers suggested by Table 5.

In addition to using $\hat{\kappa}$ and the *PABAK* coefficient to measure overall agreement, it is also advisable to describe the agreement separately in terms of those specimens that appear to be positive and those that appear to be negative. Using measures of positive agreement and negative agreement in assessing reliability is analogous to using sensitivity and specificity in assessing validity in the presence of a gold standard. Such measures can be used to help diagnose the type(s) of disagreement that may be present.

Cicchetti and Feinstein (1990) proposed indices of *average positive agreement* (p_{pos}) and *average negative agreement* (p_{neg}) for this purpose:

$$p_{\text{pos}} = \frac{n_{11}}{(n_{1.} + n_{.1})/2}$$

and

$$p_{\text{neg}} = \frac{n_{22}}{(n_{2.} + n_{.2})/2}$$

Note that the denominators of p_{pos} and p_{neg} are the average number of subjects which the two methods classify as positive and negative, respectively.

Following Graham and Bull (1998), let

$$\phi_{11} = 2/(2p_{11} + p_{12} + p_{21}) - 4p_{11}/(2p_{11} + p_{12} + p_{21})^2,$$

$$\phi_{12} = \phi_{21} = -2p_{11}/(2p_{11} + p_{12} + p_{21})^2,$$

and

$$\phi_{22} = 0.$$

Then the variance of p_{pos} can be estimated using

$$\widehat{\mathrm{Var}}(p_{pos}) = \frac{1}{n}\left(\sum_{i=1}^{2}\sum_{j=1}^{2}\phi_{ij}^{2}p_{ij} - \left(\sum_{i=1}^{2}\sum_{j=1}^{2}\phi_{ij}p_{ij}\right)^{2}\right).$$

Similarly, let

$$\gamma_{11} = 0,$$

$$\gamma_{12} = \gamma_{21} = -2p_{22}/(2p_{22} + p_{12} + p_{21})^{2},$$

and

$$\gamma_{22} = 2/(2p_{22} + p_{12} + p_{21}) - 4p_{22}/(2p_{22} + p_{12} + p_{21})^{2}.$$

Then the variance of p_{neg} can be estimated using

$$\widehat{\mathrm{Var}}(p_{neg}) = \frac{1}{n}\left(\sum_{i=1}^{2}\sum_{j=1}^{2}\gamma_{ij}^{2}p_{ij} - \left(\sum_{i=1}^{2}\sum_{j=1}^{2}\gamma_{ij}p_{ij}\right)^{2}\right). \tag{5}$$

Approximate $100(1-\alpha)\%$ confidence intervals (CIs) for the true values of p_{pos} and p_{neg} are given by $p_{pos} \pm z_{\alpha/2}\sqrt{\widehat{\mathrm{Var}}(p_{pos})}$ and $p_{neg} \pm z_{\alpha/2}\sqrt{\widehat{\mathrm{Var}}(p_{neg})}$, respectively. Simulation results due to Graham and Bull (1998) suggest that these approximate CIs provide adequate coverage for $n > 200$. For smaller n, they recommend that a bootstrap or Bayesian procedure be used to construct the CI. However, they do not provide software for implementing either of these approaches, both of which require rather extensive computer programming.

For the data in Table 5, $p_{pos} = 80/((95 + 85)/2) = 88.9\%$ and $p_{neg} = 0/((5 + 15)/2) = 0.0\%$. Thus, there is moderate overall agreement between the two observers (as measured by the *PABAK* coefficient of 0.60), "almost perfect agreement" on specimens that appear to be positive, and no agreement on specimens that appear to be negative. Hence, efforts to improve the biomarker determination process should be targeted toward those specimens that are negative.

Using the formulas given above, we obtain an approximate 95% CI for the true value of p_{pos} of $p_{pos} \pm z_{\alpha/2}\sqrt{\widehat{\mathrm{Var}}(p_{pos})} = (84.0\%, 94.7\%)$. Of course, this interval may be inaccurate since $n < 200$ (Graham and Bull, 1998). In terms of a CI for the true value of p_{neg}, note that if $p_{22} = 0$ as in Table 5, $\widehat{\mathrm{Var}}(p_{neg}) = 0$ using Eq. (5). Therefore, the asymptotic approach does not yield a meaningful CI for the true value of p_{neg} in this case.

2.3.1.2. More than two dichotomous biomarkers. The method of Fleiss (1971) can be used to calculate an overall measure of agreement among $k \geqslant 2$ dichotomous biomarkers. As described in Section 2.2.2, Cochran's Q test could also be used to test for significant disagreement among the biomarkers (what Shoukri (2004, pp. 49–51) refers to as "inter-rater bias"). Let n denote the number of biological specimens under study, and let k denote the number of biomarkers being compared. Let y_{ij} denote the determination (usually "positive" or "negative") based on the jth biomarker for the ith specimen, where $y_{ij} = 1$ for "positive" and $y_{ij} = 0$ for "negative," and let

$$y_i = \sum_{j=1}^{k} y_{ij}$$

denote the number of positive ratings on the ith specimen. Fleiss (1971) generalized Cohen's kappa to a new measure, $\hat{\kappa}_f$ as follows:

$$\hat{\kappa}_f = \frac{p_0 - \hat{p}_e}{1 - \hat{p}_e},$$

where

$$p_0 = 1 - \frac{2}{n}\sum_{i=1}^{n} \frac{y_i(k - y_i)}{k(k - 1)},$$

$$\hat{p}_e = 1 - 2\hat{\pi}(1 - \hat{\pi}),$$

and

$$\hat{\pi} = \frac{\sum_{i=1}^{n} y_i}{nk}.$$

For the hypothetical data in Table 2, $\hat{\pi} = 0.2531, \hat{p}_e = 0.6219, p_0 = 0.7343$, and $\hat{\kappa}_f = 0.30$, indicating "fair" agreement of the new biomarker with sputum cytology and chest X-ray. Of course, Cohen's kappa (or the $PABAK$ coefficient) could also be used to describe the agreement between the new biomarker and either sputum cytology or chest X-ray.

2.3.2. Continuous biomarkers

Bartczak et al. (1994) compared a high-pressure liquid chromatography (HPLC)-based assay and a gas chromatography (GC)-based assay for urinary muconic acid, both of which have been used as biomarkers to assess exposure to benzene. Their data, after omitting an outlier due to an unresolved chromatogram peak, are given in Table 6. They used Pearson's correlation coefficient r in their assessment of the agreement between the two methods (p. 255). However, at least as far back as 1973, it was recognized that r is not appropriate for assessing agreement in what are typically called "method comparison studies," i.e., studies in which neither method of measurement can be considered to be the gold standard (Westgard and Hunt, 1973). In fact, Westgard and Hunt go so far as to state that "the correlation coefficient ... is of no practical use in the statistical analysis of comparison data" (1973, p. 53).

Table 6

Data on comparison of determinations of muconic acid (ng/ml) in human urine by HPLC–diode array and GC–MS analysis

Specimen Number	HPLC (X_1)	GC–MS (X_2)	$X_1–X_2$	$(X_1 + X_2)/2$
1	139	151	−12.00	145.00
2	120	93	27.00	106.50
3	143	145	−2.00	144.00
4	496	443	53.00	469.50
5	149	153	−4.00	151.00
6	52	58	−6.00	55.00
7	184	239	−55.00	211.50
8	190	256	−66.00	223.00
9	32	69	−37.00	50.50
10	312	321	−9.00	316.50
11	19	8	11.00	13.50
12	321	364	−43.00	342.50

Source: Copyright (1994) from "Evaluation of Assays for the Identification and Quantitation of Muconic Acid, a Benzene Metabolite in Human Urine," Journal of Toxicology and Environmental Health, by A. Bartczak et al. Reproduced by permission of Taylor & Francis Group, LLC., http://www.taylorandfrancis.com.

Despite the general agreement among statisticians that r is not an acceptable measure of agreement in method comparison studies, its use in this context is still quite prevalent. Hagan and Looney (2004) found that r was used in 28% (53/189) of the method comparison studies published in the clinical research literature in 2001. The prevalence of the use of r in method comparison studies involving biomarkers was not examined separately in their study, but it is unlikely that it differed substantially from that found in the clinical research literature as a whole.

Acceptable alternatives to Pearson's r that are recommended for assessing agreement between continuous biomarkers include the coefficient of concordance (Lin, 1989, 2000), the Bland–Altman method (Altman and Bland, 1983; Bland and Altman, 1986), and Deming regression (Strike, 1996). Each of these is discussed in the sections that follow. It is interesting to note, however, that these methods are rarely used even today in method comparison studies published in the clinical research literature: Hagan and Looney (2004) found that Deming regression was used in none of the 189 method comparison studies published in 2001 and Lin's coefficient was used in only one. The Bland–Altman method was used in only 25 of the published studies (13.2%). The most commonly used method was the intra-class correlation coefficient (ICC), appearing in 118 (62.4%) of the published studies. However, the use of the ICC in method comparison studies has been criticized by several authors (e.g., Bartko, 1994; Bland and Altman, 1990; Lin, 1989; Looney, 2001) and its general use for this purpose is not recommended.

2.3.2.1. Lin's coefficient of concordance. An alternative to r that is often useful in evaluating agreement between continuous biomarkers is the *coefficient of*

concordance proposed by Lin (1989, 2000). In general, to calculate the agreement between two continuous measurements X_1 and X_2, one calculates the sample version of Lin's coefficient, denoted by r_c:

$$r_c = \frac{2s_{12}}{s_1^2 + s_2^2 + (\bar{x}_1 - \bar{x}_2)^2}, \tag{6}$$

where s_{12} is the sample covariance of X_1 and X_2, $\bar{x}_1$ the sample mean of X_1, $\bar{x}_2$ the sample mean of X_2, s_1^2 the sample variance of X_1, and s_2^2 the sample variance of X_2.

It can be shown that $r_c = 1$ if there is perfect agreement between the sample values of X_1 and X_2, $r_c = -1$ if there is perfect disagreement, and $-1 < r_c < 1$ otherwise.

The approximate standard error (SE) of Lin's coefficient is given by

$$\widehat{se}(r_c) = \sqrt{\frac{1}{n-2}\left[\left(\frac{1-r^2}{r^2}r_c^2(1-r_c^2)\right) + \left(2r_c^3(1-r_c)\frac{(\bar{x}_1-\bar{x}_2)^2}{s_1 s_2 r}\right) - r_c^4\frac{(\bar{x}_1-\bar{x}_2)^4}{2s_1^2 s_2^2 r^2}\right]}, \tag{7}$$

where r is the Pearson correlation coefficient for X_1 and X_2 and n the number of samples for which paired observations for X_1 and X_2 are obtained.

When $n \geqslant 30$, an approximate $100(1-\alpha)\%$ CI for the population value of Lin's coefficient, denoted by ρ_c, can be obtained using $r_c \pm z_{\alpha/2}\widehat{se}(r_c)$. When $n < 30$, an approximate CI based on a bootstrap approach is recommended. SAS code for calculating the bootstrap CI and the interval based on $\widehat{se}(r_c)$ can be found at http://www.ucsf.edu/cando/resources/software/linscon.sas. See Cheng and Gansky (2006) for more details.

For the data given in Table 6, $n = 12$, $\bar{x}_1 = 179.75$, $\bar{x}_2 = 191.67$, $s_1 = 137.87$, $s_2 = 134.06$, $s_{12} = 17{,}906.5455$, and $r = 0.969$. Therefore, from Eqs (6) and (7),

$$r_c = \frac{2s_{12}}{s_1^2 + s_2^2 + (\bar{x}_1 - \bar{x}_2)^2} = \frac{2(17{,}906.5455)}{(137.87)^2 + (134.06)^2 + (179.75 - 191.67)^2}$$
$$= 0.965$$

and $\widehat{se}(r_c) = 0.022$. An approximate 95% CI for ρ_c based on 1,000 bootstrap samples is given by (0.879, 0.985).

2.3.2.2. The Bland–Altman method. An alternative method for measuring agreement between two biomarkers X_1 and X_2 in which both biomarker determinations are in the same units is to apply the methodology proposed by Altman and Bland (Altman and Bland, 1983; Bland and Altman, 1986). The steps involved in this approach are as follows:

(1) Construct a scatterplot and superimpose the line $X_2 = X_1$.
(2) Plot the difference between X_1 and X_2 (denoted by d) vs. the mean of X_1 and X_2 for each subject.
(3) Perform a visual check to make sure that the within-subject repeatability is not associated with the size of the measurement, i.e., that the bias (as measured by $(X_1 - X_2)$) does not increase (or decrease) systematically as $(X_1 + X_2)/2$ increases.

(4) Perform a formal test to confirm the visual check in Step (3) by testing the hypothesis H_0: $\rho = 0$, where ρ is the true correlation between $(X_1$–$X_2)$ and $(X_1 + X_2)/2$.

(5) If there is no association between the size of the measurement and the bias, then proceed to Step (6) below. If there does appear to be significant association, then an attempt should be made to find a transformation of X_1, X_2, or both, so that the transformed data do not exhibit any association. This can be accomplished by repeating Steps (2)–(4) for the transformed data. The logarithmic transformation has been found to be most useful for this purpose. [If no transformation can be found, Altman and Bland (1983) recommend describing the differences between the methods by regressing $(X_1$–$X_2)$ on $(X_1 + X_2)/2$.]

(6) Calculate the "limits of agreement": $\bar{d} - 2s_d$ to $\bar{d} + 2s_d$, where $\bar{d}$ is the mean difference between X_1 and X_2 and s_d the standard deviation of the differences.

(7) Approximately 95% of the differences should fall within the limits in Step (6) (assuming a normal distribution). If the differences within these limits are not clinically relevant, then the two methods can be used interchangeably. However, it is important to note that this method is applicable *only* if both measurements are made in the same units.

Figure 1 shows the scatterplot of X_2 vs. X_1 with the line $X_2 = X_1$ superimposed for the data in Table 6. This plot indicates fairly good agreement except that 9 of the 12 data points are below the line of agreement.

Figure 2 shows the plot of the difference (HPLC−GC) vs. the mean of HPLC and GC for each subject. A visual inspection of Fig. 2 suggests that the within-subject repeatability is not associated with the size of the measurement, i.e., that

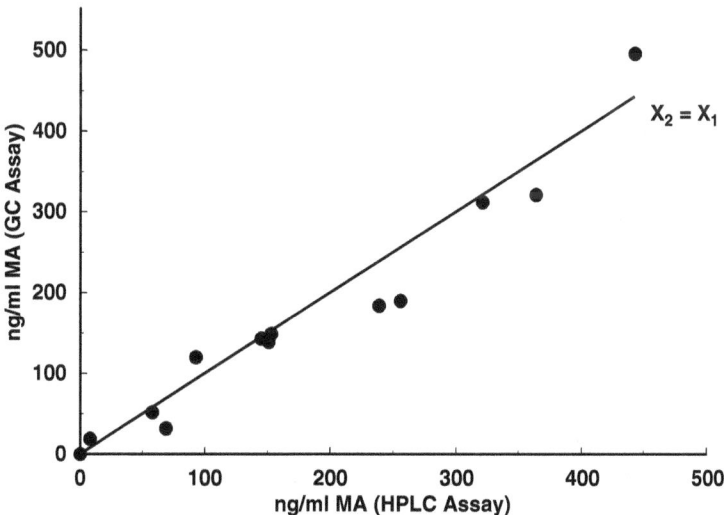

Fig. 1. Scatterplot of data on agreement between (HPLC)-based and (GC)-based assays for urinary muconic acid with the line of perfect agreement $(X_2 = X_1)$ superimposed.

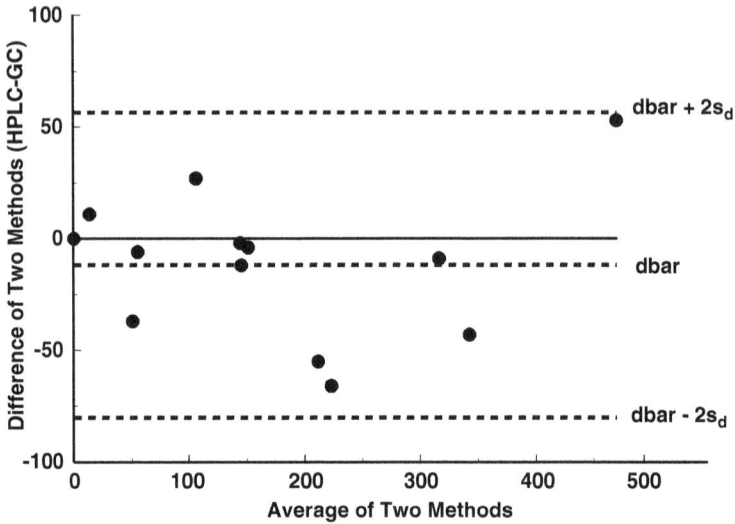

Fig. 2. Plot of difference vs. mean for data on agreement between (HPLC)-based and (GC)-based assays for urinary muconic acid.

(HPLC$-$GC) does not increase (or decrease) systematically as (HPLC$+$GC)$/2$ increases. The sample correlation between (HPLC$-$GC) and (HPLC$+$GC)$/2$ is $r = 0.113$ and the p-value for the test of H_0: $\rho = 0$ is 0.728. Therefore, the assumption of the independence between the difference and the average is not contradicted by the data. The "limits of agreement" are $\bar{d} - 2s_d = -11.9 - 2(34.2) = -80.3$ to $\bar{d} + 2s_d = -11.9 + 2(34.2) = 56.5$ and these are represented (along with $\bar{d}$) by dotted lines in Fig. 2. (Note that all of the differences fall within the limits $\bar{d} - 2s_d$ to $\bar{d} + 2s_d$.) If differences as large as 80.3 are not clinically relevant, then the two methods can be used interchangeably. Given the order of magnitude of the measurements in Table 6, it appears that a difference of 80 would be clinically important, so there is an indication of inadequate agreement between the two methods. This was not obvious from the plot in Fig. 1.

2.3.2.3. Deming regression. Strike (1996) describes an approach for determining the type of disagreement that may be present when comparing two biomarkers. These methods are most likely to be applicable when one of the methods (Method X) is a *reference* method, perhaps a biomarker that is already in routine use, and the other method (Method Y) is a *test* method, usually a new biomarker that is being evaluated. Any systematic difference (or *bias*) between the two biomarkers is relative in nature, since neither method can be thought of as representing the true exposure.

As in the Bland–Altman method described in Section 2.3.2.2, the first step is to construct a scatterplot of Y vs. X and superimpose the line $Y = X$. Any systematic discrepancy between the two biomarkers will be represented on this plot by a general shift in the location of the points away from the line $Y = X$. Strike assumes that systematic differences between the two biomarkers can be attributed to either *constant bias*, *proportional bias*, or both, and assumes the following models for each biomarker result:

$$X_i = \xi_i + \delta_i, \qquad 1 \le i \le n, \tag{8}$$
$$Y_i = \eta_i + \varepsilon_i, \qquad 1 \le i \le n,$$

where X_i is the observed value for biomarker X, ξ_i the true value of biomarker X, δ_i the random error for biomarker X, Y_i the observed value for biomarker Y, η_i the true value of biomarker Y, and ε_i the random error for biomarker Y.

Strike further assumes that the errors δ_i and ε_i are stochastically independent of each other and normally distributed with constant variance (σ_δ^2 and σ_ε^2, respectively) throughout the range of biomarker determinations in the study sample. [Strike points out that constant variance assumptions are usually unrealistic in practice and recommends a computationally intensive method for accounting for this lack of homogeneity. This method is incorporated into the MINISNAP software provided with Strike (1996).]

Strike assumes that any systematic discrepancy between Methods X and Y can be represented by

$$\eta_i = \beta_0 + \beta_1 \xi_i. \tag{9}$$

In this model, *constant bias* is represented by deviations of β_0 from 0 and *proportional bias* by deviations of β_1 from 1. [This is the same terminology used by Westgard and Hunt (1973).] If we now incorporate Eq. (9) into the equation for Y_i in Eq. (8), we have

$$Y_i = \beta_0 + \beta_1 X_i + (\varepsilon_i - \beta_1 \delta_i). \tag{10}$$

Model (2.10) is sometimes called a *functional errors-in-variables model* and assessing agreement between biomarkers X and Y requires the estimation of the parameters β_0 and β_1. Strike proposes a method that requires an estimate of the ratio of the error variances given by $\lambda = \sigma_\varepsilon^2 / \sigma_\delta^2$. This method is generally referred to in the clinical laboratory literature as "Deming regression"; however, this is somewhat of a misnomer as Deming was concerned with generalizing the errors-in-variables model to non-linear relationships. Strike points out that the method he advocates for obtaining estimates of β_0 and β_1 is actually due to Kummel (1879). The equations for estimating β_0 and β_1 are as follows:

$$\hat{\beta}_1 = \frac{(S_{yy} - \hat{\lambda} S_{xx}) + \sqrt{(S_{yy} - \hat{\lambda} S_{xx})^2 + 4\hat{\lambda} S_{xy}^2}}{2 S_{xy}}, \tag{11}$$

$$\hat{\beta}_0 = \bar{Y} - \hat{\beta}_1 \bar{X},$$

where

$$\hat{\lambda} = \frac{\hat{\sigma}_\varepsilon^2}{\hat{\sigma}_\delta^2},$$

$$S_{yy} = \sum_{i=1}^n (y_i - \bar{y})^2, \quad S_{xx} = \sum_{i=1}^n (x_i - \bar{x})^2, \quad S_{xy} = \sum_{i=1}^n (x_i - \bar{x})(y_i - \bar{y}).$$

The estimate $\hat{\lambda}$ can be obtained either from error variance estimates for each biomarker provided by the laboratory or by estimating each error variance using

$$\hat{\sigma}^2 = \frac{\sum_{i=1}^{n} d_i^2}{2n}$$

where d_i is the difference between the two determinations of the biomarker (replicates) for specimen i. (Note that the methodology proposed by Strike cannot be applied without an estimate of the ratio of error variances of the two biomarkers.)

To perform significance tests for β_0 and β_1, we need formulas for the standard errors (SEs) of $\hat{\beta}_0$ and $\hat{\beta}_1$. The approximations that Strike recommends for routine use are given by

$$\text{SE}(\hat{\beta}_1) = \left\{ \frac{\hat{\beta}_1^2 \left((1 - r^2)/r^2 \right)}{n - 2} \right\}^{1/2} \tag{12}$$

and

$$\text{SE}(\hat{\beta}_0) = \left\{ \frac{[\text{SE}(\hat{\beta}_1)]^2 \sum_{i=i}^{n} x_i^2}{n} \right\}^{1/2},$$

where

$$r^2 = \left(\frac{S_{xy}}{\sqrt{S_{xx} S_{yy}}} \right)^2$$

is the usual "R^2" value for the regression of Y on X. Tests of $H_0 : \beta_1 = 1$ and $H_0 : \beta_0 = 0$ can be performed by referring $(\hat{\beta}_1 - 1)/\text{SE}(\hat{\beta}_1)$ and $\hat{\beta}_0/\text{SE}(\hat{\beta}_0)$, respectively, to the $t(n - 2)$ distribution.

As mentioned earlier, the approach described above is based on the assumption that the error variances σ_δ^2 and σ_ε^2 are constant throughout the range of biomarker determinations in the study sample. However, as Strike points out, this assumption is usually unrealistic in practice and recommends the "weighted Deming regression" methods of Linnet (1990, 1993) for accounting for this lack of homogeneity. These methods are incorporated into the MINISNAP software provided with Strike (1996); however, replicate measurements are required for each test specimen using both biomarkers in order to apply these methods.

As an example, consider the hypothetical data in Table 7. The scatterplot for these data in Fig. 3 indicates substantial lack of agreement between X and Y and this is borne out by Lin's coefficient, which indicates substantial disagreement ($r_c = 0.102$). (Note that $r = 0.989$, indicating near-perfect linear association. This illustrates one of the major deficiencies in using r as a measure of agreement.) We apply Strike's method to gain a better understanding of the lack of agreement between X and Y.

Table 7
Hypothetical data on the agreement between biomarkers A and B

Specimen Number	Biomarker A	Biomarker B
1	31	206
2	4	28
3	17	112
4	14	98
5	16	104
6	7	47
7	11	73
8	4	43
9	14	93
10	7	57
11	10	87

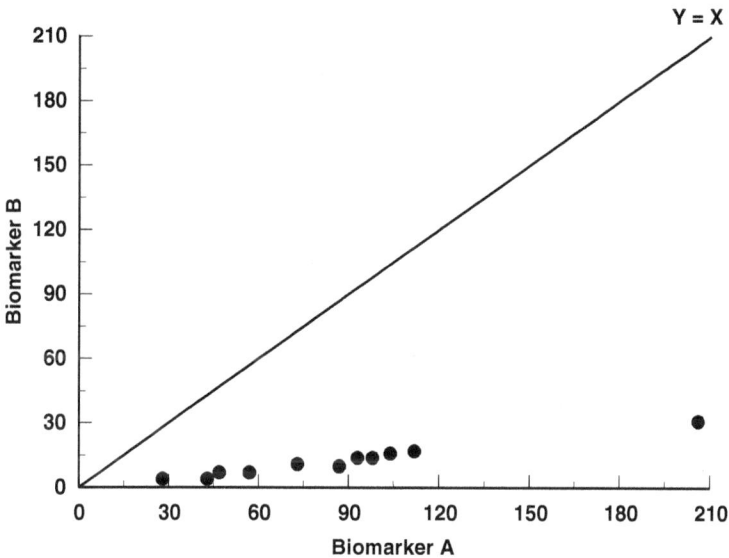

Fig. 3. Scatterplot of hypothetical data on agreement between biomarkers A and B with the line of perfect agreement ($Y = X$) superimposed.

Applying Eqs (11) and (12), we obtain $\hat{\beta}_1 = 0.158$, $\text{SE}(\hat{\beta}_1) = 0.007$, $\hat{\beta}_0 = -1.342$, and $\text{SE}(\hat{\beta}_0) = 0.614$. For the test of $H_0 : \beta_1 = 1$, this yields

$$t_{\text{cal}} = \frac{\hat{\beta}_1 - 1}{\text{SE}(\hat{\beta}_1)} = \frac{0.158 - 1}{0.007} = -129.54,$$

and using a t-distribution with $n - 2 = 9$ degrees of freedom, we find $p < 0.0001$. Therefore, there is significant proportional bias (which in this case is negative since $\hat{\beta}_1 < 1.0$). For the test of $H_0 : \beta_0 = 0$, we have

$$t_{cal} = \frac{\hat{\beta}_0}{SE(\hat{\beta}_0)} = \frac{-1.342}{0.614} = -2.19,$$

and, again using a t-distribution with 9 degrees of freedom, we have $p = 0.056$. Thus, the constant bias is not statistically significant, but just misses the usual cutoff of 0.05.

3. Statistical methods for analyzing biomarker data

3.1. Testing distributional assumptions

It is well known that violating the distributional assumption(s) underlying a statistical procedure can have serious adverse effects on the performance of the procedure (Wilcox, 1987). Therefore, it is beneficial to attempt to verify such assumptions prior to beginning data analysis. However, in many analyses of biomarker data, the underlying distributional assumptions are typically ignored and/or no attempt is made to check the distributional assumptions before proceeding with the analyses. Some authors may state something to the effect that "due to the skewed nature of the data, nonparametric statistical methods were used," but usually no formal test of the distributional assumption was ever performed. For example, in their evaluation of hemoglobin adducts as biomarkers of exposure to tobacco smoke, Atawodi et al. (1998) state that "because the distribution of HPB-Hb adduct levels was not normal, we used the nonparametric Kruskal–Wallis test ..." (p. 819); however, they offer no justification for why they concluded that the adduct levels were not normally distributed.

3.1.1. Graphical methods for assessing normality

Several graphical methods for verifying the assumption of normality have been proposed (D'Agostino, 1986). One commonly used method is the *probability plot* (Gerson, 1975), of which the quantile–quantile (Q–Q) plot is a special case. Another graphical method that is not as widely used as the probability plot is the *normal density plot* (Jones and Daly, 1995; Hazelton, 2003), which is easier to interpret than a probability plot because it is based on a direct comparison of a certain plot of the sample data vs. the familiar bell-shaped curve of the normal distribution.

While graphical examination of data can be extremely valuable in assessing a distributional assumption, the interpretation of any plot or graph is inherently subjective. Therefore, it is not sufficient to base the assessment of a distributional assumption entirely on a graphical device. Bernstein et al. (1999) evaluated the use of a bile acid-induced apoptosis assay as a measure of colon cancer risk. They determined that their apoptotic index (AI) "had a Gaussian distribution, as assessed by a box plot, quantile–quantile plot, and histogram" (p. 2354). However, each of these methods is a graphical technique, and different data analysts could interpret the plots differently. One should always supplement the graphical examination of a distributional assumption with a formal statistical test, which may itself be based on the results of the graphical device that was used. For example, correlation coefficient tests based on probability plots have been shown to have good power for detecting departures from normality against a wide variety of non-normal distributions (Looney and Gulledge, 1985). Formal tests of the distributional assumption can also be based on a normal density plot (Jones and Daly, 1995; Hazelton, 2003).

3.1.2. The Shapiro–Wilk (S–W) test

Another formal test of the assumption of normality that we recommend for general use is the Shapiro–Wilk (S–W) test (Shapiro and Wilk, 1965). Several studies have demonstrated that the S–W test has good statistical power against a wide variety of non-normal distributions (e.g., Shapiro et al., 1968). Even though the S–W test is not based directly on a graphical method for assessing normality, it is a valuable adjunct to such methods. The S–W test has been used in several studies involving biomarker data (e.g., Buckley et al., 1995; Lagorio et al., 1998; MacRae et al., 2003), although at least one author incorrectly treated the S–W test as upper-tailed, rather than lower-tailed (Buckley et al., 1995).

To perform the S–W test for normality, assume that the sample is composed of n independent and identically distributed observations $(x_1, x_2, \ldots, x_n)$ from a normal distribution with unspecified mean and variance. If $x_{[1]}, x_{[2]}, \ldots, x_{[n]}$ represents the n observations arranged in ascending sequence, the test statistic is

$$W = \frac{\left[\sum_{i=1}^{n} a_i x_{[i]} \right]^2}{\sum_{i=1}^{n} (x_i - \bar{x})^2},$$

where the a_i's represent constants that are functions of n (see Royston, 1982). The null hypothesis of normality is rejected for small values of W. Although not normally distributed under the null hypothesis (even asymptotically), W can be transformed to approximate normality when $7 \leqslant n \leqslant 2{,}000$ (Royston, 1982, 1992). For $3 \leqslant n \leqslant 6$, the methods described by Wilk and Shapiro (1968) should be used to find the lower-tailed p-value. It is especially important to account for the presence of ties when applying the S–W test (Royston, 1989). The S–W test can be performed using StatXact or the UNIVARIATE procedure within SAS.

3.1.3. Remedial measures for violation of a distributional assumption

If it has been determined that a violation of the distributional assumption underlying a statistical procedure has occurred, and that this departure is important enough to adversely affect the results of the proposed statistical analyses, at least three approaches have been recommended: (a) attempt to find a transformation of the data that will result in a new random variable that does appear to follow the assumed underlying distribution (usually the normal), (b) attempt to find a statistical procedure that is more robust to the distributional assumption, or (c) use a distribution-free test that is not dependent on the assumption of an underlying statistical distribution. Robust methods are beyond the scope of this chapter and will not be treated here; for a general treatment of these techniques, see Huber (1996). Distribution-free (also called *non-parametric*) alternatives to normal-theory-based methods for measuring association and for comparing groups are described in Sections 3.2.3.2 and 3.3, respectively. Methods for identifying an appropriate transformation for biomarker data that appear to violate a distributional assumption are discussed in the following section.

3.1.4. Choosing a transformation

A transformation based on the logarithm (usually the "natural" logarithm, $\log_e$) is commonly used in the analysis of biomarker data (e.g., Atawodi et al., 1998; MacRae et al., 2003; Strachan et al., 1990). However, authors usually provide no justification for such a transformation other than that it is commonly used in analyzing the type of data collected in the study. At the very least, the log-transformed data should be tested for normality as described in Sections 3.1.1 and 3.1.2 above. If one concludes that the log-transformed data are not normally distributed, then there are many other possible transformations that one could try. Several families of possible transformations have been proposed, including the Box–Cox family (Box and Cox, 1964), the Tukey "ladder of powers" (Tukey, 1977, pp. 88–93), the Johnson S_u family (Johnson, 1949), and the Pearson family (Stuart and Ord, 1987, pp. 210–220). The Box–Cox approach is particularly attractive, in that there is a formal statistical test for determining if the chosen transformation is "statistically significant"; however, selecting the appropriate transformation can be computationally difficult (Atkinson, 1973). (A SAS module for selecting the appropriate Box–Cox transformation parameter is available from the first author.) The Tukey "ladder of powers" is also attractive in that it requires that one consider only a small number of possible transformations. Whatever method is used to select a transformation, the transformed data should be tested for normality before proceeding to the next stage of the analysis, as was done in MacRae et al. (2003).

3.2. Analyzing cross-classified categorical data

3.2.1. Comparing two independent groups in terms of a binomial proportion

It is often of interest in the analysis of biomarker data to compare two independent groups in terms of a binomial proportion. (The comparison of dependent proportions is treated in Section 2.2.1 of this chapter.) For example, Pérez-Stable et al. (1995) compared smokers and non-smokers in terms of the proportion diagnosed with depression using the Depression Interview Schedule (DIS) (Table 8). As is commonly done with data of this type, they performed the comparison using the χ^2 test. However, this test is known to have very poor statistical properties, especially if the number of subjects in either group is small (Mehrotra et al., 2003), and is not recommended for general use. A preferred method is the "exact" version of Fisher's exact test, as implemented in StatXact or SAS. This test is described below.

Suppose that we wish to perform an exact test of the null hypothesis $H_0: \pi_1 = \pi_2$. Following the argument in Mehta and Patel (2005), denote the common probability of success for the two populations by $\pi = \pi_1 = \pi_2$. Under the null hypothesis, the probability of observing the data in Table 8 is

$$f_0(x_{11}, x_{12}, x_{21}, x_{22}) = \binom{n_1}{x_{11}} \binom{n_2}{x_{21}} \pi^{x_{11}+x_{21}}(1-\pi)^{x_{12}+x_{22}}, \tag{13}$$

Table 8
Association between dichotomized cotinine level and diagnosis of depression using the Diagnostic
Interview Survey (DIS), female subjects only

Cotinine $\geqslant 15$	DIS Diagnosis		
	Positive	Negative	Total
Yes	27	202	229
No	7	121	128
Total	34	323	357

Source: Adapted from Table 4 of Pérez-Stable et al. (1995) with permission from Elsevier.

where x_{ij} denotes the count in cell (i,j) of the 2×2 table, and n_1 and n_2 denote the
sample sizes in the two groups being compared. In order to calculate the exact
p-value for any test of H_0, we will need to calculate the probability of obtaining
a 2×2 table at least as extreme as the observed table given in Table 8. The
probability of any such table will involve the parameter π, as in Eq. (13). The
"conditional" approach to exact inference for 2×2 tables involves eliminating π
from the probability calculations by conditioning on its sufficient statistic (Cox
and Hinkley, 1974, Chapter 2). This is the approach implemented in many of the
exact statistical procedures in StatXact, and one that is recommended here. After
conditioning on the sufficient statistic for π, we find that the exact distribution of
x_{11} (the test statistic for Fisher's exact test) is hypergeometric.

For the upper-tailed alternative H_a: $\pi_1 > \pi_2$, any 2×2 table with the same
marginal row and column totals as the observed table that has a count in the (1,1)
cell that is greater than or equal to x_{11} in the observed table will be favorable
to H_a. The hypergeometric probability for each of these tables should then be
accumulated when calculating the upper-tailed p-value. The reference set under
the conditional approach is defined to be any 2×2 table with the same marginal
row and column totals as the observed table.

In Table 8, the test statistic for Fisher's exact test is $x_{11} = 27$. Then, the exact
upper-tailed p-value for the test of H_0 would be found by accumulating the
hypergeometric probabilities for all possible values in the (1,1) position that are
greater than 27, assuming that the row and column totals remain at the same
values as in Table 8. This yields an exact upper-tailed p-value of 0.0355, and a
two-tailed p-value of 0.0710.

Fisher's exact test as formulated here is known to be conservative (Agresti,
1996, pp. 41–44). That is, the hypergeometric distribution used to calculate the
exact p-values is highly discrete, especially when n_1 or n_2 is small. This means that
there will be only a small number of possible values that x_{11} can assume, leading
to a small number of possible p-values, and hence a small number of possible
significance levels, none of which may be close to 0.05. By convention, we choose
the upper-tailed significance level that is closest to, but less than or equal to
0.025. For example, for the data in Table 8, examination of the exact conditional
null distribution of x_{11} based on the hypergeometric distribution indicates
that the upper-tailed significance level closest to, but less than, 0.025 is 0.013
(obtained using a critical value of $x_{11} = 28$).

To help diminish the effect of the conservativeness of Fisher's exact test, we follow the recommendation of Agresti (2002, p. 94) that one use the *mid-p-value*, which is equal to the appropriate exact *p*-value, minus half the exact point probability of the observed value of the test statistic. For the data in Table 8, this yields a one-tailed mid-*p*-value of $0.0355 - (1/2)(0.0222) = 0.0244$. The two-tailed mid-*p*-value is $2(0.0244) = 0.0488$.

3.2.2. Testing for trend in proportions

Tunstall-Pedoe et al. (1995) examined the association between passive smoking, as measured by level of serum cotinine, and the presence or absence of several adverse health outcomes (chronic cough, coronary heart disease, etc.). Serum cotinine level was classified into four ordinal categories: "non-detectable," and 0.01–1.05, 1.06–3.97, or 3.98–17.49 ng/ml. The authors calculated odds ratios for the comparison of each serum cotinine category vs. "non-detectable" in terms of the odds of each health outcome. However, an additional analysis that we recommend for data of this type is to perform a test for trend across the serum cotinine categories in terms of the prevalence of the outcomes. Such an analysis would be especially helpful in establishing dose–response relationships between passive smoking and the adverse outcomes. Tunstall-Pedoe et al. (1995) speak in terms of a "gradient" across exposure categories, but perform no statistical test to determine if their data support the existence of such a gradient.

Recommended procedures for testing for trend include the permutation test (Gibbons and Chakraborti, 2003, Chapter 8) and the Cochran–Armitage test (Cochran, 1954; Armitage, 1955).

To perform the Cochran–Armitage (C–A) test, let k denote the number of ordinal categories for the biomarker, and suppose that a score x_i has been assigned to the ith category $(i = 1, 2, ..., k)$. Within the ith category, assume that r_i specimens out of a total of n_i have been detected as "positive" using the biomarker. Then the total sample size $n = \sum_{i=1}^{k} n_i$. Let $r = \sum_{i=1}^{k} r_i$ denote the total number of positive specimens in the sample of size n, and let

$$\bar{x} = \frac{\sum_{i=1}^{k} n_i x_i}{n}$$

denote the weighted average of the *x*-values. Then the test statistic for the C–A test for trend is given by

$$X_{trend}^2 = \frac{\left(\sum_{i=1}^{k} r_i x_i - r\bar{x} \right)^2}{p(1-p)\left(\sum_{i=1}^{k} n_i x_i^2 - n\bar{x}^2 \right)}, \tag{14}$$

where $p = r/n$ denotes the overall proportion of "positive" findings in the sample. To perform the asymptotic test for significant trend in proportions, the test statistic given in Eq. (14) is compared with a χ^2 distribution with 1 degree of freedom (upper-tailed test only). An exact test for trend based on the test statistic in Eq. (14) can be performed by using the same conditioning argument as was used for the exact version of Fisher's exact test in Section 3.2.1. The permutation test (Gibbons and Chakraborti, 2003, Chapter 8) can also be used to perform an exact test for trend in proportions across ordinal levels of a biomarker. Both the permutation test and the exact version of the C–A test are available in StatXact and the exact version of the C–A test is available in the FREQ procedure in SAS.

For the Tunstall-Pedoe et al. study described above, scores corresponding to the midpoint were assigned to each serum cotinine category (0.00, 0.53, 2.52, and 10.74 ng/ml) and then the C–A test was performed. The results indicate a highly significant increasing trend in the prevalence of "diagnosed coronary heart disease" as serum cotinine level increases ($p < 0.001$), a finding that was not reported by the authors.

One difficulty with the C–A test is that it requires preassigned fixed scores. In some cases, there may be no reasonable way to select the scores. In addition, the C–A test is more powerful when the scores and the observed binomial proportions follow a similar observed trend (Neuhäuser and Hothorn, 1999). Alternative methods that can be used without specifying scores that are robust with respect to the dose–response shape have been proposed by Neuhäuser and Hothorn (1999). However, these methods are not currently available in any widely used statistical software package, so we are unable to recommend their general use at this time.

3.2.3. Testing for linear-by-linear association

Cook et al. (1993) examined the association between the number of smokers to whom children had been exposed and their salivary cotinine measured in ng/ml. The "number of smokers" was categorized as 0, 1, 2, and $\geqslant 3$, and salivary cotinine was categorized as "non-detectable," 0.1–0.2, 0.3–0.6, 0.7–1.7, 1.8–4.0, 4.1–14.7, and > 14.7. The authors state that "salivary cotinine concentration was strongly related to the number of smokers to whom the child was usually exposed" (p. 16). However, they provide no numerical summary or statistical test to justify this assertion. One method that could be used to test for significant association between these two variables would be the linear-by-linear association test (Agresti et al., 1990). An alternative method would be to use Spearman's correlation to produce a single numerical summary of this association, and to perform a test of the null hypothesis that the population value of Spearman's correlation is different from zero.

3.2.3.1. Linear-by-linear association test. To perform the linear-by-linear association test, assume that the rows and columns of the $r \times c$ contingency table can be ordered according to some underlying variable. In the example from Cook et al. (1993) described above, there is a natural ordering in both the rows ("number of smokers") and columns (salivary cotinine level). Following the notation of Mehta and Patel (2005), let x_{ij} denote the count in the (i,j) position of the "ordered" contingency table and consider the test statistic

$$T(x) = \sum_{i=1}^{r} \sum_{j=1}^{c} u_i v_j x_{ij}, \qquad (15)$$

where u_i, $i = 1, 2, ..., r$, are row scores, and v_j, $j = 1, 2, ..., c$, are column scores. Let m_i, $i = 1, 2, ..., r$, denote the row totals, and n_j, $j = 1, 2, ..., c$, denote the column totals. Under the null hypothesis of no association between the row and column variables, the test statistic given in Eq. (15) has mean

$$E[T] = \frac{\sum_{i=1}^{r} u_i m_i \sum_{j=1}^{c} v_j n_j}{n},$$

and variance

$$Var[T] = \frac{\left[\sum_{i=1}^{r} u_i^2 m_i - \frac{\left(\sum_{i=1}^{r} u_i m_i \right)^2}{n} \right] \left[\sum_{j=1}^{c} v_j^2 n_j - \frac{\left(\sum_{j=1}^{c} v_j n_j \right)^2}{n} \right]}{n-1}$$

where

$$n = \sum_{j=1}^{c} n_j = \sum_{i=1}^{r} m_i$$

is the total sample size.

Since the test statistic given by

$$Z^* = \frac{T - E(T)}{\sqrt{Var(T)}} \tag{16}$$

has an asymptotically standard normal distribution under the null hypothesis, one can compare the calculated value of Z^* in Eq. (16) with the standard normal tables to obtain an approximate p-value. Exact p-values can be obtained for the linear-by-linear test by considering the conditional permutation distribution of the test statistic T under the null hypothesis. Consistent with our earlier discussion of exact distributions, the reference set is defined to be the set of all $r \times c$ contingency tables with the same row and column totals as the observed table.

3.2.3.2. Spearman's correlation.

There are many equivalent ways to define Spearman's correlation coefficient. (We denote the population value by ρ_s and the sample value by r_s.) One of the most useful definitions of r_s is the Pearson correlation coefficient calculated on the observations after both the x and y values have been ordered from smallest to largest and replaced by their ranks. Let $u_1, u_2, ..., u_n$ denote the ranks of the n observed values of X and let $v_1, v_2, ..., v_n$ denote the ranks of the n observed values of Y. Then Spearman's sample coefficient is defined by

$$r_s = \frac{S_{uv}}{\sqrt{S_u^2 S_v^2}}, \tag{17}$$

where S_{uv} is the sample covariance between the u's and v's, S_u^2 the sample variance of the u's, and S_v^2 the sample variance of the v's. If ties are present in the data, a modified version of Eq. (17) should be used (Gibbons and Chakraborti, 2003, pp. 429–431), although this will typically have little effect on the calculated value of r_s unless there are a large number of ties. Fisher's z transformation can be applied to Spearman's coefficient and then used to calculate approximate p-values for hypothesis tests involving ρ_s and to find approximate CIs for ρ_s. Fisher's z transformation applied to r_s is given by

$$z_s = \frac{1}{2} \ln \left(\frac{1 + r_s}{1 - r_s} \right),$$

which is approximately normally distributed with mean 0 and SE $\hat{\sigma}_s = 1.03/\sqrt{n-3}$. The exact distribution of r_s can be derived using enumeration (Gibbons and Chakraborti, 2003, pp. 424–428). Both the approximate and exact inference results for ρ_s are available in StatXact. Hypothesis tests and CIs based on the Fisher's z transformation for Spearman's coefficient are available in SAS.

For the data presented in Table 1 of Cook et al. (1993), the linear-by-linear association test indicates a strongly significant association between the "number of smokers" and salivary cotinine ($Z^* = 31.67$, $p<0.001$). Similar results were obtained for Spearman's correlation: $r_s = 0.72$, 95% CI 0.70–0.74, $p<0.001$.

3.3. Comparison of mean levels of biomarkers across groups

It is widely assumed that the optimal methods for comparing the means of normally distributed variables across groups are the t-test in the case of two groups and the analysis of variance (ANOVA) in the case of three or more groups. The proper application of both the t-test and ANOVA, as they are usually formulated, is based on two assumptions: (a) that the data in all groups being compared are normally distributed, and (b) that the population variances in all groups being compared are equal (Sheskin, 1997). In this section, we discuss the importance of these assumptions, and provide recommendations for alternative procedures to use when these assumptions appear to be violated.

3.3.1. Importance of distributional assumptions

The performance of both the t-test and ANOVA is generally robust against violations of the normality assumption; however, the presence of certain types of departures from normality can seriously affect their performance (Algina et al., 1994). If the methods for testing the assumption of normality described in Sections 3.1.1 and 3.1.2 above indicate a significant departure from normality in any of the groups being compared, we recommend that one consider applying distribution-free alternatives to the t-test and the ANOVA F-test.

For example, the Mann–Whitney–Wilcoxon (M–W–W) test has been used in biomarker studies when comparing two groups in terms of a continuous variable that appears to be non-normally distributed (e.g., Granella et al., 1996; Qiao et al., 1997). Similarly, the Kruskal–Wallis (K–W) test has been used with biomarker data when comparing more than two groups (e.g., Amorim and

Alvarez-Leite, 1997; Atawodi et al., 1998). To perform either the M–W–W or K–W tests, all of the observations are combined into one sample and ranked from smallest (1) to largest (n), where n is the combined sample size. Tied observations are assigned the midrank, i.e., the average rank of all observations having the same value. The test statistic for the M–W–W test is

$$T = \sum_{i=1}^{n_1} w_{i1},$$

where the w_{i1}'s represent the rank order of the observations in Group 1. The mean of T is

$$\mu_T = \frac{n_1(n+1)}{2},$$

and the standard deviation of T is

$$\sigma_T = \sqrt{\frac{n_1(n+1)n_2}{12}}$$

if there are no ties. If ties are present, then

$$\sigma_T = c\sqrt{\frac{n_1(n+1)n_2}{12}},$$

where

$$c = \sqrt{1 - \frac{\sum(t^3 - t)}{n(n^2 - 1)}}, \tag{18}$$

and t denotes the multiplicity of a tie and the sum is calculated over all sets of t ties.

The exact null distribution for the M–W–W test can be obtained using enumeration (or by network algorithms when enumeration is not feasible) and is available in StatXact and the NPAR1WAY procedure in SAS. Approximate p-values for the M–W–W test can be obtained by standardizing the observed value of T using μ_T and σ_T as defined above and then using the standard normal to calculate the appropriate area under the curve. This normal approximation has been found to be "reasonably accurate for equal group sizes as small as 6" (Gibbons and Chakraborti, 2003, p. 273).

To apply the K–W test (appropriate in situations in which $k \geqslant 3$ groups are being compared in terms of their biomarker determinations), let R_i denote the sum of the ranks of the observations in Group i, $i = 1, 2, \ldots, k$. Then the test statistic for the K–W test is

$$H = \frac{12}{n(n+1)} \sum_{i=1}^{k} \frac{1}{n_i} \left[R_i - \frac{n_i(n+1)}{2} \right]^2$$

if there are no ties, and $(1/c)H$, where c is given by Eq. (18), if ties are present. The exact distribution of H can be obtained using a permutation argument and is available in StatXact and the NPAR1WAY procedure in SAS. It can also be shown that H has an approximate $\chi^2(k-1)$ distribution under the null hypothesis.

One interesting feature of any distribution-free test based on ranks (of which the M–W–W and K–W tests are examples) is that applying a monotonic transformation (such as the logarithm) to the data does not affect the results of the analysis. Atawodi et al. (1998) were apparently unaware of this fact when they applied the K–W test to both the original and log-transformed data and obtained "virtually identical results" (p. 820).

It is recommended that exact p-values be used for all of the distribution-free methods mentioned in this section whenever possible; many commonly used statistical packages are able to produce only approximate p-values for distribution-free methods. This may explain the discrepancies found by Atawodi et al. (1998) when they compared the results of the K–W test for the original and log-transformed data.

A characteristic of both the M–W–W and K–W tests that is often overlooked is that these tests are most effective in detecting "shift alternatives"; i.e., the assumption is made that the populations being compared have identical shapes and the alternative hypothesis is that at least one of the populations is a "shifted" version of the others. If the "shift alternative" does not appear to be the appropriate alternative hypothesis, another method that can be used to test the null hypothesis that the parent populations are identical is the Kolmogorov–Smirnov test (Conover, 1999, pp. 428–438; Gibbons and Chakraborti, 2003, pp. 239–246). The exact version of the two-sample Kolmogorov–Smirnov test is available in both StatXact and the NPAR1WAY procedure in SAS and the exact version of the k-sample Kolmogorov–Smirnov test is available in the NPAR1WAY procedure.

3.3.2. The importance of homogeneity of variances in the comparison of means
3.3.2.1. Two-group comparisons in the presence of heterogeneity. The performance of the "usual" t-test (sometimes called the "equal variance t-test") depends very strongly on the underlying assumption of equal population variances (sometimes called *homogeneity*) between the groups (Moser et al., 1989). One approach would be to attempt to use the F-test for testing equality of population variances or another method to verify the homogeneity assumption before applying the equal variance t-test (Moser and Stevens, 1992). If the hypothesis of equal variances is not rejected, then one would apply the "usual" t-test. If the hypothesis of equal variances is rejected, then one would use an alternative approach that does not depend on the homogeneity assumption. One such alternative is the "unequal variance t-test" [sometimes referred to as the "Welch test" or "Satterthwaite approximation" (Moser and Stevens, 1992)], which is generally available in any statistical package that can perform the equal variance t-test. However, Moser and Stevens demonstrate that the preliminary F-test of equality of variances contributes nothing of value and that, in fact, the unequal variance t-test can be used any time the means of two groups are being compared since the test performs almost as well as the equal variance t-test when the population variances in the two groups are equal, and outperforms the equal variance t-test when the variances are unequal. Hence, we follow their advice and

recommend that the unequal variance t-test be used routinely whenever the means of two groups are being compared and the data appear to be normally distributed in both the groups. If the data are not normally distributed in either group, a distribution-free alternative to the t-test such as the M–W–W test (Section 3.3.1) can be used instead.

The test statistic for the unequal variance t-test recommended here is given by

$$t^* = \frac{(\bar{x} - \bar{y})}{\sqrt{(s_x^2/n_1) + (s_y^2/n_2)}}, \tag{19}$$

where $\bar{x}$, s_x^2, and n_1 denote the mean, variance, and sample size, respectively, for the biomarker levels in Group 1, and $\bar{y}$, s_y^2, and n_2 the mean, variance, and sample size, respectively, for the biomarker levels in Group 2. To perform the test of the null hypothesis that the mean biomarker level is the same in the two groups, compare the observed value of t^* in Eq. (19) with a Student's t distribution with the following degrees of freedom:

$$v = \frac{\left((1/n_1) + (u/n_2)\right)^2}{\left(1/n_1^2(n_1 - 1)\right) + \left(u^2/n_2^2(n_2 - 1)\right)}$$

where $u = s_y^2/s_x^2$.

Salmi et al. (2002) evaluated the potential usefulness of soluble vascular adhesion protein-1 (sVAP-1) as a biomarker to monitor and predict the extent of ongoing artherosclerotic processes. The investigators compared two groups: diabetic study participants on insulin treatment only ($n = 7$) vs. diabetic study participants on other treatments ($n = 41$). They used the "usual" (equal-variance) t-test to compare the mean sVAP-1 levels of the two groups: mean $\pm$ S.D. 148 ± 114 vs. 113 ± 6; $t = 2.06$, df $= 46$, one-tailed $p = 0.023$, a statistically significant result. However, they ignored the fact that the variances in the two groups they were comparing were quite different (12,996 vs. 36, $F = 361$, df $= (6,40)$, $p < 0.001$). If the unequal variance t-test is used, as recommended by Moser and Stevens (1992), one obtains $t^* = 0.81$, $v = 6$, one-tailed $p = 0.224$, a non-significant result. Given the extremely strong evidence that the two population variances are unequal, the latter results provide a more valid comparison of the two study groups.

3.3.2.2. Multiple comparisons in the presence of heterogeneity. It is often of interest to compare three or more groups in terms of the mean level of a biomarker. For example, Bernstein et al. (1999) compared the mean levels of AI across three groups: (a) "normal" subjects; that is; those with no previous history of polyps or cancer; (b) patients with a history of colorectal cancer; and (c) patients with colorectal adenomas. They used the Tukey method to perform all possible pairwise comparisons among the three groups. The Tukey method is the technique of choice if the population variances of the three groups are equal (Dunnett, 1980a); however, if they are not equal, the methods known as Dunnett's C and Dunnett's T3 are preferable (Dunnett, 1980b). These two methods are very similar to the unequal variance t-test recommended in the previous section. The Tukey, Dunnett's C, and Dunnett's T3 procedures are all available in SPSS (SPSS Inc., Chicago, IL).

Let μ_i and σ_i^2 denote the population mean and population variance, respectively, in the ith group. Let $\bar{x}_i$ denote the sample mean and let s_i^2 denote the unbiased estimate of σ_i^2 based on v_i degrees of freedom in the ith group. We wish to find a set of $100(1-\alpha)\%$ joint CI estimates for the $k(k-1)/2$ differences $\mu_i-\mu_j$, $1 \leqslant i < j \leqslant k$. Both Dunnett's C and T3 methods involve constructing joint CI estimates of the form

$$
\bar{y}_i - \bar{y}_j \pm c_{ij,\alpha,k} \sqrt{\frac{s_i^2}{n_i} + \frac{s_j^2}{n_j}},
$$

where $c_{ij,\alpha,k}$ is a "critical value" chosen so that the joint confidence coefficient is as close as possible to $1 - \alpha$.

For Dunnett's C procedure,

$$
c_{ij,\alpha,k} = \frac{\mathrm{SR}_{\alpha,k,v_{ij}^*}}{\sqrt{2}},
$$

where

$$
\mathrm{SR}_{\alpha,k,v_{ij}^*} = \frac{\left(\mathrm{SR}_{\alpha,k,v_i} s_i^2/n_i\right) + \left(\mathrm{SR}_{\alpha,k,v_j} s_j^2/n_j\right)}{\left(s_i^2/n_i\right) + \left(s_j^2/n_j\right)}
$$

and $\mathrm{SR}_{\alpha,k,v}$ denotes the upper α-percentage point of the distribution of the Studentized range of k normal variates with an estimate of the variance based on v degrees of freedom.

For Dunnett's T3 procedure,

$$
c_{ij,\alpha,k} = \mathrm{SMM}_{\alpha,k^*,\hat{v}_{ij}},
$$

where $\mathrm{SMM}_{\alpha,k^*,\hat{v}_{ij}}$ denotes the upper α-percentage point of the Studentized maximum modulus distribution of $k^* = k(k-1)/2$ uncorrelated normal variates with degrees of freedom $\hat{v}_{ij}$ given by

$$
\hat{v}_{ij} = \frac{\left((s_i^2/n_i) + (s_j^2/n_j)\right)^2}{\left(s_i^4/n_i^2(v_i)\right) + \left(s_j^4/n_j^2(v_j)\right)}.
$$

Tables of the percentage points of the SMM distribution are available in Stoline and Ury (1979). As recommended by Dunnett (1980b), percentage points of the SMM distribution for fractional degrees of freedom can be obtained by quadratic interpolation on reciprocal degrees of freedom for percentage points in the published tables.

3.4. Use of correlation coefficients in analyzing biomarker data

It is often of interest in studies involving biomarkers to examine the association between two continuous variables, at least one of which is the numerical value of a particular biomarker. For example, Salmi et al. (2002) correlated observed levels of sVAP-1 with risk factors for coronary heart disease, measures of liver dysfunction, diabetic parameter levels, etc. If both variables are normally distributed, then the appropriate measure of association to use is the Pearson correlation coefficient r. However, if the data for either variable are non-normally distributed, then a non-parametric measure of association such as Spearman's r_s should be used instead (Siegel and Castellan, 1988, pp. 224–225). In the study by Buss et al. (2003), the authors correctly used Spearman correlation in their evaluation of 3-chlorotyrosine in tracheal aspirates from preterm infants as a biomarker for protein damage by myeloperoxidase; they stated that they used Spearman's r_s "because the data were not normally distributed" (p. 5). The calculation of r_s was described in Section 3.2.3.2.

In the following sections, we consider three challenges frequently encountered when correlation coefficients are used in the analysis of biomarker data: (a) proper methods of analysis and interpretation of the results, (b) sample size determination, and (c) comparison of related correlation coefficients.

3.4.1. Proper methods of analysis and interpretation of results
Salmi et al. (2002) determined the "significance" of their correlation coefficients by testing the null hypothesis $H_0 : \rho = 0$, where ρ denotes the population correlation coefficient. However, there are several problems with this approach, the primary one being that correlations of no practical significance may be declared to be "significant" simply because the p-value is less than 0.05 (Looney, 1996). We have found the classification scheme presented by Morton et al. (1996) to be useful in interpreting the magnitude of correlation coefficients in terms of their practical significance. They classify correlations between 0.0 and 0.2 as "negligible," between 0.2 and 0.5 as "weak," between 0.5 and 0.8 as "moderate," and between 0.8 and 1.0 as "strong." In their sample of 411 Finnish men, Salmi et al. (2002) found a "significant" correlation of 0.108 between sVAP-1 and carbohydrate-deficient transferrin, a measure of liver dysfunction. While this correlation is statistically significant ($p = 0.029$), it would be considered "negligible" according to the Morton et al. criteria mentioned above, raising doubt about the practical significance of the result.

In addition to testing $H_0 : \rho = 0$, one should also construct a CI for the population correlation in order to get a sense of the precision of the correlation estimate, as well as a reasonable range of possible values for the population correlation. In the example taken from Salmi et al. (2002) mentioned above, the 95% CI for ρ is (0.01–0.20). Thus, the entire CI falls within the "negligible" range according to the Morton et al. criteria, casting further doubt on the practical significance of the observed correlation.

As discussed in Looney (1996), another problem with declaring a correlation to be significant simply because $p < 0.05$ is that smaller correlations may be declared to be "significant" even when n is fairly small, resulting in CIs that are too wide to be of any practical usefulness. In the study by Salmi et al. (2002) mentioned above, the value of r for the correlation between sVAP-1 and ketone bodies in a sample of 38 observations taken from diabetic children and adolescents was 0.34 ($p = 0.037$), a statistically significant result. However, a 95% CI for ρ is (0.02–0.60), which indicates that the population correlation could be anywhere between "negligible" and "moderate," according to the Morton et al. criteria. A CI of such large width provides very little useful information about the magnitude of the population correlation.

3.4.2. Sample size issues in the analysis of correlation coefficients
One way to avoid the difficulties described in the previous section is simply to perform a sample size calculation prior to beginning the study. There is no justification of the sample sizes used in the study by Salmi et al. (2002), so one must assume that no such calculation was done. Looney (1996) describes several approaches that typically yield sample sizes that provide more useful information about the value of the population correlation coefficient and the practical significance of the results than if one simply bases the sample size calculation on achieving adequate power for the test that the population correlation is zero. These include basing the sample size calculation on (a) the desired width of the CI for the population correlation, or (b) tests of null hypotheses other than that the population correlation is zero. (For example, one might test the null hypothesis $H_0 : \rho \leq 0.2$; rejecting this null hypothesis would indicate that the population correlation is "non-negligible.")

To perform a sample size calculation for the test of $H_0 : \rho = \rho_0$, where $\rho_0 \neq 0$, we recommend using Fisher's z-transformation applied to r as a test statistic; in other words,

$$z(r) = \frac{1}{2}\ln\left(\frac{1+r}{1-r}\right).$$

The following formula could then be used to determine the minimum sample size n required for achieving power of $100(1-\beta)\%$ for detecting an alternative correlation value of $\rho_1 > \rho_0$ using a one-tailed test of H_0 at significance level α:

$$n = 3 + \left[\frac{(z_\alpha + z_\beta)}{z(\rho_1) - z(\rho_0)}\right]^2,$$

where z_γ denotes the upper γ-percentage point of the standard normal and $z(\rho)$ the Fisher z-transform of ρ. If one wished to base the sample size calculation on the desired width of a CI for ρ, then one could use the approximate method described in Looney (1996), or the more precise method recommended by Bonett and Wright (2000).

3.4.3. Comparison of related correlation coefficients
In some studies involving biomarker data, it has been of interest to compare "related" correlation coefficients; that is, the correlation of variable X with Y vs. the correlation of variable X with Z. For example, Salmi et al. (2002) found "significant" correlations of sVAP-1 with both glucose ($r = 0.57$, $p < 0.001$) and ketone bodies ($r = 0.34$, $p = 0.037$) in their sample of 38 observations taken from

diabetic children and adolescents. They concluded that there was a "less-marked" correlation of sVAP-1 with ketone bodies than with glucose. However, they did not perform any statistical test to determine if, in fact, the corresponding population correlation coefficients were different from each other. Had they performed such a test, as described in Steiger (1980), they would have found no significant difference between the two correlations ($p = 0.093$). (SAS code for performing comparisons of related correlation coefficients is available from the first author.)

The null hypothesis for the test of dependent correlations can be stated as

$$H_0 : \rho_{uv} = \rho_{uw}, \tag{20}$$

where ρ_{uv} denotes the population correlation between the random variables U and V and ρ_{uw} the population correlation between the random variables U and W. In the example taken from Salmi et al. described above, $U = \text{sVAP-1}$, $V = \text{ketone bodies}$, and $W = \text{glucose}$. Let r_{uv} and r_{uw} denote the sample correlations between U and V and between U and W, respectively, and let $\bar{r}_{uv,uw}$ denote the mean of r_{uv} and r_{uw}. Denote by z_{uv} and z_{uw}, the Fisher's z-transforms of r_{uv} and r_{uw}, respectively. Then the test statistic recommended by Steiger (1980) for the null hypothesis in Eq. (20) is given by

$$Z^* = \frac{(z_{uv} - z_{uw})\sqrt{n - 3}}{\sqrt{2(1 - \bar{s}_{uv,uw})}}, \tag{21}$$

where $\bar{s}_{uv,uw}$ is an estimate of the covariance between z_{uv} and z_{uw} given by

$$\bar{s}_{uv,uw} = \frac{\hat{\psi}_{uv,uw}}{(1 - \bar{r}_{uv,uw}^2)^2}$$

where

$$\hat{\psi}_{uv,uw} = r_{vw}(1 - 2\bar{r}_{uv,uw}^2) - \frac{1}{2}(\bar{r}_{uv,uw}^2)(1 - 2\bar{r}_{uv,uw}^2 - r_{vw}^2).$$

The test of H_0 in Eq. (20) is performed by comparing the sample value of Z^* in Eq. (21) with the standard normal distribution. For example, using the results given in Salmi et al. (2002), $r_{uv} = 0.57$, $r_{uw} = 0.34$, $r_{vw} = 0.55$, $n = 38$, and $\bar{s}_{jk,jh} = 0.4659$, yielding $Z^* = 1.68$ and $p = 0.093$, as mentioned previously.

3.5. Dealing with non-detectable values in the analysis of biomarker data

In analyzing biomarker data, there may be samples for which the concentration of the biomarker is below the analytic limit of detection (LOD), i.e., left-censored at the LOD. These observations are commonly referred to as non-detects, or ND's. For example, Amorim and Alvarez-Leite (1997) examined the correlation between o-cresol and hippuric acid concentrations in urine samples of individuals exposed to toluene in shoe factories, painting sectors of metal industries, and printing shops. Out of 54 samples in their study, *o*-cresol concentrations were below its LOD (0.2 µg/ml) in 39. In 4 of these samples, the hippuric acid concentration was also below its LOD (0.1 mg/ml). In another study, Atawodi et al. (1998) compared 18 smokers with 52 "never smokers" in terms of their levels of hemoglobin adducts, which were being evaluated as biomarkers of exposure to tobacco smoke. In 7 of the 52 never smokers, adduct levels were below the LOD (9 fmol HPB/g Hb).

Unfortunately, methods that are commonly used in the biomarker literature for handling ND's are flawed. Perhaps the most commonly used method is to ignore the missing value(s) and analyze only those samples with complete data. This was the method used by Lagorio et al. (1998) in their examination of the correlations among the concentrations of *trans,trans* muconic acid (t,t-MA) obtained from the urine of 10 Estonian shale oil workers using three different preanalytical methods. Another commonly used method is to impute a value in place of the missing data and then apply the "usual" statistical analyses. The values commonly imputed include the LOD (Amorim and Alvarez-Leite, 1997; Atawodi et al., 1998) and LOD/2 (Cook et al., 1993).

Other methods that have been proposed for handling ND's include the "nonparametric approach," in which one treats all ND's as if they were tied at the LOD. Thus, if one wished to correlate two biomarkers, at least one of which was undetectable in some samples, one would calculate Spearman's r_s using the ranks of the entire data set, where all ND's were assigned the smallest midrank. If one wished to compare mean levels of a biomarker that was subject to ND's across two groups, one would apply the M–W–W test after computing the ranks of the two combined samples in this way. This is the method used by Atawodi et al. (1998) in their evaluation of hemoglobin adducts as biomarkers of exposure to tobacco smoke.

Recent simulation results (Wang, 2006) suggest that none of the methods described above for correlating two biomarkers that are both subject to left-censoring are satisfactory, especially if the two biomarkers are strongly correlated ($\rho \geqslant 0.5$). Instead, we recommend the maximum likelihood (ML) approach developed by Lyles et al. (2001) for estimating the correlation coefficient. A similar approach developed by Taylor et al. (2001) can be adapted to group comparisons of means and is also likely to be preferred to applying a nonparametric test to the data after replacing the ND's by the LOD. Other more advanced methods, such as multiple imputation (Scheuren, 2005), could be applied if the appropriate missing data mechanism is present. However, these methods are beyond the scope of this chapter. In this section, we briefly describe the estimation method proposed by Lyles et al. (2001).

Let X and Y denote the two biomarkers to be correlated, and denote the two fixed detection limits as L_x and L_y. Assuming a bivariate normal distribution, Lyles et al. proposed that one estimates the population parameter vector $\theta = [\mu_x, \mu_y, \sigma_x^2, \sigma_y^2, \rho]'$ using ML estimation applied to a random sample (x_i, y_i); $i = 1, \ldots, n$. In their derivation of the likelihood function, they noted that there are four types of observed pairs of (x, y) values: (1) pairs with both x and y

observed, (2) pairs with x observed and $y < L_y$, (3) pairs with y observed and $x < L_x$, and (4) pairs with $x < L_x$ and $y < L_y$. Following the notation in Lyles et al. (2001), the contribution of each pair of type 1 is given by

$$t_{i1} = (2\pi\sigma_x\sigma_{y|x})^{-1} \exp\left\{-0.5\left[\frac{(y_i - \mu_{y|x_i})^2}{\sigma_{y|x}^2} + \frac{(x_i - \mu_x)^2}{\sigma_x^2}\right]\right\},$$

where $\mu_{y|x_i} = \mu_y + \rho(\sigma_y/\sigma_x)(x_i - \mu_x)$ and $\sigma_{y|x}^2 = \sigma_y^2(1 - \rho^2)$.
   The contribution of each pair of type 2 is given by

$$t_{i2} = (2\pi\sigma_x^2)^{-1/2} \exp\left[-0.5\frac{(x_i - \mu_x)^2}{\sigma_x^2}\right] \times \Phi\left(\frac{L_y - \mu_{y|x_i}}{\sigma_{y|x}}\right),$$

where $\Phi(\cdot)$ denotes the standard normal distribution function. Similarly, the contribution of each pair of type 3 is given by

$$t_{i3} = (2\pi\sigma_y^2)^{-1/2} \exp\left[-0.5\frac{(y_i - \mu_y)^2}{\sigma_y^2}\right] \times \Phi\left(\frac{L_x - \mu_{x|y_i}}{\sigma_{x|y}}\right),$$

where $\mu_{x|y_i} = \mu_x + \rho(\sigma_x/\sigma_y)(y_i - \mu_y)$ and $\sigma_{x|y}^2 = \sigma_x^2(1 - \rho^2)$.
   Finally, each pair of type 4 contributes

$$t_4 = \int_{-\infty}^{L_y} \Phi\left\{\frac{L_x - [\mu_x + (\rho\sigma_x(y - \mu_y)/\sigma_y)]}{\sigma_x\sqrt{1 - \rho^2}}\right\}$$
$$\times (2\pi\sigma_y^2)^{-1/2} \exp\left[-0.5\frac{(y - \mu_y)^2}{\sigma_y^2}\right] dy.$$

Without loss of generality, suppose the data are ordered and indexed by i so that pairs of type 1 come first, followed by pairs of types 2, 3, and 4. Further, assume that there are n_j terms of type j ($j = 1, 2, 3, 4$) and define $n_{k\bullet} = \sum_{j=1}^{k} n_j$ for $k = 2, 3$. Then, the total likelihood can be written as

$$L(\theta|\mathbf{x}, \mathbf{y}) = \left(\prod_{i=1}^{n_1} t_{i1}\right)\left(\prod_{i=n_1+1}^{n_{2\bullet}} t_{i2}\right)\left(\prod_{i=n_{2\bullet}+1}^{n_{3\bullet}} t_{i3}\right) t_4^{n_4},$$

where $\mathbf{x}$ is the vector of observed x-values and $\mathbf{y}$ the vector of observed y-values.
   Once the ML estimates and the corresponding estimated SEs are obtained, one can construct an approximate $100(1-\alpha)\%$ Wald-type CI for ρ by using $\hat{\rho}_{ML} \pm z_{\alpha/2}\widehat{SE}(\hat{\rho}_{ML})$. Lyles et al. also considered profile likelihood CIs since Wald-type CIs are known to be potentially suspect when the sample size is small and they found that they generally performed better than the Wald-type intervals. For the data given in the study by Amorim and Alvarez-Leite (1997), the method

developed by Lyles et al. yields $\hat{\rho}_{ML} = 0.79$ and an approximate 95% CI(ρ) of (0.67, 0.91). Analyzing only the 15 cases with complete data yields $r = 0.76$ with an approximate 95% CI(ρ) of (0.40, 0.92).

4. Concluding remarks

In this chapter, we have not attempted to provide a comprehensive treatment of statistical methods that could be used in analyzing biomarker data; certainly, this entire volume could have been devoted to this task. Nor is this chapter intended to be a primer on how to perform elementary statistical analyses of biomarker data. Basic statistical methods, when properly applied, will usually suffice for this purpose. [For a good treatment of basic statistical methods and their proper application to environmental exposure data (for which biomarkers are frequently used), see Griffith et al. (1993).] Rather, we have focused our discussion on what we feel are some important analytic issues that we have encountered in our examination of biomarker data, and on some statistical techniques that we have found to be useful in dealing with those issues. It is hoped that the recommendations provided here will prove to be useful to statisticians, biomarker researchers, and other workers who are faced with the often challenging task of analyzing biomarker data.

Because of space limitations, we were unable to say very much in this chapter about power and sample size calculations. Fortunately, both StatXact and the POWER procedure within SAS are capable of carrying out power and sample size calculations for many of the procedures discussed in this chapter. Goldsmith (2001) provides a good general discussion of power and sample size considerations and provides an extensive list of references.

References

Agresti, A. (1996). *An Introduction to Categorical Data Analysis*. Wiley, New York.

Agresti, A. (2002). *Categorical Data Analysis*, 2nd ed. Wiley, Hoboken, NJ.

Agresti, A., Mehta, C.R., Patel, N.R. (1990). Exact inference for contingency tables with ordered categories. *Journal of the American Statistical Association* **85**, 453–458.

Algina, J., Oshima, T.C., Lin, W. (1994). Type I error rates for Welch's test and James's second-order test under nonnormality and inequality of variance when there are two groups. *Journal of Educational and Behavioral Statistics* **19**, 275–291.

Altman, D.G., Bland, J.M. (1983). Measurement in medicine: The analysis of method comparison studies. *The Statistician* **32**, 307–317.

Amorim, L.C.A., Alvarez-Leite, E.M. (1997). Determination of *o*-cresol by gas chromatography and comparison with hippuric acid levels in urine samples of individuals exposed to toluene. *Journal of Toxicology and Environmental Health* **50**, 401–407.

Armitage, P. (1955). Test for linear trend in proportions and frequencies. *Biometrics* **11**, 375–386.

Atawodi, S.E., Lea, S., Nyberg, F., Mukeria, A., Constantinescu, V., Ahrens, W., Brueske-Hohlfeld, I., Fortes, C., Boffetta, P., Friesen, M.D. (1998). 4-Hydroxyl-1-(3-pyridyl)-1-butanone-hemoglobin adducts as biomarkers of exposure to tobacco smoke: Validation of a method to be used in multicenter studies. *Cancer Epidemiology Biomarkers & Prevention* **7**, 817–821.

Atkinson, A.C. (1973). Testing transformations to normality. *Journal of the Royal Statistical Society Series B* **35**, 473–479.

Bartczak, A., Kline, S.A., Yu, R., Weisel, C.P., Goldstein, B.D., Witz, G. (1994). Evaluation of assays for the identification and quantitation of muconic acid, a benzene metabolite in human urine. *Journal of Toxicology and Environmental Health* **42**, 245–258.

Bartko, J.J. (1991). Measurement and reliability: Statistical thinking considerations. *Schizophrenia Bulletin* **17**, 483–489.

Bartko, J.J. (1994). General methodology II. Measures of agreement: A single procedure. *Statistics in Medicine* **13**, 737–745.

Benowitz, L. (1999). Biomarkers of environmental tobacco smoke exposure. *Environmental Health Perspectives* **107**(Suppl 2), 349–355.

Bernstein, C., Bernstein, H., Garewal, H., Dinning, P., Jabi, R., Sampliner, R.E., McCluskey, M.K., Panda, M., Roe, D.J., L'Heureux, L.L., Payne, C. (1999). A bile acid-induced apoptosis assay for colon cancer risk and associated quality control studies. *Cancer Research* **59**, 2353–2357.

Bland, J.M., Altman, D.G. (1986). Statistical methods for assessing agreement between two methods of clinical measurement. *The Lancet* (February 8, 1986), 307–310.

Bland, J.M., Altman, D.G. (1990). A note on the use of the intraclass correlation coefficient in the evaluation of agreement between two methods of measurement. *Computers in Biology and Medicine* **20**, 337–340.

Bonett, D.G., Wright, T.A. (2000). Sample size requirements for estimating Pearson, Kendall, and Spearman correlations. *Psychometrica* **65**, 23–28.

Box, G.E.P., Cox, D.R. (1964). An analysis of transformations. *Journal of the Royal Statistical Society Series B* **26**, 211–252.

Buckley, T.J., Waldman, J.M., Dhara, R., Greenberg, A., Ouyang, Z., Lioy, P.J. (1995). An assessment of a urinary biomarker for total human environmental exposure to benzo[a]pyrene. *International Archives of Occupational and Environmental Health* **67**, 257–266.

Buss, I.H., Senthilmohan, R., Darlow, B.A., Mogridge, N., Kettle, A.J., Winterbourn, C.C. (2003). 3-Chlorotyrosine as a marker of protein damage by myeloperoxidase in tracheal aspirates from preterm infants: Association with adverse respiratory outcome. *Pediatric Research* **53**, 455–462.

Byrt, T., Bishop, J., Carlin, J.B. (1993). Bias, prevalence, and kappa. *Journal of Clinical Epidemiology* **46**, 423–429.

Cheng, N.F., Gansky, S.A. A SAS macro to compute Lin's concordance correlation with confidence intervals. UCSF CAN-DO website. Accessed December 29, 2006. http://www.ucsf.edu/cando/resources/software/linscon.doc

Cicchetti, D.V., Feinstein, A.R. (1990). High agreement but low kappa: II. Resolving the paradoxes. *Journal of Clinical Epidemiology* **43**, 551–558.

Cochran, W.G. (1954). Some methods for strengthening the common χ^2 tests. *Biometrics* **10**, 417–454.

Cohen, J. (1960). A coefficient of agreement for nominal scales. *Educational and Psychological Measurement* **20**, 37–46.

Conover, W.J. (1999). *Practical Nonparametric Statistics*, 3rd ed. Wiley, New York.

Cook, D.G., Whincup, P.H., Papacosta, O., Strachan, D.P., Jarvis, M.J., Bryant, A. (1993). Relation of passive smoking as assessed by salivary cotinine concentration and questionnaire to spirometric indices in children. *Thorax* **48**, 14–20.

Cox, D.R., Hinkley, D.V. (1974). *Theoretical Statistics*. Chapman & Hall, London.

D'Agostino, R.B. (1986). Graphical analysis. In: D'Agostino, R.B., Stephens, M.A. (Eds.), *Goodness-of-Fit Techniques*. Marcel Dekker, New York, pp. 7–62.

Dunnett, C.W. (1980a). Pairwise multiple comparisons in the homogeneous variance, unequal sample size case. *Journal of the American Statistical Association* **75**, 789–795.

Dunnett, C.W. (1980b). Pairwise multiple comparisons in the unequal variance case. *Journal of the American Statistical Association* **75**, 796–800.

Feinstein, A.R., Cicchetti, D.V. (1990). High agreement but low kappa: I. The problems of two paradoxes. *Journal of Clinical Epidemiology* **43**, 543–549.

Fleiss, J.L. (1971). Measuring nominal scale agreement among many raters. *Psychological Bulletin* **76**, 378–382.

Gerson, M. (1975). The techniques and uses of probability plots. *The Statistician* **24**, 235–257.

Gibbons, J.D., Chakraborti, S. (2003). *Nonparametric Statistical Inference*, 4th ed. Marcel Dekker, New York.

Goldsmith, L.J. (2001). Power and sample size considerations in molecular biology. In: Looney, S.W. (Ed.), *Methods in Molecular Biology, Vol. 184: Biostatistical Methods*. Humana Press, Totowa, NJ, pp. 111–130.

Graham, P., Bull, B. (1998). Approximate standard errors and confidence intervals for indices of positive and negative agreement. *Journal of Clinical Epidemiology* **51**, 763–771.

Granella, M., Priante, E., Nardini, B., Bono, R., Clonfero, E. (1996). Excretion of mutagens, nicotine and its metabolites in urine of cigarette smokers. *Mutagenesis* **11**, 207–211.

Griffith, J., Aldrich, T.E., Duncan, R.C. (1993). Epidemiologic research methods. In: Aldrich, T., Griffithh, J., Cooke, C. (Eds.), *Environmental Epidemiology and Risk Assessment*. Van Nostrand Reinhold, New York, pp. 27–60.

Hagan, J.L., Looney, S.W. (2004). Frequency of use of statistical techniques for assessing agreement between continuous measurements. *Proceedings of the American Statistical Association*. American Statistical Association, Alexandria, VA, pp. 344–350.

Hazelton, M.L. (2003). A graphical tool for assessing normality. *The American Statistician* **57**, 285–288.

Huber, P.J. (1996). *Robust Statistical Procedures*, 2nd ed. Society for Industrial and Applied Mathematics, Philadelphia.

Johnson, N.L. (1949). Systems of frequency curves generated by methods of translation. *Biometrika* **36**, 149–176.

Jones, M.C., Daly, F. (1995). Density probability plots. *Communications in Statistics – Simulation and Computation* **24**, 911–927.

Kraemer, H.C. (1980). Extension of the kappa coefficient. *Biometrics* **36**, 207–216.

Kummel, C.H. (1879). Reduction of observation equations which contain more than one observed quantity. *The Analyst* **6**, 97–105.

Lagorio, S., Crebelli, R., Ricciarello, R., Conti, L., Iavarone, I., Zona, A., Ghittori, S., Carere, A. (1998). Methodological issues in biomonitoring of low level exposure to benzene. *Occupational Medicine* **8**, 497–504.

Landis, J.R., Koch, G.G. (1977). The measurement of observer agreement for categorical data. *Biometrics* **33**, 159–174.

Last, J.M. (1995). *A Dictionary of Epidemiology*, 3rd ed. Oxford University Press, New York.

Lehmann, E.L. (1975). *Nonparametrics: Statistical Methods Based on Ranks*. Holden-Day, San Francisco, pp. 267–270.

Lin, L.I. (1989). A concordance correlation coefficient to evaluate reproducibility. *Biometrics* **45**, 255–268.

Lin, L.I. (2000). A note on the concordance correlation coefficient. *Biometrics* **56**, 324–325.

Linnet, K. (1990). Estimation of the linear relationship between the measurements of two methods with proportional errors. *Statistics in Medicine* **9**, 1463–1473.

Linnet, K. (1993). Evaluation of regression procedures for methods comparison studies. *Clinical Chemistry* **39**, 424–432.

Looney, S.W. (1996). Sample size determination for correlation coefficient inference: Practical problems and practical solutions. *Proceedings of the Statistical Computing Section, American Statistical Association*. American Statistical Association, Alexandria, VA, pp. 240–245.

Looney, S.W. (Ed.) (2001). Statistical methods for assessing biomarkers. *Methods in Molecular Biology, Vol. 184: Biostatistical Methods*. Humana Press, Totowa, NJ, pp. 81–109.

Looney, S.W., Gulledge, T.R. (1985). Use of the correlation coefficient with normal probability plots. *The American Statistician* **39**, 75–79.

Lyles, R.H., Williams, J.K., Chuachoowong, R. (2001). Correlating two viral load assays with known detection limits. *Biometrics* **57**, 1238–1244.

MacRae, A.R., Gardner, H.A., Allen, L.C., Tokmakejian, S., Lepage, N. (2003). Outcome validation of the Beckman Coulter access analyzer in a second-trimester Down syndrome serum screening application. *Clinical Chemistry* **49**, 69–76.

Mehrotra, D.V., Chan, I.S.F., Berger, R.L. (2003). A cautionary note on exact unconditional inference for a difference between two independent binomial proportions. *Biometrics* **59**, 441–450.

Mehta, C., Patel, N. (2005). *StatXact 7*. CYTEL Software Corporation, Cambridge, MA.

Morton, R.F., Hebel, J.R., McCarter, R.J. (1996). *A Study Guide to Epidemiology and Biostatistics*, 4th ed. Aspen Publishers, Gaithersburg, MD, pp. 92–97.

Moser, B.K., Stevens, G.R. (1992). Homogeneity of variance in the two-sample means test. *The American Statistician* **46**, 19–21.

Moser, B.K., Stevens, G.R., Watts, C.L. (1989). The two-sample *t* test versus Satterthwaite's approximate *F* test. *Communications in Statistics Part A-Theory and Methods* **18**, 3963–3975.

Neuhäuser, M., Hothorn, L.A. (1999). An exact Cochran–Armitage test for trend when dose–response shapes are a priori unknown. *Computational Statistics and Data Analysis* **30**, 403–412.

Pérez-Stable, E.J., Benowitz, N.L., Marín, G. (1995). Is serum cotinine a better measure of cigarette smoking than self-report. *Preventive Medicine* **24**, 171–179.

Qiao, Y.-L., Tockman, M.S., Li, L., Erozan, Y.S., Yao, S., Barrett, M.J., Zhou, W., Giffen, C.A., Luo, X., Taylor, P.R. (1997). A case-cohort study of an early biomarker of lung cancer in a screening cohort of Yunnan tin miners in China. *Cancer Epidemiology, Biomarkers & Prevention* **6**, 893–900.

Royston, J.P. (1982). An extension of Shapiro and Wilk's W test for normality to large samples. *Applied Statistics – Journal of the Royal Statistical Society Series C* **31**, 115–124.

Royston, J.P. (1989). Correcting the Shapiro–Wilk *W* for ties. *Journal of Statistical Computation and Simulation* **31**, 237–249.

Royston, J.P. (1992). Approximating the Shapiro–Wilk's W test for non-normality. *Statistics and Computing* **2**, 117–119.

Salmi, M., Stolen, C., Jousilahti, P., Yegutkin, G.G., Tapanainen, P., Janatuinen, T., Knip, M., Jalkanen, S., Salomaa, V. (2002). Insulin-regulated increase of soluble vascular adhesion protein-1 in diabetes. *The American Journal of Pathology* **161**, 2255–2262.

Scheuren, F. (2005). Multiple imputation: How it began and continues. *The American Statistician* **59**, 315–319.

Shapiro, S.S., Wilk, M.B. (1965). An analysis of variance test for normality (complete samples). *Biometrika* **52**, 591–611.

Shapiro, S.S., Wilk, M.B., Chen, H.J. (1968). A comparative study of various tests for normality. *Journal of the American Statistical Association* **63**, 1343–1372.

Sheskin, D.J. (1997). *Handbook of Parametric and Nonparametric Statistical Procedures*. CRC Press, Boca Raton, FL.

Shoukri, M.M. (2004). *Measures of Interobserver Agreement*. Chapman & Hall/CRC, Boca Raton, FL.

Siegel, S., Castellan, N.J. (1988). *Nonparametric Statistics for the Behavioral Sciences*, 2nd ed. McGraw-Hill, New York.

Steiger, J.H. (1980). Tests for comparing elements of a correlation matrix. *Psychological Bulletin* **87**, 245–251.

Stoline, M.R., Ury, H.K. (1979). Tables of the studentized maximum modulus distribution and an application to multiple comparisons among means. *Technometrics* **21**, 87–93.

Strachan, D.P., Jarvis, M.J., Feyerabend, C. (1990). The relationship of salivary cotinine to respiratory symptoms, spirometry, and exercise-induced bronchospasm in seven-year-old children. *The American Review of Respiratory Disease* **142**, 147–151.

Strike, P.W. (1996). *Measurement in Laboratory Medicine: A Primer on Control and Interpretation*. Butterworth-Heinemann, Oxford, pp. 147–172.

Stuart, A., Ord, J.K. (1987). *Kendall's Advanced Theory of Statistics*. Oxford University Press, New York, pp. 210–220.

Suissa, S., Shuster, J. (1991). The 2×2 matched-pairs trial: Exact unconditional design and analysis. *Biometrics* **47**, 361–372.

Taylor, D.J., Kupper, L.L., Rappaport, S.M., Lyles, R.H. (2001). A mixture model for occupational exposure mean testing with a limit of detection. *Biometrics* **57**, 681–688.

Tockman, M.S., Gupta, P.K., Myers, J.D., Frost, J.K., Baylin, S.B., Gold, E.B., Chase, A.M., Wilkinson, P.H., Mulshine, J.L. (1988). Sensitive and specific monoclonal antibody recognition of human lung cancer antigen on preserved sputum cells: A new approach to early lung cancer detection. *Journal of Clinical Oncology* **6**, 1685–1693.

Tukey, J.W. (1977). *Exploratory Data Analysis*. Addison-Wesley, Reading, MA.

Tunstall-Pedoe, H., Brown, C.A., Woodward, M., Tavendale, R. (1995). Passive smoking by self-report and serum cotinine and the prevalence of respiratory and coronary heart disease in the Scottish heart health study. *Journal of Epidemiology and Community Health* **49**, 139–143.

Wang, H. (2006). Correlation analysis for left-censored biomarker data with known detection limits. Unpublished Masters thesis, Louisiana State University Health Sciences Center, Biostatistics Program, School of Public Health.

Westgard, J.O., Hunt, M.R. (1973). Use and interpretation of common statistical tests in method-comparison studies. *Clinical Chemistry* **19**, 49–57.

Wilcox, R.R. (1987). *New Statistical Procedures for the Social Sciences*. Lawrence Erlbaum Associates, Hillsdale, NJ.

Wilk, M.B., Shapiro, S.S. (1968). The joint assessment of normality of several independent samples. *Technometrics* **10**, 825–839.

Handbook of Statistics, Vol. 27
ISSN: 0169-7161
DOI: 10.1016/S0169-7161(07)27005-1

3

Linear and Non-Linear Regression Methods in Epidemiology and Biostatistics

*Eric Vittinghoff, Charles E. McCulloch,
David V. Glidden and Stephen C. Shiboski*

Abstract

This chapter describes a family of statistical techniques called linear and non-linear regression that are commonly used in medical research. Regression is typically used to relate an outcome (or dependent variable or response) to one or more predictor variables (or independent variables or covariates). We examine several ways in which the standard linear model can be extended to accommodate non-linearity. These include non-linear transformation of predictors and outcomes within the standard linear model framework; generalized linear models, in which the mean of the outcome is modeled as a non-linear transformation of the standard linear function of regression parameters and predictors; and fully non-linear models, in which the mean of the outcome is modeled as a non-linear function of the regression parameters. We also briefly discuss several special topics, including causal models, models with measurement error in the predictors, and missing data problems.

1. Introduction

This chapter describes a family of statistical techniques called linear and non-linear regression that are commonly used in medical research. Regression is typically used to relate an outcome (or dependent variable or response) to one or more predictor variables (or independent variables or covariates). The goal might be prediction, testing for a relationship with a single predictor (perhaps while adjusting for other predictors), or in modeling the relationship between the outcome and all the predictors. We begin with an example.

1.1. Example: Medical services utilization

The most acutely ill patients treated by a hospital system use a highly disproportionate amount of resources – often in ways that can be prevented. For example, persons without insurance may use the emergency room for non-emergency care. Sorenson et al. (2003) and Masson et al. (2004) described the utilization of medical resources in 190 patients enrolled in a randomized trial of a managed care intervention designed to improve access to healthcare. Measurements were taken at baseline, as well as at 6, 12, and 18 months after randomization. Outcomes included cost of care, number of emergency room visits, and death. Predictors included treatment group (managed care or not), gender, the Beck depression inventory (BDI), and whether the person was homeless. A primary focus was on the treatment effect, while adjusting for the effects of the other predictors. A secondary goal was to assess the impact of all the predictors on the outcomes.

1.2. Linear and non-linear regression methods

The choice of an appropriate regression model depends on both the type of outcome being modeled, which governs the random portion of the model, and how the parameters to be estimated enter the model, which governs whether it is a linear or non-linear model. In our example, cost is likely to be highly skewed right, while the logarithm of cost might be more approximately normally distributed. Death during the 18 months of follow-up is binary or could be analyzed as time to death. And number of emergency room visits is a count variable, for which we might consider a Poisson distribution appropriate. A further complication in our example is that we have repeated measurements over time on the same patient (e.g., number of emergency room visits during the preceding 6 months is collected at 6, 12, and 18 months), so that the data need to be treated as correlated.

Each of these different outcome types – continuous and skewed right, continuous and approximately normally distributed, binary, time-to-event, or count – would typically need a different style of regression analysis. Treating log(cost) at 6 months as approximately normally distributed might suggest using the usual linear regression model

$$\log \text{cost}_i = \beta_0 + \beta_1 x_{1i} + \beta_2 x_{2i} + \beta_3 x_{3i} + \beta_4 x_{4i} + \varepsilon_i, \tag{1}$$

where cost_i is the 6-month cost of medical care for patient i, x_{1i} is 1 if the patient was in the case management group and 0 otherwise, x_{2i} is 1 if the patient is female and 0 otherwise, x_{3i} is the patient's BDI at baseline, x_{4i} is 1 if the patient was homeless at baseline and 0 otherwise, and ε_i is an error term. The parameters to be estimated (the βs) enter Eq. (1) as a linear combination, hence the name *linear regression*.

Re-expressing Eq. (1) as a model for cost_i by exponentiating both sides of the equation gives

$$\begin{aligned} \text{cost}_i &= e^{\beta_0} e^{\beta_1 x_{1i}} e^{\beta_2 x_{2i}} e^{\beta_3 x_{3i}} e^{\beta_4 x_{4i}} e^{\varepsilon_i} \\ &= \gamma_0 \gamma_1^{x_{1i}} \gamma_2^{x_{2i}} \gamma_3^{x_{3i}} \gamma_4^{x_{4i}} \delta_i, \end{aligned} \tag{2}$$

where $\gamma_k = e^{\beta_k}$ and $\delta_i = e^{\varepsilon_i}$.

This is somewhat different, as we elaborate in Section 3.1, from the *non-linear regression* equation, below, which assumes (incorrectly) that cost_i is homoscedastic and normally distributed:

$$\text{cost}_i = \alpha_0 \alpha_1^{x_{1i}} \alpha_2^{x_{2i}} \alpha_3^{x_{3i}} \alpha_4^{x_{4i}} + v_i \quad \text{with} \quad v_i \sim \text{i.i.d.} \mathcal{N}(0, \sigma_v^2). \tag{3}$$

On the other hand, treating death during the 18-month follow-up period as a binary outcome would usually be handled with a *logistic regression* model, in which the probability of death is modeled in the form

$$P(D_i) = \frac{1}{1 + \exp(-[\beta_0 + \beta_1 x_{1i} + \beta_2 x_{2i} + \beta_3 x_{3i} + \beta_4 x_{4i}])}, \qquad (4)$$

where D_i is 1 if the ith patient died and 0 otherwise, and these are not the same βs as in Eq. (1). Clearly the parameters to be estimated for this model (the βs) enter in a non-linear fashion. There is no error term in this model, because the randomness is captured by the Bernoulli distribution with the appropriate probability of death given by Eq. (4).

This is an example of a *generalized linear model* (GLM) because we can transform the mean response (which is just the probability for a binary variable like D_i) to get a model that *is* linear in the parameters:

$$\log \frac{P(D_i)}{1 - P(D_i)} = \beta_0 + \beta_1 x_{1i} + \beta_2 x_{2i} + \beta_3 x_{3i} + \beta_4 x_{4i}. \qquad (5)$$

The left-hand side of Eq. (5) is the log of the ratio of the probability of death compared to the probability of survival, or the log of the *odds* of death. Therefore the logistic regression model is a linear model for the log odds and the parameters have interpretations in terms of the difference in log odds of the outcome associated with a one-unit change in the predictor (holding the other variables "constant").

The various regression models are clearly different but still share important features. The accommodation of multiple predictors and continuous or categorical predictors is similar. Techniques for adjustment by variables to control confounding and incorporate interactions, and methods for predictor selection are similar. Finally, all regression analyses are used to answer the same broad classes of practical questions involving multiple predictors.

1.3. Overview

This chapter provides a practical survey of linear and non-linear regression analysis in biomedical studies and to provide pointers to the other, more detailed chapters on special types of regression models elsewhere in this book. We start by introducing the idea of linear regression, in which the model for the mean of the outcome is a linear combination of the parameters, an example of which is Eq. (1), when the outcome is log(cost). In this context we describe inference, model checking, extensions to repeated measures data, and choice of predictors. Next, we show how building a linear model for transformations of the outcome, such as the model for log(cost), induces a non-linear model for the untransformed outcome, e.g., cost itself. Non-linear models are then developed, with identification of the important special case of generalized linear models, i.e., a model in which a transformation of the mean is a linear combination of the parameters. We also cover some models capable of handling censored data, as well as models where no transformation of the mean is linear in the parameters. Finally, we discuss recent developments such as the use of classification and regression trees (CART), generalized additive models (GAMs), and segmented and asymptotic regression, as well as computing for regression analyses.

2. Linear models

In the multiple linear regression model, the expected value of the outcome for observation i, given a set of predictors $\mathbf{x}'_i = (x_{1i}, x_{2i}, \ldots, x_{pi})$, is specified by a linear combination of the parameters $\beta_0, \beta_1, \ldots, \beta_p$:

$$E[Y_i|\mathbf{x_i}] = \beta_0 + \beta_1 x_{1i} + \beta_2 x_{2i} + \cdots + \beta_p x_{pi}. \tag{6}$$

In Eq. (6), the coefficient β_j gives the change in $E[Y_i|\mathbf{x}_i]$ for an increase of one unit in predictor x_{ji}, holding other factors in the model constant. The intercept β_0 gives the value of $E[Y|\mathbf{x}]$ if all the predictors were equal to zero. Considering all observations in the sample ($i = 1, \ldots, N$), we can write

$$E[\mathbf{Y}|\mathbf{X}] = \mathbf{X}\boldsymbol{\beta}, \tag{7}$$

where the outcomes are written as vector $\mathbf{Y}$ of order N; $\mathbf{X}$ is the *model matrix* of order N by $p+1$ with ith row $\mathbf{x}'_i$; and $\boldsymbol{\beta}$ is the vector of $p+1$ regression coefficients.

Random departures of the outcomes from their expectations may result from measurement error as well as unmeasured determinants of the outcome. Thus

$$\mathbf{Y} = \mathbf{X}\boldsymbol{\beta} + \boldsymbol{\varepsilon}, \tag{8}$$

where the vector of random errors $\boldsymbol{\varepsilon}$ has mean $\mathbf{0}$ and variance–covariance matrix $\mathbf{V}$. Note that given $\mathbf{X}$, $\mathbf{Y}$ also has variance–covariance matrix $\mathbf{V}$. In the basic form of the multiple linear regression model we usually assume that $\boldsymbol{\varepsilon} \sim \mathcal{N}(\mathbf{0}, \sigma^2\mathbf{I})$, where $\mathbf{I}$ is the identity matrix of order N; that is, the random errors are normally distributed with mean zero and constant variance σ^2, and are independent across observations.

In contrast to the outcome, no distributional assumptions are made about the predictors. However, we do formally assume that the predictors are measured without error. This is often not very realistic, and the effects of violations are the subject of ongoing statistical research. In Section 4.2, we briefly discuss the issue of measurement error.

2.1. Maximum likelihood (ML) under normality

Under the assumption that $\mathbf{Y}$ has a multivariate normal distribution – that is,

$$\mathbf{Y} \sim \mathcal{N}(\mathbf{X}\boldsymbol{\beta}, \sigma^2\mathbf{I}) \tag{9}$$

the likelihood function is

$$L = L(\boldsymbol{\beta}, \sigma^2) = \frac{\exp\left[-\frac{1}{2}(\mathbf{Y} - \mathbf{X}\boldsymbol{\beta})'(\mathbf{I}/\sigma^2)(\mathbf{Y} - \mathbf{X}\boldsymbol{\beta})\right]}{(2\pi\sigma^2)^{N/2}}. \tag{10}$$

Thus the log-likelihood is

$$l = \log L = -\frac{N}{2}\log(2\pi) - \frac{N}{2}\log\sigma^2 - \frac{1}{2}(\mathbf{Y} - \mathbf{X}\boldsymbol{\beta})'(\mathbf{Y} - X\boldsymbol{\beta})/\sigma^2 \qquad (11)$$

Setting the vector of partial derivatives of the log-likelihood with respect to the elements of $\boldsymbol{\beta}$ equal to $\mathbf{0}$ gives the *score* equation for $\boldsymbol{\beta}$:

$$\frac{\partial l}{\partial \boldsymbol{\beta}} = \frac{\mathbf{X}'\mathbf{Y} - \mathbf{X}'\mathbf{X}\boldsymbol{\beta}}{\sigma^2} = \mathbf{0} \qquad (12)$$

with solution

$$\hat{\boldsymbol{\beta}} = (\mathbf{X}'\mathbf{X})^{-1}\mathbf{X}'\mathbf{Y} \qquad (13)$$

if $(\mathbf{X}'\mathbf{X})^{-1}$ exists. See McCulloch and Searle (2000) for a full development of important cases where $\mathbf{X}$ is not full rank and generalized inverses of $\mathbf{X}'\mathbf{X}$ must be used.

For σ^2 the score equation is

$$\frac{\partial l}{\partial \sigma^2} = \frac{(\mathbf{Y} - \mathbf{X}\boldsymbol{\beta})'(\mathbf{Y} - \mathbf{X}\boldsymbol{\beta})}{2\sigma^4} - \frac{N}{2\sigma^2} = 0 \qquad (14)$$

with solution

$$\hat{\sigma}^2_{ml} = (\mathbf{Y} - \mathbf{X}\hat{\boldsymbol{\beta}})'(\mathbf{Y} - \mathbf{X}\hat{\boldsymbol{\beta}})/N \qquad (15)$$

In practice the unbiased *restricted maximum likelihood* (REML) estimate (McCulloch and Searle, 2000) is more often used. In REML, $\boldsymbol{\beta}$ is removed from the likelihood by considering the likelihood of

$$\left[\mathbf{I} - \mathbf{X}(\mathbf{X}'\mathbf{X})^{-1}\mathbf{X}'\right]\mathbf{Y}, \qquad (16)$$

in this simple case giving

$$\hat{\sigma}^2 = \frac{(\mathbf{Y} - \mathbf{X}\hat{\boldsymbol{\beta}})'(\mathbf{Y} - \mathbf{X}\hat{\boldsymbol{\beta}})}{N - (p + 1)} \qquad (17)$$

Finally, under regularity conditions, $\hat{\boldsymbol{\beta}}$ is a consistent estimator of $\boldsymbol{\beta}$, with asymptotic variance–covariance estimator $\hat{\sigma}^2(\mathbf{X}'\mathbf{X})^{-1}$ based on the Hessian of the log-likelihood – that is, the matrix of its second partial derivatives with respect to $\boldsymbol{\beta}$.

2.2. Ordinary least squares

Estimation of the regression parameters in the multiple linear regression model can also be understood in terms of *ordinary least squares* (OLS), meaning that $\hat{\boldsymbol{\beta}}$ is the value of $\boldsymbol{\beta}$ that minimizes the *residual sum of squares* under the proposed linear model:

$$\text{RSS} = (\mathbf{Y} - \mathbf{X}\boldsymbol{\beta})'(\mathbf{Y} - \mathbf{X}\boldsymbol{\beta}). \qquad (18)$$

Setting the vector of partial derivatives of Eq. (18) with respect to $\boldsymbol{\beta}$ equal to $\mathbf{0}$ gives

$$\hat{\boldsymbol{\beta}} = (\mathbf{X'X})^{-1}\mathbf{X'Y}. \tag{19}$$

Thus the OLS criterion motivates the same estimator of $\boldsymbol{\beta}$, without making distributional assumptions, as does maximum likelihood in the case where $\mathbf{Y}$ is multivariate normal.

The variance of $\hat{\boldsymbol{\beta}}$ can be written as

$$\begin{aligned}
\boldsymbol{\Sigma} &= \text{var}[(\mathbf{X'X})^{-1}\mathbf{X'Y}] \\
&= (\mathbf{X'X})^{-1}\mathbf{X'} \,\text{var}[\mathbf{Y}]\mathbf{X}(\mathbf{X'X})^{-1} \\
&= (\mathbf{X'X})^{-1}\mathbf{X'VX}(\mathbf{X'X})^{-1}
\end{aligned} \tag{20}$$

Clearly $\boldsymbol{\Sigma}$ simplifies to $\sigma^2(\mathbf{X'X})^{-1}$ when $\mathbf{V} = \sigma^2\mathbf{I}$.

If $E[\mathbf{Y}|\mathbf{X}]$ is of the form $\mathbf{X}\boldsymbol{\beta}$ and $\mathbf{X}$ is full rank, $\hat{\boldsymbol{\beta}}$ is unbiased:

$$\begin{aligned}
E[\hat{\boldsymbol{\beta}}] &= E[(\mathbf{X'X})^{-1}\mathbf{X'Y}] \\
&= (\mathbf{X'X})^{-1}\mathbf{X'}E[\mathbf{Y}] \\
&= (\mathbf{X'X})^{-1}\mathbf{X'X}\boldsymbol{\beta} \\
&= \boldsymbol{\beta}
\end{aligned} \tag{21}$$

Under the assumptions of independence and constant variance – that is, $\mathbf{V} = \sigma^2\mathbf{I}$ – the OLS estimates are minimally variable among linear unbiased estimators. They are also well-behaved in large samples when the normality assumptions concerning $\mathbf{Y}$ are not precisely met. A potentially important drawback of OLS is sensitivity to influential data points.

2.3. Tests and confidence intervals

At least in large samples, the estimates of the regression parameters have a multivariate normal distribution. This follows on theoretical grounds if the outcome $\mathbf{Y}$ is multivariate normal as in Eq. (9), regardless of sample size. Otherwise, the OLS estimators converge in distribution to multivariate normality as the sample size increases under fairly mild assumptions. If the outcome is short-tailed, then the tests and confidence intervals may be valid with as few as 30–50 observations. However, with long-tailed or skewed outcomes, samples of at least 100 may be required. Factors influencing the precision of the estimates are made clear by writing the variance of a particular $\hat{\beta}_j$ as:

$$\text{Var}(\hat{\beta}_j) = \frac{\sigma^2}{(N-1)s_{x_j}^2(1-r_j^2)}. \tag{22}$$

In Eq. (22), $s_{x_j}^2$ is the sample variance of x_j, and r_j is the multiple correlation of x_j with the other predictors; $1/(1-r_j^2)$ is known as the *variance inflation factor*. In brief, the parameter β_j is more precisely estimated when the residual variance σ^2 is small, the sample size N and sample variance of x_j are large, and x_j is minimally correlated with the other predictors in the model.

When $\mathbf{Y}$ is multivariate normal, the ratio of $\hat{\beta}_j - \beta_j$ to its standard error (defined as the square root of the estimate of Eq. (22), using Eq. (17) for σ^2) has a t-distribution with $N - (p+1)$ degrees of freedom. This reference distribution is used for Wald tests of H_0: $\beta_j = 0$, and to compute confidence intervals for β_j as

$$\hat{\beta}_j \pm t_{\alpha/2, N-(p+1)} \sqrt{\hat{\mathrm{Var}}(\hat{\beta}_j)}, \tag{23}$$

where $t_{\alpha/2, N-(p+1)}$ is the $\alpha/2$ quantile of the reference t-distribution. By extension, the variance of a linear combination $c = \mathbf{a}'\hat{\boldsymbol{\beta}}$ of the parameter estimates is $\mathbf{a}'\Sigma\mathbf{a}$, providing analogous hypothesis tests and confidence intervals for c.

The F-test is used to test composite null hypotheses involving more than one parameter, including tests for heterogeneity in the mean of the outcome across levels of multilevel categorical predictors. Suppose the categorical predictor has $k > 2$ levels and is represented by $k - 1$ indicator variables $x_{2i}, x_{3i}, \ldots, x_{ki}$, with $x_{ji} = 1$ if observation i is in category j ($j = 2, \ldots, k$) and 0 otherwise. The corresponding parameters are $\beta_2, \beta_3, \ldots, \beta_k$; x_{1i} and β_1 correspond to the reference level and are omitted. Then the F-statistic for the test of $H_0 : \beta_2 = \beta_3 = \cdots = \beta_k = 0$ is

$$F = \frac{(\mathrm{RSS}_r - \mathrm{RSS}_f)/(k-1)}{\mathrm{RSS}_f/(N-(p+1))} \tag{24}$$

where RSS_f is the residual sum of squares from the full model including the $k - 1$ indicator variables $x_2, x_3, \ldots, x_k$ and RSS_r is from the reduced model excluding these covariates. The statistic is compared to the F-distribution with $k - 1$ and $N - (p+1)$ degrees of freedom. Within the maximum likelihood framework, the F-statistic can be derived as a monotonic transformation of the likelihood-ratio statistic (McCulloch and Searle, 2000).

These exact methods for inference when $\mathbf{Y}$ is multivariate normal do not apply to non-linear models, nor to linear models used with unbalanced repeated measures data. For those cases, hypothesis testing with either maximum likelihood or restricted maximum likelihood utilizes the large sample theory of maximum likelihood estimators. Typical are Wald tests, in which the estimators divided by their standard errors are treated as approximately normal to form z-statistics. Likewise, approximate confidence intervals are based on normality by calculating the estimate ± 1.96 standard errors. Standard errors typically come from the Hessian of the log-likelihood. Kenward and Roger (1997) have suggested adjustments to improve the small sample performance of the Wald statistics in extensions of the linear model for repeated measures (see Section 2.5). Alternatively, likelihood-ratio tests and confidence regions based on the likelihood are also commonly used to form test statistics and confidence regions for $\boldsymbol{\beta}$. These are regarded as more reliable than the Wald procedures and should be used in circumstances where the two procedures give discrepant results (Cox and Hinkley, 1974).

2.4. Checking model assumptions and fit

In the multiple linear regression model (Eq. (8)), we start with assumptions that $E[\mathbf{Y}|\mathbf{X}]$ changes linearly with each continuous predictor and that the errors ε

are independently multivariate normal with mean zero and constant variance. Violations of these assumptions have the potential to bias regression coefficient estimates and undermine the validity of confidence intervals and *p*-values, and thus may motivate the use of non-linear models. Residuals are central to detecting violations of these assumptions and also assessing their severity. Model assumptions rarely hold exactly, and small departures can be benign, especially in large datasets. Nonetheless, careful attention to model assumptions can prevent us from being seriously misled, and help us to decide when non-linear methods need to be used.

Linearity. In single predictor models, checks for departures from linearity could be carried out using a non-parametric smoother, such as LOWESS (Cleveland, 1981) of the outcome on the single predictor, approximating the regression line under the weaker assumption that it is smooth but not necessarily linear. Substantial and systematic deviations of the non-parametric estimate from the linear fit indicate departures from linearity. Smoothing the residuals rather than the outcome may give a more sensitive assessment, and extends this strategy to the multiple linear regression model, providing a check on linearity after the effects of covariates have been taken into account. In this context, we smooth the residuals against each continuous predictor (*residual* vs *predictor* plots) as well as the fitted values (*residual* vs *fitted* plots). Related diagnostic plots include *component plus residual* plots (Larsen and McCleary, 1972), in which the contribution of the predictor of interest to each fitted value is added back into the corresponding residual, which is then smoothed against the predictor. In all cases, a well-behaved smoother with skillfully chosen smoothness is important for detecting non-linearity.

Departures from linearity can often be corrected using transformations of the continuous predictors causing problems. For strictly positive predictors, log transformation is useful for modeling "diminishing returns," in which the mean of the outcome changes more and more slowly as the predictor increases. In polynomial models, we may add quadratic, cubic, and even higher-order terms in the predictor. For mild non-linearities, addition of a quadratic term in the predictor is often adequate. However, for highly non-linear response patterns, polynomial models may not provide adequate flexibility, or provide it only at the cost of poor performance in the extremes of the predictor range.

In contrast to polynomial models, *splines* provide more flexibility where the predictor values are concentrated and better performance at the extremes, by fitting local polynomial models under constraints that preserve continuity and smoothness, often making the results more plausible. Simplest are *linear splines*, which model the mean response to the predictor as continuous and piecewise linear, changing slope at *knots*, or cutpoints in the range of the predictor, but linear within the intervals between knots. In the simplest cases, the knots are placed by the analyst at sample quantiles or at inflections in diagnostic smooths; however, automatic, adaptive methods are also available. *Cubic splines* are local third-order polynomials, constrained to have continuous first and second derivatives at the knots; only the third derivative is allowed to jump. *Natural cubic splines* are constrained to be linear beyond the outermost knots, for better behavior in the tails. These spline models are implemented using a linear combination of *basis* functions defined for each value of the continuous predictor, and thus remain linear in the parameters. *Smoothing splines* can be understood as cubic splines with a knot at each unique value of the predictor, but incorporating a penalty in the log-likelihood to prevent overfitting (Hastie et al., 2001). This results in shrinkage of the parameter estimates corresponding to the basis functions of the spline toward zero. The penalty parameter determining the degree of smoothness is commonly chosen by cross-validation, discussed below.

Normality. Residuals are also central to the evaluation of normality and constant variance. *Quantile–quantile* plots provide the most direct assessment of normality of the residuals; also potentially useful are histograms and non-parametric density plots. Long tails and skewness are more problematic for linear models than short-tailed distributions, with reduced efficiency the most likely result. However, both types of violation become less important with increasing sample size. In addition to diagnostic plots, which can be difficult to interpret, particularly in small samples, numerous statistical tests for non-normality are available. A disadvantage of these tests is that they lack sensitivity in small samples, where violations are relatively important, and may in contrast "detect" trivial violations in large samples.

Departures from normality can sometimes be corrected by transforming the outcome. Log and fractional power (square and cube root) transformations are commonly used for right-skewed outcome variables. Rank transformation, resulting in a uniform distribution, can be used when both tails are too long, though this incurs some loss of information. When no normalizing transformation can be found, the generalized linear models discussed in more detail below are often used.

Constant variance. Reduced efficiency as well as mistaken inferences can result from serious violations of this assumption, in particular when the mean of the outcome is being compared across subgroups of unequal size with substantially different residual variance. The OLS estimates remain unbiased but naive standard errors can be seriously misleading. In contrast to violations of the normality assumption, the adverse effects of unequal variance are not mitigated by increasing sample size.

The constant variance assumption can be checked by assessing patterns in the spread of the residuals in the residual vs. predictor and residual vs. fitted plots also used to assess linearity; similarly, the variance of the residuals within levels of categorical predictors can be compared. As for normality, tests for heteroscedasticity are available (White, 1980), but have low power in small datasets and are thus not recommended.

One often-used approach to rectifying non-constant variance is transformation of the outcome. In many situations, the variance grows approximately in proportion to the mean. In that case, the log transformation is ideal in that it will remove heteroscedasticity. Often, other model assumptions hold on the transformed scale, although this is not guaranteed.

Alternatively, if the variance matrix of the errors is known, inference can proceed by weighted least squares, which will produce unbiased and efficient point estimates of $\hat{\beta}$. However, the required variance matrix is usually unknown. For that case, a variety of asymptotic estimators, variants of the robust or "sandwich" variance estimator (Huber, 1967) explained in more detail below, are consistent in the presence of heteroscedasticity. In this case $\mathbf{V}$ in Eq. (20) is a diagonal matrix with element v_{ii} estimated by some function of $e_i = (Y_i - \mathbf{x}'_i\hat{\boldsymbol{\beta}})$, the residual for observation i. While the various estimators are asymptotically equivalent, their behavior in small sample sizes can vary considerably. In extensive simulations, Long and Ervin (2000) show that the basic robust HC0 estimator, with $\hat{v}_{ii} \equiv e_i^2$, performs poorly in samples as large as 250 observations. They find that the more conservative HC3 estimator developed by MacKinnon and White (1985) has the best properties and should be used when subject-matter knowledge or exploratory data analysis suggests heteroscedasticity. In the HC3 estimator, $\hat{v}_{ii} = (e_i/(1 - h_{ii}))^2$, where h_{ii} is the ith diagonal element of the *hat* or *projection* matrix $\mathbf{H} = \mathbf{X}(\mathbf{X}'\mathbf{X})^{-1}\mathbf{X}'$.

Influential points. We would mistrust regression results – which purport to summarize the information in the entire dataset – if they change substantively when one or a few observations are omitted from the analysis. This can happen when *high-leverage* observations with extreme values of one or more of the predictors, or an anomalous combination of predictor values, also have large residuals. Especially in small datasets, the OLS coefficient estimates may unduly reflect minimization of the contribution of these observations to RSS. In linear models it is easy to compute the exact changes in each of the regression coefficient estimates, called *DFBETAs*, when each of the N observations is omitted; in logistic regression and other GLMs easily computed approximations are available. Boxplots of these *DFBETA* statistics for each predictor can then be used to identify influential points. Statistics that summarize the influence of each observation on all coefficient estimates include *DFITS* (Welsch and Kuh, 1977), *Cook's distance* (Cook, 1977), and *Welsch distance* (Welsch, 1982). Identifying influential *sets* of observations that are influential in combination but not necessarily individually remains a difficult computational problem.

2.5. Repeated measures

It is not unusual to collect repeated measurements on the same individuals, at the same centers, or from the same doctors. For example, in the medical services utilization example, measurements were taken on the same person at baseline, 6, 12, and 18 months after randomization. Outcomes measured on the same person, center, or doctor (sometimes called a cluster) are almost certain to be correlated and this needs to be accommodated in the analysis. Another feature of such data is that predictors can be measured at the observation level (e.g., length of time post-randomization or whether the person was homeless a majority of the preceding 6 months) or at the cluster level (gender, treatment group).

Consider an elaboration of the introductory model to accommodate the repeated measures:

$$Y_{it} = \log \text{cost}_{it} = \beta_0 + \beta_1 x_{1i} + \beta_2 x_{2i} + \beta_3 x_{3it} + \beta_4 x_{4it} + \delta_{it}, \tag{25}$$

where cost_{it} is the cost of medical care during the previous 6 months for $t = 6, 12$, or 18, x_{1i} is 1 if the patient was in the case management group and 0 otherwise,

x_{2i} is 1 if the patient is female and 0 otherwise, x_{3it} is the patient's BDI at time t, x_{4it} is 1 if the patient was homeless a majority of the past six months and 0 otherwise, and δ_{it} is an error term.

So far there is nothing in the model to incorporate the potential correlation among measurements within a subject. One method is to directly assume a correlation among the error terms:

$$\text{var} \begin{pmatrix} \delta_{i6} \\ \delta_{i12} \\ \delta_{i18} \end{pmatrix} = \Sigma_\delta = \begin{pmatrix} \sigma_{\delta,6,6} & \sigma_{\delta,6,12} & \sigma_{\delta,6,18} \\ \sigma_{\delta,12,6} & \sigma_{\delta,12,12} & \sigma_{\delta,12,18} \\ \sigma_{\delta,18,6} & \sigma_{\delta,18,6} & \sigma_{\delta,18,18} \end{pmatrix}. \tag{26}$$

Another common strategy is to induce a variance–covariance structure by hypothesizing the existence of random effects. Essentially we decompose the error term, δ_{it} into two pieces, a subject-specific term, b, and an observation-specific term, ε:

$$\delta_{it} = b_i + \varepsilon_{it}, \tag{27}$$

with $b_i \sim$ i.i.d. $\mathcal{N}(0, \sigma_b^2)$ independent of $\varepsilon_{it} \sim$ i.i.d. $\mathcal{N}(0, \sigma_\varepsilon^2)$. The b_i are called *random effects* since we have assigned them a distribution. In this case, (25) would be called a *mixed model*, since it would include random effects as well as the usual *fixed* effects x_1, ..., x_4.

From this model is it easy to calculate the covariance between two observations on the same subject: $\text{cov}(Y_{it}, Y_{is}) = \text{cov}(\delta_{it}, \delta_{is}) = \sigma_b^2$. Note that this result holds without needing the assumption of normality of b_i or ε_{it}. In a similar manner it is straightforward to calculate the variance of Y_{it} or Y_{is} as $\sigma_b^2 + \sigma_e^2$ and the correlation between them as $\sigma_b^2/(\sigma_b^2 + \sigma_e^2)$.

So Eq. (27) corresponds to a special case of Eq. (26) with

$$\Sigma_\delta = \mathbf{I}\sigma_\varepsilon^2 + \mathbf{J}\sigma_b^2 = \begin{pmatrix} \sigma_\varepsilon^2 + \sigma_b^2 & \sigma_b^2 & \sigma_b^2 \\ \sigma_b^2 & \sigma_\varepsilon^2 + \sigma_b^2 & \sigma_b^2 \\ \sigma_b^2 & \sigma_b^2 & \sigma_\varepsilon^2 + \sigma_b^2 \end{pmatrix}, \tag{28}$$

where $\mathbf{J}$ is a matrix of all ones.

2.5.1. Estimation
Whether we formulate the model as Eq. (26) or the special case of Eq. (27), how should we fit the model and conduct statistical inference? OLS does not accommodate the correlated data. If the variance–covariance matrix, $\mathbf{V}$, were known, then weighted least squares could be used, weighting by the inverse of the variance–covariance matrix. This would yield:

$$\hat{\beta}_V = (\mathbf{X}'\mathbf{V}^{-1}\mathbf{X})^{-1}\mathbf{X}'\mathbf{V}^{-1}\mathbf{Y}. \tag{29}$$

Or with a full parametric specification (i.e., that the data are multivariate normal) a logical method is maximum likelihood or a variant mentioned earlier, restricted maximum likelihood.

Consider a general model for the situation with correlated data and a linear model for the mean:

$$\mathbf{Y} \sim \mathcal{N}(\mathbf{X}\boldsymbol{\beta}, \mathbf{V}). \tag{30}$$

For the medical utilization example, if each of the N subjects had exactly three observations that followed model (26), and if the data vector $\mathbf{Y}$ were ordered by subject, then $\mathbf{V} = \mathbf{I}_N \otimes \boldsymbol{\Sigma}_\delta$, with $\otimes$ denoting a Kronecker product, i.e., $\mathbf{A} \otimes \mathbf{B}$ is a partitioned matrix with entries $a_{ij}\mathbf{B}$. In particular $\mathbf{V} = \mathbf{I}_N \otimes \boldsymbol{\Sigma}_\delta$ implies that $\mathbf{V}$ is block diagonal with $\boldsymbol{\Sigma}_\delta$ on the diagonal.

It is easy to show that the OLS estimator is unbiased, even in the presence of correlated data: Eq. (21) remains valid in this case. It is also straightforward to show that its variance is given by Eq. (20); in this case, of course, $\mathbf{V}$ does not simplify to $\sigma^2\mathbf{I}$. Similar calculations show that the weighted least squares estimator, Eq. (29), which is optimal under normality, is also unbiased and has variance equal to $(\mathbf{X}'\mathbf{V}^{-1}\mathbf{X})^{-1}$. Interestingly the OLS estimator often retains nearly full efficiency compared to the weighted least squares estimator (Diggle et al., 2002).

In practical situations the variance–covariance matrix of the data is never known and must be estimated. Typically $\mathbf{V}$ is a function of parameters θ, and as long as the parameters θ are not functionally related to $\boldsymbol{\beta}$, the ML equations for $\boldsymbol{\beta}$ take the form:

$$\hat{\boldsymbol{\beta}}_{\hat{V}} = (\mathbf{X}'\hat{\mathbf{V}}^{-1}\mathbf{X})^{-1}\mathbf{X}'\hat{\mathbf{V}}^{-1}\mathbf{Y}, \tag{31}$$

where $\hat{\mathbf{V}}$ is the ML estimator of $\mathbf{V}$, i.e., $\mathbf{V}$ with the ML estimator of θ substituted for θ (McCulloch and Searle, 2000).

The ML equations for θ are considerably more complicated and depend on the specific parametric form of $\mathbf{V}$ so we will not elaborate here, but refer the reader to McCulloch and Searle (2000) or Searle et al. (1992). Often the REML log-likelihood based on Eq. (16), and introduced in Section 2.1, is maximized to find an estimate of θ, which is then used in Eq. (31). Again, see Searle et al. (1992) for details.

2.5.2. Prediction

One of the advantages of the random effects approach, Eq. (27), is the ability to generate predicted values for each of the random effects, b_i, which we do not get to observe directly. Mixed models are used, for example, in rating the perform-ance of hospitals or doctors (Normand et al., 1997; Hofer et al., 1999). In such a situation the outcome is a performance measure for the hospital, e.g., average log cost, and the random effects would represent, after adjustment for the fixed factors in the model, how a particular hospital or doctor deviated from the average.

Predicted values from random effects models are so-called shrinkage estima-tors because they are typically closer to a common value than estimates based on raw or adjusted averages. The shrinkage factor depends on the random effects variance and the sample size per cluster. When there is little variation from cluster to cluster and/or when the sample sizes are small, the shrinkage is greatest, reflecting the facts that clusters with extreme outcome values are likely to be due to chance in those circumstances. On the other hand, with sufficient data per cluster or evidence that clusters are quite different, the predicted values exhibit little shrinkage and are closer to raw or adjusted averages. So with varying sample sizes per cluster, estimates based on smaller sample sizes will show more shrinkage. Shrinkage predictions can be shown theoretically (Searle et al., 1992) to give more accurate predictions than those derived from the raw data. This occurs, especially with small cluster sizes, because information from other clusters is used to improve the prediction; this is sometimes called "borrowing strength" from the other clusters.

2.5.3. Robust and sandwich variance estimators

The fact that the OLS estimator is unbiased and often fairly efficient suggests that it could be used in practice. The problem with using the usual OLS regression packages is that they get the standard errors and hence tests and confidence intervals wrong by assuming all the data are independent.

In the case of longitudinal data, where we have independent data on M different subjects, a direct estimator of the true variance of the OLS estimator, Eq. (20) can be formed. Let $\mathbf{Y}_i$ denote the n_i outcomes for the ith subject, so that the number of observations $N = \sum_{i=1}^{M} n_i$. Then the model for the ith subject, using a corresponding model matrix $\mathbf{X}_i$, is

$$
\mathbf{Y}_i = \mathbf{X}_i \boldsymbol{\beta} + \varepsilon_i \quad i = 1, \ldots, M
$$
$$
\text{var}[\varepsilon_i] = \mathbf{V}_i. \tag{32}
$$

In this case the OLS estimator $\hat{\boldsymbol{\beta}} = (\mathbf{X}'\mathbf{X})^{-1}(\mathbf{X}'\mathbf{Y})$ can be written as

$$
\left(\sum_i \mathbf{X}_i'\mathbf{X}_i \right)^{-1} \left(\sum_i \mathbf{X}_i'\mathbf{Y}_i \right) \tag{33}
$$

with variance

$$
\left(\sum_i \mathbf{X}_i'\mathbf{X}_i \right)^{-1} \left(\sum_i \mathbf{X}_i'\mathbf{V}_i\mathbf{X}_i \right) \left(\sum_i \mathbf{X}_i'\mathbf{X}_i \right)^{-1}. \tag{34}
$$

A crude estimator of $\mathbf{V}_i$ can be formed as $\hat{\mathbf{V}}_i = (\mathbf{Y}_i - \mathbf{X}_i\hat{\boldsymbol{\beta}})(\mathbf{Y}_i - \mathbf{X}_i\hat{\boldsymbol{\beta}})'$ giving

$$
\hat{\text{var}}[\hat{\boldsymbol{\beta}}] = \left(\sum_i \mathbf{X}_i'\mathbf{X}_i \right)^{-1} \left(\sum_i \mathbf{X}_i'\hat{\mathbf{V}}_i\mathbf{X}_i \right) \left(\sum_i \mathbf{X}_i'\mathbf{X}_i \right)^{-1} \tag{35}
$$

Even though $\hat{\mathbf{V}}_i$ is a crude estimator, Eq. (35) is often a good estimator of the variance of $\hat{\boldsymbol{\beta}}$ due to the averaging over the M subjects and the "averaging" that takes place when pre- and post-multiplying by $\mathbf{X}_i$. This is called the "sandwich" estimator due to the sandwiching of the $\mathbf{X}'\mathbf{V}^{-1}\mathbf{X}$ piece between $(\mathbf{X}'\mathbf{X})^{-1}$ terms and is a robust estimator in the sense that it is asymptotically (as $M \to \infty$) valid without making assumptions about the variance–covariance structure. As such, it is quite useful for sensitivity checks against model assumptions. When M is not large, inferences based on the robust variance estimator may be liberal. This is consistent with the results cited in Section 2.4 for the HC0 estimator, to which Eq. (35) reduces when there is only one outcome per subject (see Kauermann and Carroll, 2001).

2.5.4. Repeated measures ANOVA

Correlated data analyses can sometimes be handled by repeated measures analysis of variance (ANOVA). When the data are balanced and appropriate for ANOVA, statistics with exact null hypothesis distributions (as opposed to asymptotic, likelihood based) are available for testing. However, the variance–covariance structure is typically estimated by the method of moments, which may be less efficient than maximum likelihood. For unbalanced data, tests are approximate, and, even though approximations have been developed (e.g., the Geisser–Greenhouse correction; Greenhouse and Geisser, 1959), may not achieve nominal significance levels. Also, in the specification of approximate F-statistics, it is not always straightforward to specify a denominator mean square (i.e., what is the "right" error term?).

Maximum likelihood estimation generates test statistics relatively automatically and gives better predictions of the random effects. Maximum likelihood methods also generalize naturally to non-normally distributed outcomes (see, e.g., McCulloch and Searle, 2000), unlike repeated measures ANOVA. See McCulloch (2005) for further discussion.

2.6. Model selection

Many more potential predictor variables are commonly measured than can reasonably be included in a multivariable regression model. In the introductory example, many factors in addition to gender, the BDI, and homelessness are likely to influence medical services utilization, including having health insurance and the range of health conditions driving the need for such services. The difficult problem of how to select predictors can be resolved to serve three distinct uses of regression. First, *prediction*: Can we identify which types of patients will use the most medical resources? Regression is a powerful and general tool for using multiple measured predictors to make useful predictions for future observations. Second, *isolating the effect of a single predictor*: What is the effect of the case management treatment on use of the emergency room, after adjusting for whether the patients in the two treatment groups (although randomized) differ with regard to gender, depression, or homeless status? Regression is a method to isolate the effect of one predictor (treatment) while adjusting for other differences. And third, *understanding multiple predictors*: Are the homeless at an increased risk of mortality and does the case management especially help the homeless? Regression is a method for understanding the joint and combined associations of all the predictors with the outcome.

2.6.1. Prediction

Here the primary issue is minimizing prediction error rather than causal interpretation of the predictors in the model. *Prediction error* (*PE*) measures how well
the model is able to predict the outcome for a new, randomly selected observation that was not used in estimating the parameters of the prediction model.
In this context, inclusive models that minimize confounding may not work as
well as models with smaller numbers of predictors. This can be understood in
terms of the *bias-variance trade-off*. Bias is often reduced when more variables are
included, but as less important covariates are added, precision may suffer without commensurate decreases in bias. The larger models may be *overfitted* to the
data, reflecting random error to such an extent that they are less able to predict
new observations than models with fewer predictors that give slightly biased
estimates but are less reflective of randomness in the current data.

Because R^2, the proportion of variance explained, increases with each additional covariate, even if it adds minimal information about the outcome, a model
that maximizes R^2 is unlikely to minimize *PE*. Alternative measures include
adjusted R^2, which works by penalizing R^2 for the number of predictors in the
model. Thus when a variable is added, adjusted R^2 increases only if the increment
in R^2 outweighs the added penalty. Mallow's C_p, the Akaike information criterion (AIC), and the Bayesian information criterion (BIC) are analogs which
impose respectively stiffer penalties for each additional variable, and thus lead
to selection of smaller models. Measures of concordance of the observed and
predicted outcomes for the logistic and Cox models include the *c*-statistic
and Somer's D (Harrell et al., 1996), as well as adaptations of the Brier score
(Graf et al., 1999).

More direct estimates of *PE* are based on *cross-validation* (CV), a class of
methods that work by using distinct sets of observations to estimate the model
and to evaluate *PE*. The most straightforward example is the learning set/test set
(LS/TS) approach, in which the parameter estimates are obtained from the
learning set and then used to evaluate *PE* in the test set. In linear regression,
computing *PE* is straightforward, using $\hat{\beta}$ from the learning set to compute the
predicted value $\hat{y}$ and corresponding residual for each observation in the test set.
The learning and test sets are sometimes obtained by splitting a single dataset,
often with two-thirds of the observations randomly assigned to the learning set.
However, using an independent sample as the test set may give more general-
izable estimates of *PE*, since the test set is generally not sampled from exactly the
same population as the learning set.

An alternative to LS/TS is leave-one-out or *jackknife* methods, in which all but
one observation are used to estimate the model, and then *PE* is evaluated for the
omitted observation; this is done in turn for each observation. In linear regression models, the resulting predicted residual sum of squares (PRESS) can be
computed for the entire dataset with minimal extra computation. In logistic and
Cox models, fast one-step approximations are available.

Midway between LS/TS and the jackknife is *h-fold cross-validation* (hCV). The
dataset is divided into h mutually exclusive subsets and a measure of *PE* is
evaluated in each subset, using parameter estimates obtained from the remaining

observations. A global estimate of *PE* is then found by averaging over the *h* subset estimates. Typically values of *h* from 5 to 10 are used.

Bootstrap methods provide a potentially more efficient alternative to cross-validation for estimating prediction error (Efron, 1986; Harrell et al., 1996). Prediction models are developed using the methods employed with the original data but applied to bootstrap samples, and then evaluated using both the bootstrap and original data. The estimated prediction error of the rule both developed and evaluated using the original data is then corrected by the average difference between the two prediction error estimates for the bootstrap datasets.

Modern computing power makes it possible to use CV or the bootstrap not just to validate a prediction model using independent data but to guide iterative predictor selection procedures. Among them, Breiman (2001) describes modern methods that do not follow the paradigm motivated by the bias-variance trade-off that smaller models are better for prediction. The newer methods tend to keep all the predictors in play, while using various methods to avoid overfitting and control variance; cross-validation plays a central role throughout.

The so-called shrinkage procedures also play an important role in prediction, especially those made on the basis of small datasets. In this approach over-fitting is avoided and prediction improved by shrinking the estimated regression coefficients toward zero, rather than eliminating weak predictors from the model. Variants of shrinkage include the *non-negative garrote* (Breiman, 1995) and the *LASSO* method, short for *least absolute shrinkage and selection operator* (Tibshirani, 1997). An alternative to direct shrinkage implements *penalties* in the fitting procedure against coefficient estimates which violate some measure of smoothness. This achieves something like shrinkage of the estimates and thus better predictions; see Le Cessie and Van Houwelingen (1992) and Verweij and Van Houwelingen (1994) for applications to logistic and Cox regression. These methods derive from *ridge regression* (Hoerl and Kennard, 1970), a method for obtaining slightly biased but stabler estimates in linear models with highly correlated predictors.

Finally, Altman and Royston (2000) give an excellent discussion of validating prediction models from a broader perspective, focusing on the ways in which these models may or may not be useful in clinical and other practical applications.

2.6.2. Isolating the effect of a single predictor

In observational data, the main problem in evaluating a predictor of primary interest is to rule out non-causal explanations of an association between this predictor and the outcome as persuasively as possible – that is, *confounding* of the association by the true causal factors, or correlates of such factors. Confounders are associated with the predictor of interest and independently associated with the outcome, and thus may explain all or part of the unadjusted association of the primary predictor and the outcome. As a result, addition of the confounder to the model typically affects the estimate for the primary predictor; in most cases, the adjusted estimate is smaller. Potential confounders to be considered include factors identified in previous studies or hypothesized to matter on substantive grounds, as well as variables that behave like confounders by the statistical measures. Two classes of covariates would not be considered for inclusion in the model: covariates which are essentially alternative measures of either the outcome or the predictor of interest, and those hypothesized to *mediate* its effect – that is, to lie on a causal pathway between the predictor of interest and the outcome.

To rule out confounding more effectively, a liberal criterion of $p < 0.2$ for inclusion of covariates in the model makes sense (Maldonado and Greenland, 1993). A comparably effective alternative is to retain variables if removing them changes the coefficient for the predictor of interest by more than 10% or 15% (Greenland, 1989; Mickey and Greenland, 1989). These inclusive rules are particularly important in small datasets, where even important confounders may not meet the usual criterion for statistical significance. Among the common procedures that could be used to select covariates, backward selection (that is, starting with the full model and sequentially eliminating the least important remaining variable) has the advantage that *negatively confounded* variables are less likely to be omitted from the final model (Sun et al., 1999). Negatively confounded variables appear *more* important when they are included in the model together, in contrast to the more common case in which addition of a confounder to the model attenuates the estimate for the predictor of interest.

Randomized experiments including clinical trials represent a special case where the predictor of primary interest is the intervention; confounding is not usually an issue, but covariates are sometimes included in the model for other reasons. These include design variables in stratified experiments, including clinical center in multicenter randomized trials, necessary for obtaining valid standard errors, *p*-values, and confidence intervals. In linear models inclusion of important prognostic variables can also substantially reduce residual error and thus increase power; Hauck et al. (1998) emphasize, however, that the adjusted model should be pre-specified in the study protocol. Furthermore, adjustment in experiments with binary or failure time outcomes can avoid attenuation of treatment effect estimates in logistic (Neuhaus and Jewell, 1993; Neuhaus, 1998) and Cox models (Gail et al., 1984; Schmoor and Schumacher, 1997; Henderson and Oman, 1999). Hypothesis tests remain valid when there is no treatment effect (Gail et al., 1988), but power is lost in proportion to the importance of the omitted covariates (Lagakos and Schoenfeld, 1984; Begg and Lagakos, 1993). Note, however, that adjustment for *im*balanced covariates can potentially increase as well as decrease the treatment effect estimate, and can erode both precision and power. Finally, adjusted or de-attenuated treatment effect estimates are more nearly interpretable as *subject-specific* – in contrast to *population-averaged* (Hauck et al., 1998).

2.6.3. Understanding multiple predictors
This is the most difficult case, and one in which both causal interpretation and statistical inference are most problematic. When the focus is on isolating the effect of a single predictor, covariates are included in order to obtain a minimally confounded estimate. However, broadening the focus to multiple important predictors of an outcome can make selecting a single best model considerably

more difficult. For example, inferences about most or all of the predictors retained in the model are now of primary interest, so overfitting and false-positive results are more of an issue, particularly for novel and seemingly implausible associations. Interaction – that is, the dependence of the effect of one predictor on the value of another – will usually be of interest, but systematically assessing the large number of possible interactions can easily lead to false-positive findings, some at least not easily rejected as implausible. It may also be difficult to choose between alternative models that each include one variable from a collinear pair or set. Mediation is also more difficult to handle, to the extent that both the overall effect of a predictor as well as its direct and indirect effects may be of interest. In this case, models which both exclude and include the mediator may be required to give a full picture. Especially in the earlier stages of research, modeling these complex relationships is difficult, prone to error, and likely to require considerable re-analysis in response to input from subject-matter experts.

2.6.4. Number of predictors

The rationale for inclusive predictor selection rules, whether we are isolating the effect of single predictor or trying to understand multiple predictors, is to obtain minimally confounded estimates. However, this can make regression coefficient estimates less precise, especially for highly correlated predictors. At the extreme, model performance can be severely degraded by the inclusion of too many predictors. Rules of thumb have been suggested for number of predictors that can be safely included as a function of sample size or number of events. A commonly used guideline prescribes ten observations for each predictor; with binary or survival outcomes the analogous guideline specifies ten events per predictor (Peduzzi et al., 1995, 1996; Concato et al., 1995). The rationale is to obtain adequately precise estimates, and in the case of the logistic and Cox models, to ensure that the models behave properly.

However, such guidelines are too simple. Their primary limitation is that the precision of coefficient estimates depends on other factors as well as the number of observations or events per predictor. In particular, the variance of a coefficient estimate in a linear model (Eq. (22)) depends on the residual variance of the outcome, which is generally reduced by the inclusion of important covariates. Precision also depends on the multiple correlation between a predictor of interest and other variables in the model, which figures in the denominator of Eq. (22). Thus addition of covariates that are at most weakly correlated with the primary predictor but explain substantial outcome variance can actually improve the precision of the estimate for the predictor of interest. In contrast, addition of just one collinear predictor can degrade its precision unacceptably. In addition, the allowable number of predictors depends on effect size, with larger effects being more robust to multiple adjustments than smaller ones.

In many contexts where these guidelines might be violated, power is low, in which case misleading inferences can usually be avoided if confidence intervals are used to interpret negative findings (Hoenig and Heisey, 2001). However, when statistically significant associations are found despite the inclusion of more predictors than this rule allows – with 5 or more events per variable – only a modest degree of extra caution appears to be warranted (Vittinghoff and McCulloch, 2007).

2.6.5. Model selection complicates inference

Underlying the confidence intervals and *p*-values which play a central role in interpreting regression results is the assumption that the predictors to be included in the model were specified a priori without reference to the data. In *confirmatory* analyses in well-developed areas of research, including phase-III clinical trials, prior determination of the model is feasible and important. In contrast, at earlier stages of research, data-driven predictor selection and checking are reasonable, even obligatory, and certainly widely used. However, some of the issues raised for inference include the following:

- The chance of at least one type-I error can greatly exceed the nominal level used to test each term.
- In small datasets precision and power are often poor, so important predictors may be omitted from the model, especially if a restrictive inclusion criterion is used.
- Parameter estimates can be biased away from the null, owing to selection of estimates that are large by chance (Steyerberg et al., 1999).
- Choices between predictors can be poorly motivated, especially between collinear variables, and are potentially sensitive to addition or deletion of a few observations. Altman and Andersen (1989) propose bootstrap methods for assessing this sensitivity.

Breiman (2001) is skeptical of modeling causal pathways using such procedures, and argues that computer-intensive methods validated strictly in terms of prediction error not only give better predictions but may also be more reliable guides to "variable importance" – another term for understanding multiple predictors, and with implications for assessing isolating the effect of a single predictor.

Finally, we note that these issues in predictor selection apply broadly, to non-linear as well as linear models.

3. Non-linear models

3.1. Introduction: A salary analysis

One of us recently completed an analysis of salary data for the compensation plan at our university to check for inequities in pay between males and females. Not surprising, the salary data is highly skewed right with a few extreme salaries (mostly MDs who generate large amounts of clinical income). The traditional method of handling such data is to consider a log transformation of the outcome, which made the data approximately normally distributed. Here is an overly simplistic version of the analysis to illustrate the basic points, adjusting only for faculty rank before looking for a gender effect. The model uses a reference group of assistant professor and is given by

$$\log(\text{salary}_i) = \beta_0 + \beta_1 x_{1i} + \beta_2 x_{2i} + \beta_3 x_{3i} + \varepsilon_i, \tag{36}$$

where salary$_i$ is the monthly salary of the ith faculty member, and x_{1i}, x_{2i}, and x_{3i} are the indicator functions for the faculty member being an associate professor, being a full professor, and being male, respectively.

The gender effect, β_3, was estimated to be 0.185 with a 95% confidence interval of (0.116, 0.254). How do we interpret this result? It is unsatisfying to interpret log(dollars) so the inclination is to back transform both sides of Eq. (36) giving

$$
\begin{aligned}
\text{salary}_i &= \exp\{\beta_0 + \beta_1 x_{1i} + \beta_2 x_{2i} + \beta_3 x_{3i} + \varepsilon_i\} \\
&= e^{\beta_0} e^{\beta_1 x_{1i}} e^{\beta_2 x_{2i}} e^{\beta_3 x_{3i}} e^{\varepsilon_i} \\
&= \gamma_0 \gamma_1^{x_{1i}} \gamma_2^{x_{2i}} \gamma_3^{x_{3i}} \delta_i,
\end{aligned}
\tag{37}
$$

here $\gamma_j = e^{\beta_j}$ and $\delta_i = e^{\varepsilon_i}$. Ignoring the error term, δ, for the moment, and taking the ratio of the model equation, Eq. (37), for males and females of the same rank gives

$$
\gamma_3 = \frac{\gamma_0 \gamma_1^{x_1} \gamma_2^{x_2} \gamma_3^1}{\gamma_0 \gamma_1^{x_1} \gamma_2^{x_2} \gamma_3^0}
\tag{38}
$$

In words, males make, on average, $e^{0.185} = 1.203$ or about 20% more with a confidence interval of (1.123, 1.289).

Being more careful, in Eq. (38), we have taken the ratio of values of $\exp\{E[\log(\text{salary})]\}$, which is not the same as $E[\text{salary}]$. However, if the log transformation makes the errors, ε_i, normally distributed (or, more generally symmetrically distributed) as it did in this example, then the mean and the median are the same. So we can also interpret the model as a model for median log(salary). Since

$$
\exp\{\text{median}[\log(\text{salary})]\} = \exp\{\log(\text{median}[\text{salary}])\} = \text{median}[\text{salary}]
\tag{39}
$$

we can interpret γ_3 in terms of median salaries. In particular, males have a median salary that is, on average, about 20% higher than females.

This is a very reasonable interpretation and is, in many cases, preferred to a model for mean salary, which is sensitive to the few extreme salaries. Furthermore, the ratio interpretation (20% more for males) is a common way of thinking about salaries as opposed to an additive one (e.g., $1,800 more per month) since, for example, raises are often decided on a percentage basis.

However, what about the medical center administrator in charge of making sure the compensation plan generates enough revenue to pay all the faculty? Clearly, she is concerned with *mean* salary since the total revenue has to exceed the mean salary times the number of faculty. What models are available if we require a model for mean salary?

The ratio form of the model, but for the mean salary, could be retained by fitting a model of the form

$$
\text{salary}_i = \gamma_0^* \gamma_1^{* x_{1i}} \gamma_2^{* x_{2i}} \gamma_3^{* x_{3i}} + \varepsilon_i^*,
\tag{40}
$$

Non-linear least squares could be used and would give consistent estimates even though we would not feel comfortable assuming that the ε_i^* were homoscedastic and normally distributed. So confidence intervals or tests for γ_3 based on normality assumptions would be suspect but inferences could still be achieved, e.g., through bootstrapping. Fitting model (40) to the salary data gave $\hat{\gamma}_3^* = 1.165$ with a bootstrap confidence interval of $(1.086, 1.244)$.

But it might be more satisfying to make mild, but reasonable assumptions about the form of the distribution, for example that the salaries had a gamma distribution with mean μ_i given by a multiplicative model and constant coefficient of variation:

$$\text{salary}_i \sim \text{Gamma}(\mu_i)$$
$$\log(\mu_i) = \beta_0^{**} + \beta_1^{**} x_{1i} + \beta_2^{**} x_{2i} + \beta_3^{**} x_{3i}. \tag{41}$$

Fitting this model gives an estimate $\exp\{\hat{\beta}_3^{**}\} = 1.223$ with a model based confidence interval of $(1.138, 1.314)$ and a bootstrap confidence interval of $(1.142, 1.310)$.

Models (40) and (41) differ from (36) in that they model the mean salary rather than the median salary and by the fact that they are non-linear in the parameters. Model (41) differs from (40) in that it is a generalized linear model: a known transformation of the mean is linear in the parameters ($\log(\mu_i)$ is linear in the β_j^{**} whereas the log of the mean of model (40) is not linear in the γ_j^*). In the next section, we present a model for survival times which is analogous to model (41) but can also be written as a linear model with a log-transformed outcome and non-normal errors.

3.2. The accelerated failure time model

Consider examining the effect of the managed care intervention on survival among homeless patients. Survival times typically have a right-skewed distribution; hence we might use a model similar to the last model (41) proposed for faculty salaries:

$$\text{survival}_i \sim \text{exponential}(\mu_i)$$
$$\log(\mu_i) = \beta_0 + \beta x_{1i} + \beta_2 x_{2i} + \beta_3 x_{3i} \tag{42}$$

In Eq. (42), x_{1i} is the intervention indicator, x_{2i} is the BDI, and x_{3i} indicates if the subject is homeless. The exponential distribution is an important special case for survival data because the so-called hazard function is constant under this model.

However, an important difference between the salary and survival time outcome variables is that many subjects either drop out prior to or survive past the end of the study, so we only know that their actual survival times are greater than their observed follow-up time Y_i. In the salary example, this would amount to knowing only that some of the faculty were earning more than, say, \$500,000 per year. These survival times are said to be *right-censored*.

The *accelerated failure time* (AFT) model can be written in terms of the so-called survival function, $S_i(t) = P(\text{survival}_i > t)$. Under the AFT,

$$P(\text{survival}_i > t | \mathbf{x}_i) = S_i(t) = S_0\left(t \ \exp(\mathbf{x}_i'\boldsymbol{\beta})\right) \tag{43}$$

where $S_0(t) = P(\text{survival}_i > t | \mathbf{x}_i = 0)$ is the baseline survival function. The baseline survival function plays the role of the intercept β_0 in other regression models, and represents the survival function for a subject with all covariate values equal to 0; this can be made interpretable by centering covariate values. The effect of the covariates in the model is to multiply t by $\exp(\mathbf{x}_i'\boldsymbol{\beta})$, in some sense speeding up or slowing down time, depending on the sign of $\mathbf{x}_i'\boldsymbol{\beta}$. The interpretation is similar to the equivalence of 1 dog and 7 human years – for the dog, time is accelerated.

The AFT model can also be written as a linear model with log-transformed outcome:

$$\log(\text{survival}_i) = -\mathbf{x}_i'b + \varepsilon_i \tag{44}$$

where ε_i follows some distribution. In particular, if survival$_i$ follows an exponential distribution, then ε_i follows the extreme-value distribution. When the distribution of ε (or, equivalently $S_0(\cdot)$) is parametrically specified, maximum likelihood estimation of $\boldsymbol{\beta}$ is straightforward. The likelihood of the possibly censored follow-up time Y_i has the form

$$f_i(Y_i)^{\Delta_i} S_i(Y_i)^{(1-\Delta_i)} \tag{45}$$

where $f_i(t) = -\partial S_i(t)/\partial t$ is the density function, and Δ_i is 0 if subject i is censored and 1 otherwise. Intuitively, the likelihood contribution for a censored observation is just $P(\text{survival}_i > t_i)$.

For example, under the exponential AFT model, with baseline survival function $S_0(t) = \exp(-\lambda t)$, the log-likelihood based on Eq. (45) is

$$\sum_{i=1}^{N} \Delta_i \{\log \lambda + \mathbf{x}_i'\boldsymbol{\beta} - \lambda Y_i \exp(\mathbf{x}_i'\boldsymbol{\beta})\} + (1 - \Delta_i)\{-\lambda Y_i \exp(\mathbf{x}_i'\boldsymbol{\beta})\}. \tag{46}$$

This simplifies to

$$\sum_{i=1}^{N} \Delta_i(\log \lambda + \mathbf{x}_i'\boldsymbol{\beta}) - \lambda Y_i \exp(\mathbf{x}_i'\boldsymbol{\beta}) \tag{47}$$

and is straightforward to maximize numerically.

In general, AFT models have proved useful in industrial applications and have been advocated for biomedical research (Wei, 1992). However, when the distribution of ε is unspecified, estimation becomes a complex problem. Considerable interest has centered on rank-based estimation in the semi-parametric case where ε follows an unspecified distribution. Estimation there has proven difficult due to non-monotone, non-differentiable estimation functions (Lin and Geyer, 1992). Recently, more computationally feasible approaches have been developed (Jin et al., 2003).

3.3. Generalized linear models

We return to the example of Section 1.1 on utilization of health resources. Recall that interest focused on an intervention to reduce health care costs, number of emergency room visits, and death. How should we model the outcome of number of emergency room visits as a function of the predictors: intervention group, gender, baseline depression score, and homeless status?

This outcome is a count variable and skewed to the right. Furthermore, in subsets of the data in which the mean value is higher (e.g., among homeless persons) the variability is higher. Both of these features make a linear regression model assuming normality and homoscedasticity of the outcome an unattractive strategy.

We might consider a transformation of the outcome to try to make it more approximately normally distributed and to achieve variance homogeneity. This strategy will not work in cases where a large percentage of observations are zero, as they were for this dataset. The most a transformation will do is move the large percentage of data exactly equal to zero to a different value. For example the square root transformation, a common transformation for count data, would leave the same large percentage of zeros at zero.

The typical linear regression model for the mean is also unattractive for this example. The mean number of emergency room visits for any particular configuration of the predictors must be positive, but a linear regression model will not be so constrained.

3.3.1. Modeling a transformation of the mean

A solution is to separately define the distribution of the data and then model some function of the mean instead of the mean itself. For simplicity we will consider just the first measurement (at 6 months) and accordingly define Y_i as the number of emergency room visits for patient i between the baseline and 6-month visits.

Since the data are counts, we might consider a Poisson distribution as a first step. With a small mean value, this may accurately model the large percentage of zeroes. A common and useful function of the mean to model is the logarithm, which we will justify later. That leads us to

$$
\begin{aligned}
Y_i &\sim \text{indep. Poisson}(E[Y_i]) \\
\log E[Y_i] &= \beta_0 + \beta_1 x_{1i} + \beta_2 x_{2i} + \beta_3 x_{3i} + \beta_4 x_{4i}.
\end{aligned}
\tag{48}
$$

where x_{1i}, x_{2i}, and x_{3i} are the indicators for being in the case management group, female, and homeless, respectively, and x_{4i} is the patient's BDI at baseline.

Back transforming the mean in Eq. (48) gives the following non-linear regression equation relating the mean rate in 6 months to the predictors:

$$
\begin{aligned}
E[Y_i] &= \exp\{\beta_0 + \beta_1 x_{1i} + \beta_2 x_{2i} + \beta_3 x_{3i} + \beta_4 x_{4i}\} \\
&= e^{\beta_0} e^{\beta_1 x_{1i}} e^{\beta_2 x_{2i}} e^{\beta_3 x_{3i}} e^{\beta_4 x_{4i}} \\
&\equiv \gamma_0 \gamma_1^{x_{1i}} \gamma_2^{x_{2i}} \gamma_3^{x_{3i}} \gamma_4^{x_{4i}},
\end{aligned}
\tag{49}
$$

with $\gamma_k \equiv e^{\beta_k}$.

Although many of the data points are zero (and hence not acceptable to log transform) the mean value will not be exactly zero, allowing the use of the log function. Also, the exponential in Eq. (49) keeps the mean value positive, allowing flexible linear models for $\log E[Y_i]$.

Model (49) is clearly a multiplicative model in the parameters and the coefficients have a ratio interpretation. As an example we calculate the ratio of the means, holding intervention group, gender, and homeless status as fixed and evaluating the BDI at the values $x^* + 1$ and x^*:

$$
\frac{E[Y|x_4 = x^* + 1]}{E[Y|x_4 = x^*]} = \frac{\exp\{\beta_0 + \beta_1 x_1 + \beta_2 x_2 + \beta_3 x_3 + \beta_4(x^* + 1)\}}{\exp\{\beta_0 + \beta_1 x_1 + \beta_2 x_2 + \beta_3 x_3 + \beta_4 x^*\}}
$$
$$
= \exp\{\beta_4\} \tag{50}
$$
$$
= \gamma_4.
$$

So γ_4 has the interpretation as the relative rate of emergency room visits (per 6 months) when BDI is increased by 1. The other coefficients are interpreted similarly, for example, γ_3 is the relative rate for homeless compared to non-homeless. So we see that modeling the log transformation of the mean, called using a log *link*, has two attractive features: it keeps the mean values positive and provides a relative rate interpretation.

It has a different, more subtle advantage. This is a model for the number of emergency room visits per half year. What if the subject is followed for only 2 months before dying? Let t_i be the amount of time that subject i is followed. Then we would like to build a model for the rate of emergency room visits per unit time, namely, $E[Y_i]/t_i$. When using the log link the model then can be rearranged to

$$
\log\left(E[Y_i]/t_i\right) = \beta_0 + \beta_1 x_{1i} + \beta_2 x_{2i} + \beta_3 x_{3i} + \beta_4 x_{4i},
$$
$$
\log E[Y_i] = \beta_0 + \beta_1 x_{1i} + \beta_2 x_{2i} + \beta_3 x_{3i} + \beta_4 x_{4i} + \log t_i. \tag{51}
$$

Notably, we can still model the mean of a Poisson variate (Y_i/t_i is not Poisson distributed since it can take non-integer values) as long as we include a term, $\log t_i$, on the right-hand side of the equation. This is not quite a predictor or covariate because it has no coefficient multiplying it and so it is called an *offset*. Statistical analysis programs that fit such models usually allow the specification of an offset so the program does not estimate an associated coefficient.

3.3.2. A log link binary data model

We now consider a similar model, but for binary data. Recall that in Section 1.1 we posited a logistic regression model for the binary outcome of death. This model had multiplicative interpretations in terms of odds so that exponentiating a coefficient gave the odds ratio of death associated with increasing the predictor by 1. But some analysts find odds ratios hard to interpret and instead prefer *relative risks*, namely the ratio of the risk of death under two different scenarios. We now investigate the consequences of using a log link for binary outcome data:

$$
Y_i = 1 \quad \text{if subject } i \text{ dies in the first 6 months and 0 otherwise}
$$
$$
Y_i \sim \text{indep. Bernoulli}(E[Y_i]) \tag{52}
$$
$$
\log E[Y_i] = \beta_0 + \beta_1 x_{1i} + \beta_2 x_{2i} + \beta_3 x_{3i} + \beta_4 x_{4i}.
$$

Using arguments the same as in Eq. (50) we see that $\gamma_3 = e^{\beta_3}$ gives the relative risk of death for homeless compared to non-homeless.

The log link is not as attractive in this scenario as it is for the Poisson model. While the log link keeps the model for the mean (which is the probability of the outcome for a binary data model) positive, as is required, it does not constrain the probabilities to be less than 1 (which the logistic model does). So Eq. (52) is mainly useful when the outcome is rare and probabilities near or above 1 will not be estimated in a reasonable range of the model; otherwise the model can be unstable to fit.

3.3.3. A general approach

Models like the one developed in this section are called *generalized linear models* because a model that is linear in the parameters is assumed to hold for a known function of the mean of the outcome. Besides the generality gained by using a different function of the mean, this approach has the advantage of separating the decision as to the distribution of the outcome and what sort of model to create for the mean. In particular, we illustrated two possible models for the Bernoulli distribution, using either a logit or log link.

The key to use of a generalized linear model program is the specification of the relationship of the variance to the mean. As examples, the Poisson distribution assumes the mean (μ) and variance (σ^2) are equal; the Bernoulli assumes $\sigma^2 = \mu(1 - \mu)$; and the Gamma assumes $\sigma \propto \mu$. Most programs use this information as input to an iteratively re-weighted least squares algorithm and base inferences on a quasi-likelihood (which does not require specification of a full probabilistic model). The variance-to-mean relationship may be implied by the distribution (as with a binary outcome), inferred from past experience (e.g., if lipid measures are known to have standard deviation proportional to the mean), or assessed using the data, for example by plotting subgroup standard deviations against their means.

Generalized linear models have been extended to accommodate correlated data using two main approaches. The first is by including random effects along with likelihood estimation (e.g., McCulloch and Searle, 2000). The second approach is the use of the robust variance estimate (as in Section 2.5.3) using so-called generalized estimating equations (Diggle et al., 2002).

3.4. Transformations of predictors resulting in non-linear models

In the generalized linear models just described, a function of $E[Y_i|\mathbf{x_i}]$ is specified by a linear combination of the regression parameters, and thus is similar to a linear model. And in a previous section we described spline models which, despite using elaborate transformations of continuous predictors, nonetheless retain this property. However, some methods of transforming predictors induce models which are intrinsically non-linear, in that no transformation of the mean of the outcome can be represented as a linear function of the regression parameters. These include *segmented regression models*, *GAMs*, *CART*, and other non-linear models.

Segmented regression models. With segmented regression models, we postulate that the mean of the outcome is a series of connected line segments (much like linear regression splines). However, in segmented regression the general form is specified, but with knots as well as slopes unknown. Segmented regression is thus useful in problems where inference on the placement of the knots is of interest. The technique has been used to examine if there were trends in cancer diagnosis over time and, if so, which were the years of the change points (Hankey et al., 1999). Such problems are not linear because the mean cannot be represented as a linear function of the knots.

Generalized additive models (GAMs). An interesting class of models, termed GAMs (Hastie and Tibshirani, 1990) relax the assumptions of the classic generalized linear model. These models take the form

$$g(E[y|x]) = f_0 + f_1(x_1) + \cdots + f_p(x_p) \tag{53}$$

where $g(\cdot)$ is known but the $f_j(\cdot)$ are unspecified but smooth functions. These models make it possible to examine the response as a non-linear function of the predictors. The approach is useful for simultaneous non-parametric exploration of the effects of predictors on the outcome. A description of the effect of the jth covariate is given in the form of $\hat{f}_j$.

Classification and regression trees (CART) (Breiman et al., 1984) divide the predictor space into a series of mutually exclusive and exhaustive subsets. Given the subsets, the model can be written as linear in a series of indicator functions. The splits (or nodes) defined by CART are arrived at by recursive partitioning of the predictor space based on a splitting criterion which measures homogeneity within the nodes (e.g., the sum of the squared residuals). The approach is appealing because it seamlessly handles many different predictor types and missing values, automatically detects interactions and avoids distributional assumptions. *Pruning* of the tree based on cross-validation is commonly used to avoid over-fitting.

3.5. Other non-linear models

In many situations, scientific knowledge about a biological phenomenon of interest suggests an appropriate form for the regression relationship between outcome and predictors. Because many such models cannot be reduced to the linear additive form familiar from conventional regression, alternate techniques for estimation and inference are often required. An example is provided by analyses of left ventricular pressure data aimed at estimating clinically relevant features indicative of cardiac performance (Takeuchi et al., 1991). The basic data are in the form of pressure data obtained from cardiac catheterization, and are in the form of *loops* corresponding to individual heartbeats. A typical example is illustrated in Fig. 1. The points represent the observed data for a single beat, and the line gives the theoretical pressure curve. The latter cannot be observed directly because in a typical ventricular contraction, the heart valves release before maximum pressure is attained and observed pressure drops accordingly. The labeled quantity P_{max} represents the maximum pressure that the ventricular contraction can theoretically generate. The goal of the analysis is to fit a plausible model to the observed data (typically using multiple beats for a given individual), and use it to estimate P_{max}. A model for pressure, $P(t)$, as a function of time, t, has been proposed by Takeuchi et al. (1991), which takes the following form:

$$P(t) = 1/2P_{max}[1 - \cos(\omega t + C)] + \text{EDP}. \tag{54}$$

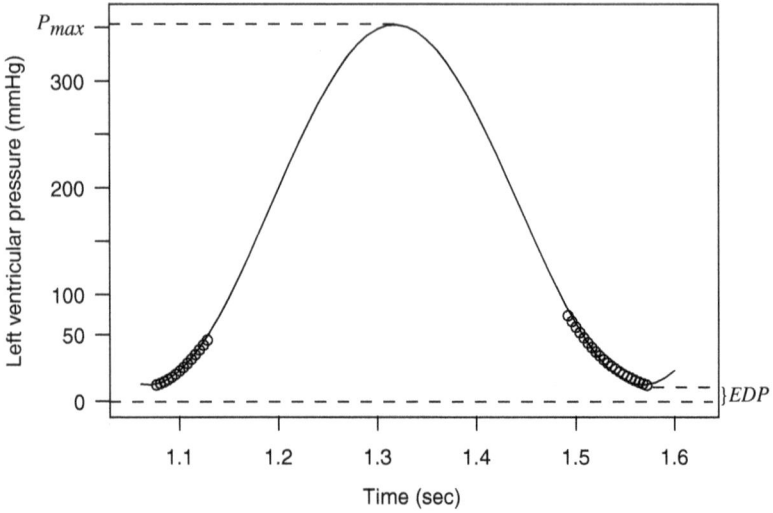

Fig. 1. Ventricular pressure data for a single heart beat.

Here, $P_{\max}$, ω, and C represent the amplitude, angular frequency, and phase shift angle of the theoretical pressure curve, respectively. EDP refers to end-diastolic ventricular pressure, which is defined as the distance from the lowest point of the curve to the horizontal axis in the figure. The angular frequency $\omega = 2\pi/T$, where T is the duration of the approximated pressure curve. The quantities ω and EDP are typically obtained from separate measurements, leaving C and $P_{\max}$ as the primary unknown parameters to be estimated from the observed pressure data.

The model (55) can be viewed as a special case of the following general non-linear regression model:

$$Y_i = f(\mathbf{x}_i; \boldsymbol{\theta}) + \varepsilon_i \quad i = 1, \ldots, N, \tag{55}$$

where f is a non-linear function of predictor variables $\mathbf{x}$, $\boldsymbol{\theta}$ is a vector of parameters, and the errors ε are typically assumed to be i.i.d. normally distributed. Estimation is typically performed via non-linear least squares, where the estimate $\hat{\boldsymbol{\theta}}$ is obtained as the minimizer of the following equation:

$$\hat{\boldsymbol{\theta}} = \operatorname{argmin} \sum_{i=1}^{N} (Y_i - f(\mathbf{x}_i; \boldsymbol{\theta}))^2 \tag{56}$$

When the errors ε are normally distributed this yields the maximum likelihood estimate of $\boldsymbol{\theta}$. Even in situations where this is not the case, estimation is typically based on Eq. (56). For the data presented in Fig. 1, the estimates (approximate standard errors) for $P_{\max}$ and C were 337.2 (6.87) and -7.3 (0.007).

The *asymptotic regression* model, Eq. (57), provides another example of an inherently non-linear model:

$$Y_i = \beta_0 + \beta_2 e^{\beta_2 x_i} \tag{57}$$

For negative values of β_2, Y reaches the asymptote β_0 as x increases. This model is commonly applied in analyses of growth curves.

Additional examples arise in a number of applications where models of biological phenomena exist. For instance, studies of pharmacokinetic properties of drugs often focus on quantities such as the rate of drug metabolism as a function of applied dose. This relationship can frequently be described using simple differential equation models, the parameters of which are useful in summarizing characteristics of the drug. The *Michaelis–Menten* model is an example (Pinheiro and Bates, 2000). Other examples include models of carcinogenesis (Day, 1990) and of infectious disease spread (Becker, 1989). Techniques for estimation and inference for such models are reviewed in a number of books, including Seber and Wild (2003) and Bates and Watts (1988).

4. Special topics

4.1. Causal models

Regression models used to isolate the effect of a predictor or understand multiple predictors often have the implicit goal of assessing possible causal relationships with the outcome. The difficulties of achieving this goal are clearly recognized in epidemiology as in other fields relying on observational data: in particular the requirement that all confounders must have been measured and adequately adjusted for in the model. The superiority of experiments, including clinical trials, for determining causation stems from random assignment to treatment or experimental condition, more or less ensuring that all other determinants of the outcome are balanced across the treatment groups, and thus could not confound treatment assignment. In contrast, treatment actually received could be confounded; estimating the causal effect of treatment in trials with poor adherence poses problems similar to those posed by inherently observational data.

Propensity scores (Rosenbaum and Rubin, 1983) attempt to avoid potential difficulties in adequately adjusting for all confounders of a non-randomized treatment by adjusting instead for an estimate of the probability of receiving the treatment, given the full range of confounders (that is, the propensity score); related strategies are to stratify by or match on the scores (D'Agostino, 1998). Closely related *inverse probability of treatment weighted* (IPTW) models weight observations in inverse proportion to the estimated probability of the treatment actually received (Hernan et al., 2001; Robins et al., 2000). Propensity scores are most clearly an improvement over conventional regression adjustment when the outcome is binary and rare, limiting our ability to adjust adequately, but treatment is relatively common, so that the propensity score is relatively easy to model. However, this approach does not avoid the crucial requirement that all confounders are measured. Moreover, variability in the effect of treatment across levels of the propensity score, as well as gross dissimilarity between the treated and untreated subsamples, can invalidate the analysis (Kurth et al., 2005).

Instrumental variables are an alternative method for estimating causal effects from observational data (Greenland, 2000). An instrumental variable is associated with the treatment received, but uncorrelated with the outcome after controlling for treatment received. Because treatment assignment meets these criteria, instrumental variable arguments can be used to motivate a well-known estimator of the causal effect of treatment in trials with all-or-nothing adherence in which the observed treatment–control difference in the mean value of the outcome is inflated by the inverse of the proportion adherent. In observational settings, identification and validation of the instrumental variable is of course crucial.

4.2. Measurement error and misclassification

Data collected in many experimental and observational studies in epidemiology and medicine are based on measurements subject to error. Errors may occur in both the outcome and predictors of regression models, and may arise from a number of sources, including laboratory instruments and assays, medical devices and monitors, and from participant responses to survey questions. The presence of measurement error raises a legitimate concern that estimates from fitted regression models may be biased, and that associated inferences may be incorrect.

There is a wealth of published research on the impacts of measurement error in predictors in the context of linear models (Fuller, 1987). Most of this relies on the *classical error model*, in which the observed (and error prone) predictor W is related to the actual predictor X via the additive model

$$W = X + U, \tag{58}$$

in which U is a random variable with conditional (given X and other predictors measured without error) mean zero and variance σ_u^2. In the linear regression model (8) with a single predictor X, regression of the outcome Y on the error-contaminated W in Eq. (58) yields an attenuated estimate β^* of the true coefficient β, defined as $E[Y|X = x + 1] - E[Y|X = x]$. The degree of attenuation is described by the multiplicative factor

$$\frac{\sigma_\varepsilon^2}{\sigma_\varepsilon^2 + \sigma_u^2} < 1. \tag{59}$$

An additional impact of this type of measurement error is inflation of the residual variance of the outcome, resulting in reduced precision of estimates. In practice, the impact of measurement error in this context depends on a number of factors, including the nature of the assumed measurement error model, presence of additional predictors, and bias in W as an estimate of X.

In the case of non-linear models (e.g., generalized linear models with links other than the identity), the effects of measurement error are more complex than in the situation just described. Although these are usually manifested as attenuation in estimated coefficients and inflation of associated variances, the nature of the bias depends on the model, the type of parameter, and the assumed error model. The book by Carroll et al. (2006) provides broad coverage of this topic for non-linear models.

Measurement error can also occur in the outcome variable Y. In the case of linear models, this is generally handled via modifications of the conditional error distribution. Approaches for non-linear models are discussed in Carroll et al. (2006) and illustrated in Magder and Hughes (1997).

4.3. Missing data

For the medical services utilization example, consider a regression model for the effect of depression on the cost of care. It is possible that some subjects may have missing values for cost and/or depression, as measured by the BDI. The possible causes for these missing values could be missed visits or declining to fill out a sensitive item on a questionnaire. When the fact that the data are missing is related to the outcomes of interest, loss of efficiency or serious distortion of study results can occur. Therefore it is useful to classify the mechanism of missing data to understand these relationships and to inform analytic approaches. An exhaustive treatment is given by Little and Rubin (1986).

Denote the complete data as $\mathbf{Y}_{\text{full}}$. In the example, this would be the values of depression and cost of care on all subjects. The available values of cost and depression are denoted by $\mathbf{Y}_{\text{obs}}$ while the missing values are denoted as $\mathbf{Y}_{\text{miss}}$. The variable $\mathbf{R}_i$ indicates the pattern of missing data for subject i; in particular, $\mathbf{R}_i = (0,0)$ if both cost and BDI are available, $(1, 0)$ if only cost is missing; $(0, 1)$ if only BDI is missing; and $(1, 1)$ if both are missing. Let $g(\mathbf{R};\gamma)$ denote the distribution of $\mathbf{R}$.

Missing data fall into three broad classes. Data are said to be *missing completely at random* (MCAR) if the distribution of $\mathbf{R}$ depends on neither $\mathbf{Y}_{\text{miss}}$ nor $\mathbf{Y}_{\text{obs}}$: that is, $g(\mathbf{R}|\mathbf{Y}_{\text{miss}}, \mathbf{Y}_{\text{obs}}; \gamma) = g(\mathbf{R};\gamma)$. If the data are *missing at random* (MAR) the distribution of $\mathbf{R}$ does not depend on $\mathbf{Y}_{\text{miss}}$ after conditioning on $\mathbf{Y}_{\text{obs}}$. Formally, this implies that $g(\mathbf{R}|\mathbf{Y}_{\text{miss}}, \mathbf{Y}_{\text{obs}}; \gamma) = g(\mathbf{R}|\mathbf{Y}_{\text{obs}}; \gamma)$. Both of these are *ignorable* missing data mechanisms, in the sense, explained in more detail below, that we can consistently estimate the regression parameters of interest without loss of efficiency while ignoring $g(\mathbf{R}|\mathbf{Y}_{\text{obs}}; \gamma)$. Otherwise, the data are said to have a non-ignorable missing data mechanism, or to be missing not at random (MNAR).

It can be shown that if data are MCAR, then naive approaches which just delete observations with missing values (so-called complete case analyses) will yield unbiased estimates. However, this can be quite inefficient if the number of omitted observations is large. Further, the MCAR assumption is not credible in many practical situations. Fortunately, it can be shown that for data which are MAR, likelihood-based methods will yield correct inferences. This is because the likelihood

$$f(\mathbf{Y}_{\text{obs}}; \theta) = \int f(\mathbf{Y}_{\text{obs}}, \mathbf{Y}_{\text{miss}}, \theta)\mathrm{d}\mathbf{Y}_{\text{miss}} \qquad (60)$$

is proportional to the full data log-likelihood

$$f(\mathbf{R}, \mathbf{Y}_{\mathrm{obs}}; \boldsymbol{\theta}) = \int f(\mathbf{Y}_{\mathrm{obs}}, \mathbf{Y}_{\mathrm{miss}}, \boldsymbol{\theta}) g(\mathbf{R}|\mathbf{Y}, \mathbf{Y}_{\mathrm{obs}}, \mathbf{Y}_{\mathrm{miss}}; \gamma) d\mathbf{Y}_{\mathrm{miss}} \qquad (61)$$

which under the MAR mechanism is then

$$\int f(\mathbf{Y}_{\mathrm{obs}}, \mathbf{Y}_{\mathrm{miss}}; \boldsymbol{\theta}) g(\mathbf{R}|\mathbf{Y}_{\mathrm{obs}}; \gamma) d\mathbf{Y}_{\mathrm{miss}} \qquad (62)$$

which simplifies to the observed data likelihood

$$f(\mathbf{Y}_{\mathrm{obs}}, \boldsymbol{\theta}) g(\mathbf{R}|\mathbf{Y}_{\mathrm{obs}}; \gamma) \qquad (63)$$

Provided there are no common elements in the parameter vectors $\boldsymbol{\theta}$ and γ, we can safely maximize Eq. (60) while ignoring $g(\mathbf{R}|\mathbf{Y}_{\mathrm{obs}}; \gamma)$. Many statistical approaches are likelihood-based and thus can easily handle MAR data without modeling the missing data mechanism.

In some cases, it is difficult to calculate or maximize the likelihood for the observed data; however, it would be easy to calculate the likelihood estimates for the complete data. In such cases, the EM algorithm (Dempster et al., 1977) is a useful approach to ML estimation. The EM algorithm alternates between an E (expectation) step and an M (maximization) step. In the E-step, we calculate the expected values of the sufficient statistics (i.e., the data or data summaries) of the complete data log-likelihood, conditional on the observed data and current parameter estimates. Then in the M-step the parameters of the complete data log-likelihood are maximized, using the expected values from the E-step. The algorithm is iterated to convergence and produces parameter estimates which can be shown to maximize the observed data log-likelihood.

To see how the EM algorithm might work, consider the exponential AFT model for censored survival times presented in Section 3.2. When the survival times are censored, the observed data consist of $(\mathbf{Y}, \boldsymbol{\Delta}, \mathbf{X})$, where $Y_i = T_i$, the actual survival time, only for uncensored subjects (i.e. $\Delta_i = 1$), and $\mathbf{X}$ is the familiar matrix of predictors. In contrast, the full data are just $(\mathbf{T}, \mathbf{X})$. The log-likelihood for the full data is

$$\sum_{i=1}^{n} \log \lambda + \mathbf{x}_i' \boldsymbol{\beta} - \lambda T_i \exp(\mathbf{x}_i' \boldsymbol{\beta}) \qquad (64)$$

The more complicated log-likelihood for the observed data, Eq. (46), could be maximized by repeated maximization of Eq. (64) using the EM algorithm. In the pth iteration of the E-step, we calculate $\widetilde{\mathbf{T}}^{(p)}$, the expected value of $\mathbf{T}$, given the observed data and the current parameter estimates $(\hat{\lambda}^{(p)}, \hat{\boldsymbol{\beta}}^{(p)})$. Under the exponential AFT,

$$\tilde{T}_i^{(p)} = E\left(T_i | Y_i, \Delta_i, \mathbf{x}_i; \hat{\lambda}^{(p)}, \hat{\boldsymbol{\beta}}^{(p)}\right)$$

$$= \begin{cases} Y_i & \Delta_i = 1 \\ Y_i + \exp\left(-\mathbf{x}_i' \hat{\boldsymbol{\beta}}^{(p)}\right)/\hat{\lambda}^{(p)} & \Delta_i = 0 \end{cases} \qquad (65)$$

In the pth iteration of the M-step, updated parameter estimates $(\hat{\lambda}^{(p+1)}, \hat{\boldsymbol{\beta}}^{(p+1)})$ are obtained by maximizing Eq. (64) over the parameters, using $\widetilde{\mathbf{T}}^{(p)}$ in place of $\mathbf{T}$. The two-step algorithm is iterated to convergence, yielding estimates $(\hat{\lambda}_{em}, \hat{\boldsymbol{\beta}}_{em})$ that maximize Eq. (46).

An alternative approach is to augment the data by *multiple imputation* (Rubin, 1987; Schafer, 1999). In this method, we sample the missing values from $f\{\mathbf{Y}_{\text{full}}|\mathbf{Y}_{\text{obs}}\}$, resulting in several "completed" datasets, each of which is analyzed using complete-data methods. Summary parameter estimates are found by averaging over the estimates from each of the imputations; in addition, the averaged standard errors are inflated by a function of the between-imputation variability in the parameter estimates, to reflect that fact that some of the data are imputed, not observed, and thus only known approximately. This approach can be used in settings where the E-step is difficult to calculate analytically, as well as in MNAR problems where the missingness mechanism can be specified.

Many techniques discussed in this chapter (e.g., generalized estimating equations) are not likelihood based. Robins et al. (1994) proposed an approach in which an explicit model for the missingness is postulated. Weights inversely proportional to the estimated probability that each subject is observed are then incorporated explicitly in the analysis. This approach is adapted from classic methods for survey sampling developed by Horvitz and Thompson (1952). By incorporating the inverse weights, non-likelihood based methods such as GEE are valid for MAR data.

Analysis of MNAR data requires detailed specification of the missing data mechanism. Two alternative approaches stem from different decompositions of the full-data likelihood. The decomposition Eq. (61) represents a so-called selection model (Little, 1995), because the missingness or selection mechanism is specified by $g(\mathbf{R}|\mathbf{Y}_{\text{obs}}, \mathbf{Y}_{\text{miss}}; \gamma)$; results are known to be sensitive to this specification (Kenward, 1998). Under the alternative *pattern mixture model*, the complete data likelihood is decomposed as

$$f(\mathbf{R}, \mathbf{Y}_{\text{obs}}; \theta) = \int f^*(\mathbf{Y}_{\text{obs}}, \mathbf{Y}_{\text{miss}}|\mathbf{R}; \theta^*) g^*(\mathbf{R}; \gamma^*) d\mathbf{Y}_{\text{miss}} \qquad (66)$$

(Little, 1993). In this case summary parameter estimates are weighted averages over the various missing data patterns. The two strategies are closely related but pattern mixture models typically are more computationally feasible (Schafer and Graham, 2002).

As an example of the pattern mixture model, consider a randomized placebo-controlled trial of clopidogrel, an antiplatelet agent, administered in the first 24 hours following a mild stroke. One objective of the trial is to assess the effect of clopidogrel on cognitive function, as measured by the Digit Symbols Substitution Test (DSST). The DSST will be administered at enrollment, 1 month, and 3 months. Denote the DSST values for subject i by $\mathbf{Y}_i' = (Y_{0i}, Y_{1i}, Y_{2i})$. Pattern mixture models specify the distribution of $\mathbf{Y}$ conditional on the pattern of missing data. Nearly all subjects will have a baseline DSST, so missing data will involve missing values of Y_1 and Y_2. We again denote patterns of missing data by $\mathbf{R}_i$, the vector of missing data indicators, with values $(0, 1, 0)$, $(0, 0, 1)$, or $(0, 1, 1)$, when the second, third, or both follow-up DSST values are missing, respectively. We index those three patterns of missing data as $M = 1, 2, 3$, respectively; subjects with complete data (i.e., $R = (0, 0, 0)$) are indexed as pattern $M = 0$.

Then the pattern mixture model is the product of a multinomial model for M and a model for $f(\mathbf{Y}|M)$. One possibility might be to estimate $\mu = E(\mathbf{Y})$ and $\mathbf{\Sigma} = \mathrm{cov}(\mathbf{Y})$, the mean and variance of $\mathbf{Y}$, the first of which can be expressed as

$$\mu = \sum_{m=0}^{3} \mu^{(m)} P(M = m). \tag{67}$$

where $\mu^{(m)} = E(Y|M = m)$. The pattern mixture approach obtains MLEs of μ through likelihood-based estimates of the parameters of the mixture model (68).

The MLEs of $P(M = m)$ are just the observed frequencies of the missing data patterns. However, the parameters $\mu^{(m)}$ are under-identified by this model. For instance, there are no data on Y_2 in the subsample with $M = 2$, so $\mu_2^{(2)} = E(Y_2|M = 2)$ cannot be estimated. To estimate all parameters, *identifying restrictions* must be imposed. For example, we might assume that the trend over time is the same for $M = 2$ as for $M = 1$. Other potential restrictions encompass the familiar MCAR and MAR assumptions; if the data are MCAR, the parameterization is simplified because $\mu^{(m)}$ and $\mathbf{\Sigma}^{(m)}$ are identical for all patterns. It is also possible to specify pattern mixture models which allow for more general ignorable and non-ignorable missingness mechanisms (Little, 1993). An important advantage of these models, especially compared with selection models, is the fact that the identifying restrictions are explicitly specified. Furthermore, the likelihoods for these models are straightforward to maximize as compared to those for selection models.

The weighting approach described earlier can also be applied to MNAR data; see Bang and Robins (2005) for a review. This approach is related to selection models, but handles missingness using a weighted analysis. As before, data points are weighted in inverse proportion to the estimated probability of being observed.

4.4. Computing

Regression problems have been one of the major driving forces in many of the recent advances in numerical computing. Books by Gentle (2005), Monahan (2001), and Thisted (1988) cover many of these, and provide details on computational techniques used in many of the methods covered here.

The continued expansion in the number of software tools to perform statistical analyses coupled with increases in the processing speed and capacity of modern computer hardware has made what were once considered insurmountable tasks practical even for many desktop machines. Major commercial statistical software packages with extensive facilities for many of the regression methods described here include SAS (SAS Institute Inc., 2005), Stata (StataCorp LP., 2005), SPSS (SPSS Inc., 2006), and S-PLUS (Insightful Corporation, 2006). The R statistical programming language (R Development Core Team, 2005) is public domain

Table 1
Regression features of several major statistical software packages

Regression Technique	SAS	Stata	SPSS	S-PLUS	R
Linear	X	X	X	X	X
Generalized linear	X	X	X	X	X
Non-linear	X	X	X	X	X
Mixed effects linear	X	X	X	X	X
Mixed effects non-linear	X	X	–	X	X
Non-parametric	X	X	–	X	X

software most similar to S-PLUS. Despite substantial overlap in regression-oriented features, these packages are quite different in terms of programming style and user interface. SAS, SPSS, and Stata have generally more developed and "user friendly" interfaces, while S-PLUS and R are more akin to interpreted programming languages that provide many "canned" procedures, but also allow great flexibility in user-defined functions (including support for linking with external routines written in compiled languages such as C and FORTRAN).

Table 1 summarizes capabilities for many of the methods covered here. Although all offer similar features for standard regression methods and generalized linear models, the depth of coverage of more specialized techniques varies considerably. In the area of mixed-effects regression, the *MIXED* and *NLMIXED* procedures in SAS are more fully featured than competitors. Stata is distinguished by the implementation of generalized estimating equation and robust variance methods as an option with most of the included regression commands. In addition, methods for bootstrap, jackknife, and permutation testing are implemented in a very accessible way. Because of their extensibility and the availability of a large range of procedures written by researchers, S-PLUS and R tend to have more functionality in the areas of non-parametric regression, smoothing methods, alternative variable selection procedures, and approaches for dealing with missing data and measurement error.

In addition to the major packages covered here, there are a number of specialized software offerings that target particular regression methods or related numerical computations. These include CART (Steinberg and Colla, 1995) software for classification and regression tree methods and the LogXact (Mehta and Patel, 1996) program for exact logistic regression. Additional packages that focus more generally on numerical computation, but that also provide more limited regression capabilities (and also support user-defined regression functions) include Matlab (MathWorks, 2006), Mathematica (Wolfram Research Inc., 2005), and Maple (Maplesoft, 2003).

References

Altman, D.G., Andersen, P.K. (1989). Bootstrap investigation of the stability of the Cox regression model. *Statistics in Medicine* **8**, 771–783.
Altman, D.G., Royston, P. (2000). What do we mean by validating a prognostic model? *Statistics in Medicine* **19**, 453–473.

Bang, H., Robins, J.M. (2005). Doubly robust estimation in missing data and causal inference models. *Biometrics* **61**, 962–973.

Bates, D., Watts, D. (1988). *Nonlinear Regression Analysis and its Applications*. Wiley, Chichester, New York.

Becker, N. (1989). *Analysis of Infectious Disease Data*. Chapman & Hall/CRC, London.

Begg, M.D., Lagakos, S. (1993). Loss in efficiency caused by omitted covariates and misspecifying exposure in logistic regression models. *Journal of the American Statistical Association* **88**(421), 166–170.

Breiman, L. (1995). Better model selection using the nonnegative garrote. *Technometrics* **37**, 373–384.

Breiman, L. (2001). Statistical modeling: The two cultures. *Statistical Science* **16**(3), 199–231.

Breiman, L., Friedman, J.H., Olshen, R.A., and Stone, C.J. (1984). *Classification and Regression Trees*. Statistics/Probability Series. Wadsworth Publishing Company, Belmont, CA.

Carroll, R., Rupprt, D., Stefanski, L., Crainiceanu, C. (2006). *Measurement Error in Nonlinear Models: A Modern Perspective*, 2nd ed. Chapman & Hall/CRC, London.

Cleveland, W.S. (1981). Lowess: A program for smoothing scatterplots by robust locally weighted regression. *The American Statistician* **35**, 45–54.

Concato, J., Peduzzi, P., Holfold, T.R. (1995). Importance of events per independent variable in proportional hazards analysis. I. background, goals, and general strategy. *Journal of Clinical Epidemiology* **48**, 1495–1501.

Cook, R.D. (1977). Detection of influential observations in linear regression. *Technometrics* **19**, 15–18.

Cox, D.R., Hinkley, D.V. (1974). *Theoretical Statistics*. Chapman & Hall, London, New York.

D'Agostino, R.B. (1998). Propensity score methods for bias reduction in the comparison of a treatment to a non-randomized control group. *Statistics in Medicine* **17**, 2265–2281.

Day, N. (1990). The Armitage-Doll multistage model of carcinogenesis. *Statistics in Medicine* **83**, 677–689.

Dempster, A.P., Laird, N., Rubin, D. (1977). Maximum-likelihood from incomplete data via the em algorithm. *Journal of the Royal Statistical Society, Series B* **39**(1–38).

Diggle, P., Heagerty, P., Liang, K.-Y., Zeger, S.L. (2002). *Analysis of Longitudinal Data*, 2nd ed. Oxford University Press, Oxford.

Efron, B. (1986). Estimating the error rate of a prediction rule: Improvement on cross-validation. *Journal of the American Statistical Association* **81**, 316–331.

Fuller, W. (1987). *Measurement Error Models*, 2nd ed. Wiley, New York.

Gail, M.H., Tan, W.Y., Piantodosi, S. (1988). Tests for no treatment effect in randomized clinical trials. *Biometrika* **75**, 57–64.

Gail, M.H., Wieand, S., Piantodosi, S. (1984). Biased estimates of treatment effect in randomized experiments with nonlinear regressions and omitted covariates. *Biometrika* **71**, 431–444.

Gentle, J. (2005). *Elements of Computational Statistics*, 1st ed. Springer, New York.

Graf, E., Schmoor, C., Sauerbrei, W., Schumacher, M. (1999). Assessment and comparison of prognostic classification schemes for survival data. *Statistics in Medicine* **18**, 2529–2545.

Greenhouse, S.W., Geisser, S. (1959). On methods in the analysis of profile data. *Psychometrika* **32**, 95–112.

Greenland, S. (1989). Modeling and variable selection in epidemiologic analysis. *American Journal of Public Health* **79**(3), 340–349.

Greenland, S. (2000). An introduction to instrumental variables for epidemiologists. *International Journal of Epidemiology* **29**, 722–729.

Hankey, B.F., Feuer, E.J., Clegg, L.X., Hayes, R.B., Legler, J.M., Prorok, P.C., Ries, L.A., Merrill, R.M., Kaplan, R.S. (1999). Cancer surveillance series: Interpreting trends in prostate Cancer. Part I: Evidence of the effects of screening in recent prostate cancer incidence, mortality, and survival rates. *Journal of the National Cancer Institute* **91**, 1017–1024.

Harrell, F.E., Lee, K.L., Mark, D.B. (1996). Multivariable prognostic models: Issues in developing models, evaluating assumptions and adequacy, and measuring and reducing errors. *Statistics in Medicine* **15**, 361–387.

Hastie, T., Tibshirani, R. (1990). *Generalized Additive Models*. Chapman & Hall, New York.

Hastie, T., Tibshirani, R., Friedman, J.H. (2001). *The Elements of Statistical Learning: Data Mining, Inference, and Prediction*. Springer, New York.

Hauck, W.W., Anderson, S., Marcus, S.M. (1998). Should we adjust for covariates in nonlinear regression analyses of randomized trials? *Controlled Clinical Trials* **19**, 249–256.

Henderson, R., Oman, P. (1999). Effect of frailty on marginal regression estimates in survival analysis. *Journal of the Royal Statistical Society, Series B, Methodological* **61**, 367–379.

Hernan, M.A., Brumback, B., Robins, J.M. (2001). Marginal structural models to estimate the joint causal effect of nonrandomized treatments. *Journal of the American Statistical Association* **96**, 440–448.

Hoenig, J.M., Heisey, D.M. (2001). The abuse of power: The pervasive fallacy of power calculations for data analysis. *The American Statistician* **55**(1), 19–24.

Hoerl, A.E., Kennard, R.W. (1970). Ridge regression: Biased estimates for nonorthogonal problems. *Technometrics* **12**, 55–67.

Hofer, T., Hayward, R., Greenfield, S., Wagner, E., Kaplan, S., Manning, W. (1999). The unreliability of individual physician "report cards" for assessing the costs and quality of care of a chronic disease. *Journal of the American Medical Association* **281**, 2098–2105.

Horvitz, D.G., Thompson, D.J. (1952). A generalization of sampling without replacement from a finite universe. *Journal of the American Statistical Association* **47**, 663–685.

Huber, P.J. (1967). The behaviour of maximum likelihood estimates under nonstandard conditions. In: Le Cam, L., Neyman, J. (Eds.), *The Fifth Berkeley Symposium in Mathematical Statistics and Probability*. University of California Press, Berkeley.

Insightful Corporation. (2006). *S-PLUS version 7.0 for Windows*. Seattle, Washington.

Jin, Z., Lin, D.Y., Wei, L.J., Ying, Z. (2003). Rank-based inference for the accelerated failure time model. *Biometrika* **90**, 341–353.

Kauermann, G., Carroll, R.J. (2001). A note on the efficiency of sandwich covariance matrix estimation. *Journal of the American Statistical Association* **96**(456), 1387–1396.

Kenward, M.G. (1998). Selection models for repeated measurements with non-random dropout: An illustration of sensitivity. *Statistics in Medicine* **17**, 2723–2732.

Kenward, M.G., Roger, J.H. (1997). Small sample inference for fixed effects from restricted maximum likelihood. *Biometrics* **53**, 983–997.

Kurth, T., Walker, A.M., Glynn, R.J., Chan, K.A., Gaziano, J.M., Berger, K., Robins, J.M. (2005). Results of multivariable logistic regression, propensity matching, propensity adjustment, and propensity-based weighting under conditions of nonuniform effect. *American Journal of Epidemiology* **163**, 262–270.

Lagakos, S.W., Schoenfeld, D.A. (1984). Properties of proportional-hazards score tests under misspecified regression models. *Biometrics* **40**, 1037–1048.

Larsen, W.A., McCleary, S.J. (1972). The use of partial residual plots in regression analysis. *Technometrics* **14**, 781–790.

Le Cessie, S., Van Houwelingen, J.C. (1992). Ridge estimators in logistic regression. *Applied Statistics* **41**, 191–201.

Lin, D.Y., Geyer, C.J. (1992). Computational methods for semiparametric linear regression with censored data. *Journal of Computational and Graphical Statistics* **1**, 77–90.

Little, R.J.A. (1993). Pattern-mixture models for multivariate incomplete data. *Journal of the American Statistical Association* **88**, 125–134.

Little, R.J.A. (1995). Modeling the drop-out mechanism in longitudinal studies. *Journal of the American Statistical Association* **90**, 1112–1121.

Little, R.J.A., Rubin, D.B. (1986). *Statistical Analysis with Missing Data*. Wiley, New York.

Long, J.S., Ervin, L.H. (2000). Using heteroscedasticity consistent standard errors in the linear regression model. *The American Statistician* **54**, 217–224.

MacKinnon, J.G., White, H. (1985). Some heteroskedasticity consistent covariance matrix estimators with improved finite sample properties. *Journal of Econometrics* **29**, 53–57.

Magder, L., Hughes, J. (1997). Logistic regression when the outcome is measured with uncertainty. *American Journal of Epidemiology* **146**, 195–203.

Maldonado, G., Greenland, S. (1993). Simulation study of confounder-selection strategies. *American Journal of Epidemiology* **138**, 923–936.

Maplesoft. (2003). *Maple 9 Getting Started Guide*. Waterloo, ON, Canada.

Masson, C., Sorensen, J., Phibbs, C., Okin, R. (2004). Predictors of medical service utilization among individuals with co-occurring HIV infection and substance abuse disorders. *AIDS Care* **16**(6), 744–755.

MathWorks. (2006). *MATLAB version 7.2*. Natick, MA.

McCulloch, C.E. (2005). Repeated measures ANOVA, R.I.P.? *Chance* **18**, 29–33.

McCulloch, C.E., Searle, S.R. (2000). *Generalized, Linear, and Mixed Models.* Wiley, Chichester, New York.

Mehta, C., Patel, N. (1996). *LogXact for Windows.* Cytel Software Corporation, Cambridge, MA.

Mickey, R.M., Greenland, S. (1989). The impact of confounder selection on effect estimation. *American Journal of Epidemiology* **129**(1), 125–137.

Monahan, J. (2001). *Numerical Methods of Statistics*, 1st ed. Cambridge University Press, Cambridge.

Neuhaus, J. (1998). Estimation efficiency with omitted covariates in generalized linear models. *Journal of the American Statistical Association* **93**, 1124–1129.

Neuhaus, J., Jewell, N.P. (1993). A geometric approach to assess bias due to omitted covariates in generalized linear models. *Biometrika* **80**, 807–815.

Normand, S.-L.T., Glickman, M.E., Gatsonis, C.A. (1997). Statistical methods for profiling providers of medical care: Issues and applications. *Journal of the American Statistical Association* **92**, 803–814.

Peduzzi, P., Concato, J., Feinstein, A.R. (1995). Importance of events per independent variable in proportional hazards regression analysis. II. Accuracy and precision of regression estimates. *Journal of Clinical Epidemiology* **48**, 1503–1510.

Peduzzi, P., Concato, J., Kemper, E., Holford, T.R., Feinstein, A.R. (1996). A simulation study of the number of events per variable in logistic regression analysis. *Journal of Clinical Epidemiology* **49**, 1373–1379.

Pinheiro, J., Bates, D. (2000). *Mixed-effects models in S and S-PLUS.* Springer, New York.

R Development Core Team. 2005. *R: A Language and Environment for Statistical Computing.* R Foundation for Statistical Computing, Vienna, Austria. ISBN 3-900051-07-0.

Robins, J.M., Hernan, M.A., Brumback, B. (2000). Marginal structural models and causal inference in epidemiology. *Epidemiology* **11**, 550–560.

Robins, J.M., Rotnitzky, A., Zhao, L.P. (1994). Estimation of regression coefficients when some regressors are not always observed. *Journal of the American Statistical Association* **89**, 846–866.

Rosenbaum, P.R., Rubin, D.B. (1983). The central role of the propensity score in observational studies for causal effects. *Biometrika* **70**, 41–55.

Rubin, D.B. (1987). *Multiple Imputation for Nonresponse in Surveys.* Wiley, Chichester, New York.

SAS Institute Inc. (2005). *SAS/STAT Software, Version 9.* Cary, NC.

Schafer, J.L. (1999). Multiple imputation: A primer. *Statistical Methods in Medical Research* **8**, 3–15.

Schafer, J.L., Graham, J.W. (2002). Missing data: Our view of the state of the art. *Psychological Methods* **7**, 147–177.

Schmoor, C., Schumacher, M. (1997). Effects of covariate omission and categorization when analysing randomized trials with the Cox model. *Statistics in Medicine* **16**, 225–237.

Searle, S.R., Casella, G., McCulloch, C.E. (1992). *Variance Components.* Wiley, Chichester, New York.

Seber, G., Wild, C. (2003). *Nonlinear Regression*, 2nd ed. Wiley, Chichester, New York.

Sorensen, J., Dilley, J., London, J., Okin, R., Delucchi, K., Phibbs, C. (2003). Case management for substance abusers with HIV/AIDS: A randomized clinical trial. *The American Journal of Drug And Alcohol Abuse* **29**, 133–150.

SPSS Inc. (2006). *SPSS for Windows, Rel. 14.0.* Chicago, IL.

StataCorp LP. (2005). *Stata Statistical Software: Release 9.* College Station, TX.

Steinberg, D., Colla, P. (1995). *CART: Tree-Structured Nonparametric Data Analysis.* Salford Systems, San Diego, CA.

Steyerberg, E.W., Eijkemans, M.J.C., Habbema, J.D.F. (1999). Stepwise selection in small datasets: a simulation study of bias in logistic regression analysis. *Journal of Clinical Epidemiology* **52**, 935–942.

Sun, G.W., Shook, T.L., Kay, G.L. (1999). Inappropriate use of bivariable analysis to screen risk factors for use in multivariable analysis. *Journal of Clinical Epidemiology* **49**, 907–916.

Takeuchi, M., Igarashi, Y., Tomimoto, S., Odake, M., Hayashi, T., Tsukamoto, T., Hata, K., Takaoka, H., Fukuzaki, H. (1991). Single-beat estimation of the slope of end-systolic pressure-volume relation in the human left ventricle. *Circulation* **83**, 202–212.

Thisted, R. (1988). *Elements of Statistical Computing: Numerical Computation*, 1st ed. Chapman & Hall, New York.

Tibshirani, R. (1997). The LASSO method for variable selection in the Cox model. *Statistics in Medicine* **16**, 385–395.

Verweij, P.J.M., Van Houwelingen, H.C. (1994). Penalized likelihood in Cox regression. *Statistics in Medicine* **13**, 2427–2436.

Vittinghoff, E., McCulloch, C.E. (2007). Relaxing the rule of ten events per variable in logistic and Cox regression. *American Journal of Epidemiology* **165**(6), 710–718.

Wei, L.J. (1992). The accelerated failure time model: A useful alternative to the Cox regression model in survival analysis. *Statistics in Medicine* **11**, 1871–1879.

Welsch, R.E. (1982). Influence functions and regression diagnostics. In: Launer, R.L., Siegel, A.F. (Eds.), *Modern Data Analysis*. Academic Press, New York, pp. 149–169.

Welsch, R.E., Kuh, E. (1977). Linear Regression Diagnostics. Technical report 923-77, Sloan School of Management, Massachusetts Insititute of Technology, Cambridge, MA.

White, H. (1980). A heteroskedastic-consistent covariance matrix estimator and a direct test of heteroskedasticity. *Econometrica* **48**, 817–838.

Wolfram Research Inc. (2005). *Mathematica Version 5.2*. Champaign, IL.

Handbook of Statistics, Vol. 27
ISSN: 0169-7161
DOI: 10.1016/S0169-7161(07)27007-5

4

Count Response Regression Models

Joseph M. Hilbe and William H. Greene

Abstract

Count response regression models refer to regression models having a count as the response; e.g., hospital length of stay, number of bacterial pneumonia cases per zip code in Arizona from 2000 to 2005. Poisson regression is the basic model of this class. Having an assumption of the equality of the distributional mean and variance, Poisson models are inappropriate for many count-modeling situations. Overdispersion occurs when the variance exceeds the nominal mean. The negative binomial (NB2) is commonly employed to model overdispersed Poisson data, but NB models can themselves be overdispersed. A wide variety of alternative count models have been designed to accommodate overdispersion in both Poisson and NB models; e.g., zero-inflated, zero-truncated, hurdle, and sample selection models. Data can also be censored and truncated; specialized count models have been designed for these situations as well. In addition, the wide range of Poisson and NB panel and mixed models has been developed. In the chapter we provide an overview of the above varieties of count response models, and discuss available software that can be used for their estimation.

1. Introduction

Modeling counts of events can be found in all areas of statistics, econometrics, and throughout the social and physical sciences. Some familiar applications include:

- the incidence of diseases in specific populations,
- numbers of patents applied for,
- numbers of regime changes in political units,
- numbers of financial 'incidents' such as defaults or bankruptcies,
- numbers of doctor visits,
- numbers of incidents of drug or alcohol abuse, and so on.

The literatures in all these fields and many more are replete with applications of models for counts. The signature feature of all of these is that familiar linear regression techniques that would relate the measured outcomes to appropriate covariates – smoking and disease or research and development to patents for examples – would not be applicable because the response variable is discrete, not continuous. Nonetheless, a related counterpart to the familiar regression model is a natural departure point. The Poisson regression model has been used through-out the research landscape to model counts in applications such as these. The Poisson model is a nonlinear, albeit straightforward and popular modeling tool. It is ubiquitous enough that estimation routines are built into all well-known contemporary computer programs. This chapter will survey models and methods for analyzing counts, beginning with this basic tool.

The Poisson model provides the platform for modeling count data. Practical issues in 'real' data have compelled researchers to extend the model in several directions. The most fundamental extension involves augmenting the model to allow a more realistic treatment of variation of the responses variable. The Poisson model, at its heart, describes the mean of the response. A consequence of the specification is that it implies a wholly unsatisfactory model for the variance of the response variable. Models such as the NB model are designed to accommodate a more complete description of the distribution of observed outcomes. Observed data often present other forms of 'nonPoissonness.' An important example is the 'excess zeros' case. Survey data often contain more zero responses (or more of some other responses) than would be predicted by a Poisson or a NB model. For example, the incidence of hypertension in school age children, or credit card default, are relatively rare events. The count response is amenable to modeling in this framework; however, an unmodified Poisson model will underpredict the zero outcome. In another interesting application, Poisson-like models are often used to model family size; however, family size data in Western societies will often display excess twos in the number of children, where, once again, by 'excess' we mean in excess of what would typically be predicted by a Poisson model. Finally, other data and situation-driven applications will call for more than one equation in the count model. For example, in modeling health care system utilization, researchers often profitably employ 'two part models' in which one part describes a decision to use the health care system and a second equation describes the intensity of system utilization given the decision to use the system at all.

This chapter will survey these count models. The analysis will proceed as follows: Section 2 details the fundamental results for the Poisson regression model. Section 3 discusses the most familiar extension of models for counts, the NB model. Section 4 considers the types of broad model extensions suggested above including the important extensions to longitudinal (panel) data. Section 5 presents several additional more specialized model extensions. Section 5 describes some of the available software tools for estimation. Rather than collecting an extended example in one place at the end of the survey, we will develop some applications as part of the ongoing presentations. Our analyses are done with LIMDEP statistical software. Section 5 describes this and a few other packages in some more detail. Section 6 concludes.

2. The Poisson regression model

The Poisson model derives from a description of how often events occur per unit of time. Consider, for example, a service window at a bank, or an observer watching a population for the outbreak of diseases. The 'interarrival time' is the amount of time that elapses between events, for example, the duration between arrivals of customers at the teller window or the amount of time that passes between 'arrivals' of cases of a particular disease. If the interarrival time is such that the probability that a new incident will occur in the next instant of time is independent of how much time has passed since the last one, then the process is said to be 'memoryless.' The exponential distribution is used to describe such processes. Now, consider not the interarrival time, but the number of arrivals that occur in a fixed length interval of time. Under the assumptions already made, if the length of time is short, then the 'Poisson' distribution will be an appropriate distribution to use to model the number of arrivals that occur during a fixed time interval.[1]

More formally, suppose the process is such that the expected interarrival time does not vary over time. Say θ is this value. Then, the number of arrivals that can be expected to arrive per unit of time is $\lambda = 1/\theta$. The distribution of the number of arrivals, Y, in a fixed interval is the Poisson distribution

$$f(Y) = Prob[Y = y] = \frac{\exp(-\lambda)\lambda^y}{y!}, \quad y = 0, 1, \ldots; \quad \lambda > 0. \tag{1}$$

The Poisson model describes the number of arrivals per single unit of time. Suppose that the observer observes T consecutive intervals. Then, the expected number of arrivals would naturally be λT. Assuming the process is not changing from one interval to the next, the appropriate distribution to model a window of length T, rather than 1, would be

$$f(Y) = Prob[Y = y] = \frac{\exp(-\lambda T)(\lambda T)^y}{y!}, \quad y = 0, 1, \ldots; \quad \lambda > 0. \tag{2}$$

One can imagine a sampling process such that successive observers watched the population or process for different amounts of time. The appropriate model for the number of observed events in such a sample would necessarily have to account for the different lengths of time. A sample of observations would be $(y_1, T_1), \ldots (y_N, T_N)$. The joint observations would consist of an observed count variable and an observed 'exposure' variable. (For reasons that are far from obvious, such a variable is often called an 'offset' variable – see, e.g., the

---

[1] Another way to develop the Poisson model from first principles is to consider a Bernoulli sampling process in which the success probability, π, becomes small while the number of trials, T, becomes large such that πT is constant. The limiting process of this binomial sampling scheme is the Poisson model. By treating the 'draws' as specific short intervals of time, we can view this as an alternative view of the exponential model suggested earlier.

documentation for *Stata* or *SAS*.) An analogous process would follow if the observation were designed so that each observation was based on a count of occurrences in a group of size T_i, where T_i is allowed to differ from one observation to another. Larger groups would tend to produce larger counts, not because the process had changed, but because of the increased 'exposure' to the same process.

The Poisson random variable has mean

$$E[Y] = \lambda T \tag{3}$$

and variance

$$\text{Var}[Y] = \lambda T. \tag{4}$$

These are derived for the case $T = 1$ in any basic statistics book. For convenience at this point, we will focus on that case as well. Where necessary, we will reinstate the exposure as part of the model for a particular sampling process. Note, in particular, that the variance equals the mean, a fact that will become important in the next section of this survey.

To extend this model to a regression context, consider once again the health application. For any group observed at random in a population in a given time interval, suppose the Poisson model, is appropriate. To consider a concrete example, suppose we observe new cancer cases per unit of time or per group. The overall average number of cases observed per unit of time may be well described with a fixed mean, λ. However, for the assumed case, three significant comorbidity factors, age, weight, and smoking, stand out as possible explanatory variables. For researchers observing different populations in different places, one might surmise that the parameter, λ, which is the mean number of new cases per unit of time, would vary substantively with these covariates. This brings us to the point of 'model' building, and, in particular, since we have surmised that the mean of the distribution is a function of the covariates, regression modeling.

Precisely, how the covariates in the model should enter the mean is an important question. Suppose we denote average age, average weight, and percent who smoke in the different observed groups suggested by the example, for convenience, as (x_1, x_2, x_3), it would be tempting to write the mean of the random variable as

$$\lambda = \beta_0 + \beta_1 x_1 + \beta_2 x_2 + \beta_3 x_3. \tag{5}$$

However, a crucial feature of the model emerges immediately. Note in (1), and for obvious reasons, $\lambda > 0$. This is the mean of a nonnegative random variable. It would not be possible to insure that the function in (5) is positive for all values of the parameters and any data. The constraint is more important yet in view of (4). The commonly accepted solution, and the conventional approach in modeling count data, is to use

$$\lambda = \exp(\boldsymbol{\beta}'\mathbf{x}), \tag{6}$$

where the vector notation is used for convenience, and $\boldsymbol{\beta}$ and $\mathbf{x}$ are assumed to include a constant term.[2]

To summarize, then, the Poisson regression model that is typically used to model count data is

$$f(Y|\mathbf{x}) = Prob[Y = y] = \frac{\exp(-\lambda T)(\lambda T)^y}{y!}, \quad y = 0, 1, \ldots;$$

$$\lambda = \exp(\boldsymbol{\beta}'\mathbf{x}) > 0. \tag{7}$$

This is a nonlinear regression which has conditional mean function

$$E[Y|\mathbf{x}] = \lambda = \exp(\boldsymbol{\beta}'\mathbf{x}) \tag{8}$$

and heteroskedastic conditional variance

$$\text{Var}[Y|\mathbf{x}] = \lambda. \tag{9}$$

2.1. Estimation of the Poisson model

The parameters of the nonlinear Poisson regression model, $\boldsymbol{\beta}$, can, in principle, be estimated by nonlinear least squares by minimizing the conventional sum of squares. With a sample of N observations, $(y_1, \mathbf{x}_1), \ldots, (y_N, \mathbf{x}_N)$, we would minimize

$$\text{SS}(\boldsymbol{\beta}) = \sum_{i=1}^{N} [y_i - \exp(\boldsymbol{\beta}'\mathbf{x}_i + \log T_i)]^2. \tag{10}$$

However, maximum likelihood estimation is the method of most common choice for this model. The log-likelihood function for a sample of N observations may be characterized as

$$\log L(\boldsymbol{\beta}) \sum_{i=1}^{N} y_i(\boldsymbol{\beta}'\mathbf{x}_i + \log T_i) - \exp(\boldsymbol{\beta}'\mathbf{x}_i + \log T_i) - \log(y_i!). \tag{11}$$

Note how the exposure variable enters the model, as if it were a covariate having a coefficient of one. As such, accommodating data sets that are heterogeneous in this respect does not require any substantial modification of the model or the estimator. For convenience in what follows, we will assume that each observation is made in an interval of one period (or one observation unit; $T_i = 1$; $\ln T_i = 0$). As noted earlier, this is a particularly straightforward model to estimate, and it is available as a built-in option in all modern software.

---

[2] This implies that the model is a 'log-linear' model in the development of McCullagh and Nelder (1983) – indeed, in the history of log-linear modeling, the Poisson model might reasonably be regarded as *the* log-linear model. The Poisson model plays a central role in the development of the theory. As we will not be exploring this aspect of the model in any depth in this review, we note this feature of the model at this point only in passing.

The conditional mean function for the Poisson model is nonlinear

$$E[y|\mathbf{x}] = \exp(\boldsymbol{\beta}'\mathbf{x}). \tag{12}$$

For inference purposes, e.g., testing for the significance of average weight in the incidence of disease, the coefficients, β, provide the appropriate metric. For analysis of the behavior of the response variable, however, one typically examines the partial effects

$$\boldsymbol{\delta}(\mathbf{x}) = \frac{\partial E[y|\mathbf{x}]}{\partial \mathbf{x}} = \exp(\boldsymbol{\beta}'\mathbf{x}) \times \boldsymbol{\beta}. \tag{13}$$

As in any regression model, this measure is a function of the data point at which it is evaluated. For analysis of the Poisson model, researchers typically use one of the two approaches: The marginal effects, computed at the mean, or the center of the data are

$$\boldsymbol{\delta}(\bar{\mathbf{x}}) = \frac{\partial E[y|\bar{\mathbf{x}}]}{\partial \bar{\mathbf{x}}} = \exp(\boldsymbol{\beta}'\bar{\mathbf{x}}) \times \boldsymbol{\beta}, \tag{14}$$

where $\bar{\mathbf{x}} = (1/N)\Sigma_{i=1}^{N}\mathbf{x}_i$ is the sample mean of the data. An alternative, commonly used measure is the set of average partial effects,

$$\bar{\boldsymbol{\delta}}(\mathbf{X}) = \frac{1}{N}\sum_{i=1}^{N}\frac{\partial E[y|\mathbf{x}_i]}{\partial \mathbf{x}_i} = \frac{1}{N}\sum_{i=1}^{N}\exp(\boldsymbol{\beta}'\mathbf{x}_i) \times \boldsymbol{\beta}. \tag{15}$$

Although the two measures will generally not differ by very much in a practical setting, the two measures will not converge to the same value as the sample size increases. The estimator in (15) will converge to that (13) plus a term that depends on the higher order moments of the distribution of the covariates.

We note two aspects of the computation of partial effects that are occasionally overlooked in applications. Most applications of count models involve individual level data. The typical model will involve dummy variables, for example, sex, race, education, marital status, working status, and so on. One cannot differentiate with respect to a binary variable. The proper computation for the partial effect of a binary variable, say z_i is

$$\Delta(z_i) = E[y|\mathbf{x}, z = 1] - E[y|\mathbf{x}, z = 0].$$

In practical terms, the computation of these finite differences will usually produce results similar to those that use derivatives – the finite difference is a crude derivative. Nonetheless, the finite difference presents the more accurate picture of the desired result. Second, models often include nonlinear functions of the independent variables. In our applications below, for example, we have a tezrm $\beta_1\text{AGE} + \beta_2\text{AGE}^2$. In this instance, neither coefficient, nor the associates marginal effect, is useful by itself for measuring the impact of education. The appropriate computation would be

$$\delta(\text{AGE}) = \exp(\boldsymbol{\beta}'\mathbf{x}_i)[\beta_1 + 2\beta_2\text{AGE}].$$

2.2. Statistical inference

For basic inference about coefficients in the model, the standard trinity of likelihood-based tests, likelihood ratio, Wald and Lagrange multiplier (LM), are easily computed.[3] For testing a hypothesis, linear or nonlinear, of the form

$$H_0 : \mathbf{c}(\boldsymbol{\beta}) = \mathbf{0}, \tag{16}$$

the likelihood-ratio statistic is the obvious choice. This requires estimation of β subject to the restrictions of the null hypothesis, for example, subject to the exclusions of a null hypothesis that states that certain variables should have zero coefficients – that is, that they should not appear in the model. Then, the likelihood-ratio statistic is

$$\chi^2[J] = 2(\log L - \log L_0), \tag{17}$$

where $\log L$ is the log-likelihood computed using the unrestricted estimator, $\log L_0$ the counterpart based on the restricted estimator and the degrees of freedom, J, the number of restrictions (an example appears below).

   Each predictor, including the constant, can have a calculated Wald statistic, defined as $[\beta_j/\mathrm{SE}(\beta_j)]^2$, which is distributed as χ^2. $[\beta_j/\mathrm{SE}(\beta_j)]$ defines both the t or z statistic, respectively distributed as t or normal. For computation of Wald statistics, one needs an estimate of the asymptotic covariance matrix of the coefficients. The Hessian of the log-likelihood is

$$\frac{\partial^2 \log L}{\partial\boldsymbol{\beta}\partial\boldsymbol{\beta}'} = -\sum_{i=1}^{N} \lambda_i \mathbf{x}_i \mathbf{x}_i', \tag{18}$$

where $\lambda_i = \exp(\boldsymbol{\beta}'\mathbf{x}_i)$. Since this does not involve the random variable, y_i, (18) also gives the expected Hessian. The estimated asymptotic covariance matrix for the maximum likelihood, based on the Hessian, is

$$\mathbf{V}_{\mathrm{H}} = \mathrm{Est.Asy.Var}[\hat{\boldsymbol{\beta}}_{\mathrm{MLE}}] = \left[\sum_{i=1}^{N} \hat{\lambda}_i \mathbf{x}_i \mathbf{x}_i'\right]^{-1}, \tag{19}$$

where $\hat{\lambda}_i = \exp(\hat{\boldsymbol{\beta}}'\mathbf{x}_i)$. Although in practice, one normally uses the variance matrices discussed in Section 2.4, a commonly used alternative estimator based on the first derivatives is the BHHH, or outer products estimator,

$$\mathbf{V}_{\mathrm{OPG}} = \mathrm{Est.Asy.Var}[\hat{\boldsymbol{\beta}}_{\mathrm{MLE}}] = \left[\sum_{i=1}^{N} (y_i - \hat{\lambda}_i)^2 \mathbf{x}_i \mathbf{x}_i'\right]^{-1}. \tag{20}$$

   Researchers often compute asymptotic standard errors for their estimates of the marginal effects. This is a moderately complicated exercise in some cases. The

---

[3] The presentation here is fairly terse. For more detailed derivations of these results, the reader may refer many of the sources that develop this model in detail, including Hilbe (2007), Winkelmann (2003), or Greene (2003, Chapter 21).

most straightforward case is based on (14). To use the delta method to estimate the asymptotic covariance matrix for $\hat{\delta}(\bar{\mathbf{x}})$, we would require the Jacobian,

$$\hat{\mathbf{G}} = \frac{\partial \hat{\delta}(\bar{\mathbf{x}})}{\partial \hat{\boldsymbol{\beta}}} = \hat{\lambda}(\bar{\mathbf{x}})(I + \hat{\boldsymbol{\beta}}\bar{\mathbf{x}}'). \tag{21}$$

Then, the desired asymptotic covariance matrix is computed using

$$\text{Est.Asy.Var}[\hat{\delta}(\bar{\mathbf{x}})] = \hat{\mathbf{G}}\mathbf{V}\hat{\mathbf{G}}'. \tag{22}$$

The analogous computation can be done for the average partial effect in (15). To do this, note that in the sample mean computed there, all N terms are based on the same estimator of β. As such, the computation of an asymptotic analogous to (22) must have N^2 terms. The result will be

$$\text{Est.Asy.Var}[\hat{\bar{\delta}}(\mathbf{X})] = \frac{1}{N^2}\sum_{i=1}^{N}\sum_{j=1}^{N}\hat{\mathbf{G}}_i\mathbf{V}\hat{\mathbf{G}}_j'. \tag{23}$$

An alternative method of computing an asymptotic covariance matrix for such a function of the estimated parameters suggested by Krinsky and Robb (1986) is to sample from the estimated asymptotic variance distribution of and compute $\hat{\boldsymbol{\beta}}$ the empirical variance of the observations on $\hat{\delta}(\bar{\mathbf{x}})$. This method does not appear to be widely employed in this setting.

To compute a LM statistic, also referred to as a score test, we note that the bracketed matrix (uninverted) in either (18) or (19) is an estimator of the asymptotic covariance matrix of the score vector

$$\mathbf{g}(\boldsymbol{\beta}) = \frac{\partial \log L}{\partial \boldsymbol{\beta}} = \sum_{i=1}^{N} e_i\mathbf{x}_i, \tag{24}$$

where e_i is the generalized (as well as the simple) residual, $e_i = y_i - \exp(\boldsymbol{\beta}'\mathbf{x}_i)$. The LM statistics for tests of restrictions are computed using the χ^2 statistic

$$\text{LM} = \mathbf{g}(\hat{\boldsymbol{\beta}}_0)'[\mathbf{V}_0]^{-1}\mathbf{g}(\hat{\boldsymbol{\beta}}_0), \tag{25}$$

where $\hat{\boldsymbol{\beta}}_0$ is the estimator of $\boldsymbol{\beta}$ with the restrictions imposed, and $\mathbf{V}_0$ is either of the matrices in (18) or (19) evaluated at $\hat{\boldsymbol{\beta}}_0$ (not $\boldsymbol{\beta}$). In view of (24), the LM statistic based on (19) has an interesting form

$$\begin{aligned}\text{LM} &= \left(\sum_{i=1}^{N} e_i\mathbf{x}_i\right)'\left(\sum_{i=1}^{N} e_i^2\mathbf{x}_i\mathbf{x}_i'\right)\left(\sum_{i=1}^{N} e_i\mathbf{x}_i\right)\\ &= \mathbf{i}'\mathbf{X}^*(\mathbf{X}^{*'}\mathbf{X}^*)^{-1}\mathbf{X}^*\mathbf{i}, \end{aligned} \tag{26}$$

where $\mathbf{i}$ is a column of ones and $\mathbf{X}^*$ a matrix of derivatives; each row is one of the terms in the summation in (24). This is the NR^2 in a linear regression of a column of ones on the first derivatives, $\mathbf{g}_i = e_i\mathbf{x}_i$.

2.3. Fit and prediction in the Poisson model

Like any nonlinear model, the Poisson regression specification does not imply an obvious counterpart to R^2 for measuring the goodness of fit of the model to the data. One measure that has become very popular is the

$$\text{Pseudo} - R^2 = \frac{1 - \log L_0}{\log L}, \tag{27}$$

where $\log L_0$ is the log-likelihood for a model that contains only a constant and $\log L$ the log-likelihood for the model as a whole. Note that for this measure to 'work,' the latter must actually contain a constant term. As happens in the linear model as well, if the regression does not contain a constant, then fit measures, such as these, can be negative or larger than one, depending on how they are computed. By construction, the pseudo$-R^2$ is between zero and one, and increases toward one as variables are added to a model. Beyond that, it is difficult to extend the analogy to the R^2 in a linear model, since the maximum likelihood estimation (MLE) in the Poisson model is not computed so as to maximize the fit of the model to the data, nor does it correspond to a proportion of variation explained. Nonetheless, it is current practice to report this statistic with one's other results.

Two other statistics related to the lack of fit of the model are often computed. The deviance measure is

$$G^2 = 2 \sum_{i=1}^{N} y_i \log\left(\frac{y_i}{\hat{\lambda}_i}\right) \tag{28}$$

(where it is understood that $0 \times \log 0 = 0$). The Pearson goodness-of-fit statistic is

$$C^2 = \sum_{i=1}^{N} \frac{(y_i - \hat{\lambda}_i)^2}{\hat{\lambda}_i}. \tag{29}$$

The second of these resembles the familiar fit measure in discrete response analysis

$$C_*^2 = \sum_{i=1}^{N} \frac{(\text{Observed}_i - \text{Expected}_i)^2}{\text{Expected}_i}. \tag{30}$$

Both of these statistics have limiting χ^2 distributions. They can be translated to aggregate fit measures by dividing each by the counterpart measure that uses the simple mean as the prediction. Thus,

$$R_{\text{Deviance}}^2 = 1 - \frac{\sum_{i=1}^{N} y_i \log(y_i/\hat{\lambda}_i)}{\sum_{i=1}^{N} y_i \log(y_i/\bar{y})} \tag{31}$$

and

$$R^2_{\text{Pearson}} = 1 - \frac{\sum\limits_{i=1}^{N}(y_i - \hat{\lambda}_i)^2/\hat{\lambda}_i}{\sum\limits_{i=1}^{N}(y_i - \bar{y})^2/\bar{y}}. \tag{32}$$

We note, although there is no obvious counterpart to R^2 in the linear model, with regard to 'explained variation,' one can compute the correlation between the actual and fitted values in the Poisson model easily enough by using the conditional mean function as the prediction. The statistic would be

$$r_{y,\hat{\lambda}} = \frac{\sum\limits_{i=1}^{N}(y_i - \bar{y})(\hat{\lambda}_i - \bar{y})}{\sqrt{\sum\limits_{i=1}^{N}(y_i - \bar{y})^2 \sum\limits_{i=1}^{N}(\hat{\lambda}_i - \bar{y})^2}} \tag{33}$$

(where we have made use of the first-order condition, $\bar{\hat{\lambda}} = \bar{y}$).

The Wald, likelihood ratio and LM tests developed in Section 2.2 are used to analyze the specification of the conditional mean function by testing restrictions on the parameters. Nonnested (and nested) models are often compared on the basis of the 'information criteria' statistics, which are, in the realm of maximum likelihood estimation, rough counterparts to adjusted R^2s. A frequently used statistic is the Akaike information criterion (AIC),

$$\text{AIC} = \frac{-2\log L + 2K}{N}, \tag{34}$$

where K is the full number of parameters in the model (see Hardin and Hilbe, 2007; McCullagh and Nelder, 1989).

2.4. Specification testing and robust covariance matrix estimation

A crucial part of the specification of the Poisson model, the assumption that the conditional mean and variance are equal (to λ_i), cannot be tested in this fashion. Nonetheless, this is generally viewed as the fundamental shortcoming of the model, and is always subjected to close scrutiny. There are several ways of addressing the question of over- (or under-) dispersion. Section 3 considers a direct approach of specifying a more general model. Alternatively, one can begin the analysis by examining the estimated Poisson model itself to ascertain whether it satisfies the assumption. In the same manner that the squares of OLS regression residuals can be examined for evidence of heteroskedasticity, the squared residuals in the Poisson model can provide evidence of overdispersion. Cameron and Trivedi (1990) suggested a pair of statistics to examine this relationship. In the linear regression of $z_i = [(y_i - \hat{\lambda}_i)^2 - y_i]/\hat{\lambda}\sqrt{2}$ on $w_i = g(\hat{\lambda}_i)/\hat{\lambda}_i\sqrt{2}$, if the equidispersion assumption of the model is correct, then the coefficient on w_i should be close to zero, regardless of the choice of $g(.)$. The authors suggest two candidates for $g(\hat{\lambda}_i)$, $\hat{\lambda}_i$, and $\hat{\lambda}_i^2$. A simple t-test of the restriction that the coefficient is zero is equivalent to a test of the equidispersion hypothesis. (The literature contains many other suggested tests, most based on this idea. See Hilbe (2007) or Winkelmann (2003) for discussion of some others.)

Another concern about the estimator of the model parameters is their robustness to failures of the assumption of the model. Specifically, if the specification of the Poisson model is incorrect, what useful information can be retained from the MLE? For a certain failure of the assumptions, namely the equidispersion restriction, the Poisson maximum likelihood estimator remains consistent. However, the estimated asymptotic covariance matrix based on (18) or (19) may missestimate the appropriate matrix. An estimator based on both (18) and (19) – now colorfully called the 'sandwich estimator' – solves the problem. The robust covariance matrix based on this result is

$$\text{Est.Asy.Var}[\hat{\boldsymbol{\beta}}_{\text{MLE}}] = \left[\sum_{i=1}^{N} \hat{\lambda}_i \mathbf{x}_i \mathbf{x}_i'\right]^{-1} \left[\sum_{i=1}^{N} (y_i - \hat{\lambda}_i)^2 \mathbf{x}_i \mathbf{x}_i'\right] \left[\sum_{i=1}^{N} \hat{\lambda}_i \mathbf{x}_i \mathbf{x}_i'\right]^{-1}.$$

(35)

We emphasize, this is not a cureall for all possible model misspecification, and if we do use (35), then the likelihood-ratio and LM tests in Section 2.2 are no longer valid. Some, such as endogeneity of the covariates, missing variables, and many others, render the MLE inconsistent. In these cases, 'robust' covariance matrix is a moot point.

A related issue that gets considerable attention in the current literature is the so-called 'cluster effects.' Suppose observations in the sample of N are grouped in sets of N_i in some fashion such that observations within a group are correlated with each other. Once again, we have to assume that in spite of this, the (now, pseudo-) MLE remains consistent. ['pseudo-' is used since the cluster nature of the data violates the *iid* assumption of likelihood theory.] It will follow once again that the estimated asymptotic covariance matrix is inaccurate. A commonly used alternative to (18) or (19) is related to (32). In the clustering case, the center matrix in (35) is replaced with

$$\mathbf{C} = \left[\sum_{r=1}^{G} \sum_{i=1}^{N_g} (\mathbf{g}_{ir} - \bar{\mathbf{g}}_r)(\mathbf{g}_{ir} - \bar{\mathbf{g}}_r)'\right]$$

(36)

where there are G groups or clusters, the number of observations in cluster 'r' is N_r, $\mathbf{g}_{ir} = e_{ir}\mathbf{x}_{ir}$, and $\bar{\mathbf{g}}_r = (1/N_r)\sum_{i=1}^{N_r}\mathbf{g}_{ir}$.

2.5. An application

To illustrate this model (and several extensions), we will employ the data used in the study by Ripahn et al. (2003). The raw data are published on the *Journal of Applied Econometrics* data archive website, http://qed.econ.queensu.ca/jae/ [4] The .zip file contains the single data file **rwm.data**.[5] The data file contains raw data on variables (original names) (Table 1).

---

[4] The URL for the data file is http://qed.econ.queensu.ca/jae/2003-v18.4/riphahn-wambach-million/ This URL provides links to a text file which describes the data, http://qed.econ.queensu.ca/jae/2003-v18.4/riphahn-wambach-million/readme.rwm.txt and the raw data, themselves, which are in text form, zipped in the file http://qed.econ.queensu.ca/jae/2003-v18.4/riphahn-wambach-million/rwm-data.zip.
[5] Data handling and aspects of software usage are discussed in Section 5.

Table 1
Data used in applications

id	person – identification number
female	female = 1; male = 0
year	calendar year of the observation
age	age in years
hsat	health satisfaction, coded 0 (low) – 10 (high)
handdum	handicapped = 1; otherwise = 0
handper	degree of handicap in percent (0–100)
hhninc	household nominal monthly net income in German marks/ 1000
hhkids	children under age 16 in the household = 1; otherwise = 0
educ	years of schooling
married	married = 1; otherwise = 0
haupts	highest schooling degree is high school; degree = 1; else = 0
reals	highest schooling degree is college degree = 1; else = 0
fachhs	highest schooling degree is technical degree = 1; else = 0
abitur	highest schooling degree is trade school = 1; otherwise = 0
univ	highest schooling degree is university degree = 1; otherwise = 0
working	employed = 1; otherwise = 0
bluec	blue collar employee = 1; otherwise = 0
whitec	white collar employee = 1; otherwise = 0
self	self employed = 1; otherwise = 0
beamt	civil servant = 1; otherwise = 0
docvis	number of doctor visits in last three months
hospvis	number of hospital visits in last calendar year
public	insured in public health insurance = 1; otherwise = 0
addon	insured by add-on insurance = 1; otherwise = 0

The data file contains 27,326 observations. They are an unbalanced panel, with group sizes ranging from 1 to 7 with frequencies T: 1 = 1525, 2 = 2158, 3 = 825, 4 = 926, 5 = 1051, 6 = 1000, and 7 = 987. Additional variables created in the data set included year dummy variables, sex = female + 1, and $age^2/1000$. For the purpose of this illustration, we are interested in the count variable DOCVIS, which is the number of doctor visits in the last three months. A histogram of this variable appears in Fig. 1.

The model in Table 2 is based on the authors' specification in the paper. The estimator of the asymptotic covariance matrix is based on the second derivatives, as in (18). The likelihood-ratio test of the hypothesis that all of the coefficients are zero is computed using the log-likelihood for the full model, −89,431.01, and the log-likelihood for the model that contains only the constant term, −108,662.1. The χ^2 statistic of 38,462.26 is far larger than the 95% critical value for the χ^2 distribution with 16 degrees of freedom, 26.29. There are two alternative methods of testing this hypothesis. The Wald statistic will be computed using

$$W = (\hat{\boldsymbol{\beta}}_0 - \mathbf{0})[\text{Est.Asy. Var}(\hat{\boldsymbol{\beta}}_0 - \mathbf{0})]^{-1}(\hat{\boldsymbol{\beta}}_0 - \mathbf{0}), \qquad (37)$$

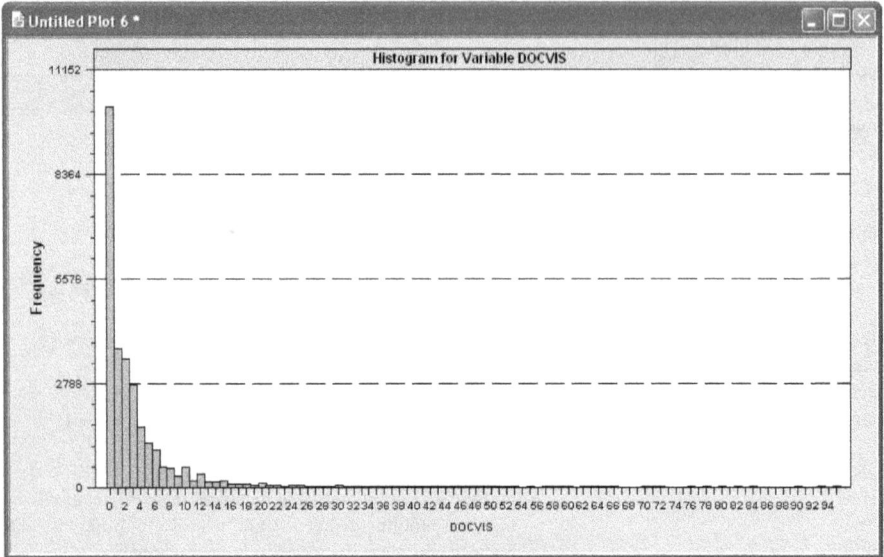

Fig. 1. Histogram of doctor visits.

where $\hat{\boldsymbol{\beta}}_0$ is all coefficients save the intercept (the latter 16 of them) and Est.Asy.Var$(\hat{\boldsymbol{\beta}}_0 - \mathbf{0})$ is the 16×16 part of the estimated covariance matrix that omits the constant term. The result is 41,853.37, again with 16 degrees of freedom. As before, this is far larger than the critical value, so the hypothesis is rejected. Finally, the LM statistic is computed according to (18) and (23), giving a value of 44,346.59. As is typical, the three statistics are reasonably close to one another.

The coefficient estimates are shown at the left of the table. Standard tests of the hypothesis that each is zero are shown in the third column of results. Most of the individual significance tests decisively reject the hypothesis that the coefficients are zero, so the conclusions drawn above about the coefficient vector as a whole are not surprising. The partial effects reported at the right of the table are average partial effects, as defined in (15), with standard errors computed using (22). As these are a straightforward multiple of the original coefficient vector, conclusions drawn about the impacts of the variables on the response variable follow those based on the estimate of $\boldsymbol{\beta}$. The multiple, 3.1835 is, in fact, the sample mean of the response variable. (This is straightforward to verify. The necessary condition for maximization of $\log L$ in (24) implies that $\Sigma_i e_i = \Sigma_i(y_i - \lambda_i) = 0$ at the MLE. The claimed result follows immediately. Note that this does not occur if the model does not contain a constant term – the same result that occurs in a linear regression setting.) As noted earlier, since AGE enters this model nonlinearly, neither the coefficients nor the partial effects for AGE or AGESQ give the right measure for the impact of AGE. The partial effects evaluated at the means would be

$$\delta(\bar{\mathbf{x}}, \overline{\text{AGE}}) = (\beta_3 + 2\beta_4\overline{\text{AGE}}/1000) \times \exp(\boldsymbol{\beta}'\bar{\mathbf{x}}), \qquad (37a)$$

which we compute at the mean of age of 43.5256898. The resulting estimate is 0.012924. In order to compute a standard error for this estimator, we would use

Table 2
Estimated Poisson regression model

	Coeff.	Std. Err.	b/Std. Err.	Robust SE	Cluster SE	Partial Effect	SE Partial[a]
Constant	2.48612758	.06626647	37.517	.17631321	.21816313	0.	0.
FEMALE	.28187106	.00774175	36.409	.02448327	.03106782	.89734351	.03529496**
AGE	−.01835519	.00277022	−6.626	.00804534	.00983497	−.05843420	.01121654**
AGESQ	.26778487	.03096216	8.649	.09134073	.11183550	.85249979	.12576669**
HSAT	−.21345503	.00141482	−150.871	.00449869	.00497983	−.67953940	.01375581**
HANDDUM	.09041129	.00963870	9.380	.02960213	.02873540	.28782659	.03917770**
HANDPER	.00300153	.00017626	17.029	.00057489	.00073815	.00955544	.00073483**
MARRIED	.03873812	.00881265	4.396	.02752875	.03325271	.12332377	.03558146**
EDUC	−.00342252	.00187631	−1.824	.00489031	.00639244	−.01089568	.00756284
HHNINC	−.16498398	.02291240	−7.201	.06072932	.07060708	−.52523061	.09283605**
HHKIDS	−.09762798	.00862042	−11.325	.02555567	.03154185	−.31080111	.03519498**
SELF	−.23243199	.01806908	−12.864	.05225385	.06470690	−.73995303	.07402117**
BEAMT	.03640374	.01921475	1.895	.04994140	.06426340	.11589220	.07745533
BLUEC	−.01916882	.01006783	−1.904	.02922716	.03577130	−.06102440	.04058392
WORKING	.00041819	.00941149	.044	.02808178	.03266767	.00133132	.03792298
PUBLIC	.14122076	.01565581	9.020	.03926803	.04593042	.44957981	.06360250**
ADDON	.02584454	.02544319	1.016	.05875837	.06596606	.08227672	.10253177

[a] ** indicates the ratio of estimate to standard error as larger than 2.0.

Diagnostic Statistics for Poisson Regression

Number of observations	27,326
Log-likelihood function	−89,431.01
Restricted log-likelihood	−10,8662.1
χ^2	38,462.26
Akaike information criterion	6.54673
McFadden pseudo R^2	.176981
χ^2 based on Pearson residuals	184,919.711
R^2 based on Pearson residuals	.3345
G^2 based on deviance	25,823.429
R^2 based on deviance	.2341
Overdispersion test: $g = \lambda_i$	22.899
Overdispersion test: $g = \lambda_i^2$	23.487

the delta method. The required derivatives are $(g_1, g_2, \ldots, g_{17})$, where all 17 components equal $\delta(\bar{\mathbf{x}}, \overline{\mathrm{AGE}})$ times the corresponding element of $\bar{\mathbf{x}}$ save for the third and fourth (corresponding to the coefficients on AGE and $\mathrm{AGE}^2/1000$, which are

$$g_3 = \partial\delta(\bar{\mathbf{x}}, \overline{\mathrm{AGE}})/\partial\beta_3 = \lambda(\bar{\mathbf{x}}, \overline{\mathrm{AGE}}) + \delta(\bar{\mathbf{x}}, \overline{\mathrm{AGE}}) \times \overline{\mathrm{AGE}} \qquad (37b)$$

$$g_4 = \partial\delta(\bar{\mathbf{x}}, \overline{\mathrm{AGE}})\partial\beta_4 = \lambda(\bar{\mathbf{x}}, \overline{\mathrm{AGE}}) + 2\overline{\mathrm{AGE}}/1000$$
$$+ \delta(\bar{\mathbf{x}}, \overline{\mathrm{AGE}}) \times \overline{\mathrm{AGE}}^2/1000. \qquad (37c)$$

The estimated standard error is 0.001114. (There is a large amount of variation across computer packages in the ease with which this kind of secondary computation can be done using the results of estimation.)

These data are a panel, so, in fact, the motivation for the cluster robust covariance matrix in (32) or (33) would apply here. These alternative estimates of the standard errors of the Poisson regression coefficients are given in Table 2. As is clearly evident, these are substantially larger than the 'pooled' counterparts. While not a formal test, these results are strongly suggestive that the Poisson model as examined so far should be extended to accommodate these data.

The two Cameron and Trivedi tests of overdispersion also strongly suggest that the equidispersion assumption of the Poisson model is inconsistent with the data. We will pursue this now, in the next section. Together, these results are convincing that the specification of the Poisson model is inadequate for these data. There are two directions to be considered. The overdispersion tests suggest that a model that relaxes this restriction, such as the NB model discussed below, should be considered. The large increase in the standard errors implied by the cluster corrected estimator would motivate this researcher to examine a formal panel data specification, such as those detailed in Section 4.

3. Heterogeneity and overdispersion

The test results in the preceding example that suggest overdispersion in the Poisson model are typical – indeed it is rare not to find evidence of over- (or under-) dispersion in count data. The equidispersion assumption of the model is a fairly serious shortcoming. One way to approach the issue directly is to allow the Poisson mean to accommodate unmeasured heterogeneity in the regression function. The extended model appears

$$E[y|\mathbf{x}, \varepsilon] = \exp(\boldsymbol{\beta}'\mathbf{x} + \varepsilon), \qquad \mathrm{Cov}[\mathbf{x}, \varepsilon] = \mathbf{0}, \tag{38}$$

where the unmeasured ε plays the role of a regression disturbance. More to the point here, it plays the role of the unmeasured heterogeneity in the Poisson model. How the model evolves from here depends crucially on what is assumed about the distribution of ε. In the linear model, a normal distribution is typically assumed. That is possible here as well (see ESI, 2007), however, most contemporary applications use the log-gamma density to produce an empirically manageable formulation. With the log-gamma assumption, as we show below, the familiar NB model emerges for the unconditional (on the unobserved ε) distribution of the observed variable, y. The NB model has become the standard device for accommodating overdispersion in count data since its implementation into commercial software beginning with *LIMDEP* (1987), *Stata* Corp. (1993), and *SAS* (1998).

3.1. The negative binomial model

The Poisson model with log-gamma heterogeneity may be written

$$f(y_i|\mathbf{x}_i, u_i) = Prob[Y = y_i|\mathbf{x}_i, u_i]$$
$$= \frac{\exp(-\lambda_i u_i)(\lambda_i u_i)^{y_i}}{y_i!}, \qquad y = 0, 1, \ldots. \tag{39}$$

The log-gamma assumption for ε implies that $u_i = \exp(\varepsilon_i)$ has a gamma distribution. The resulting distribution is a Poisson-gamma mixture model. The gamma noise, which is mixed with the Poisson distribution, is constrained to have a mean of one. The conditional mean of y_i in (38), given the gamma heterogeneity, is therefore given as $\lambda_i u_i$ rather than the standard Poisson mean, λ_i. (We can thus see that this will preserve the Poisson mean, λ_i, but induce additional variation, which was the purpose.) In order to estimate the model parameters (and use the model), it must be written in terms of the observable variables (so that we can construct the likelihood function). The unconditional distribution of y_i is obtained by integrating u_i out of the density. Thus,

$$f(y_i|\mathbf{x}_i) = \int_n f(y_i|\mathbf{x}_i, u_i)g(u_i)\,\mathrm{d}u_i$$
$$= \int_u \frac{\exp(-\lambda_i u_i)(\lambda_i u_i)^{y_i}}{y_i!} g(u_i)\,\mathrm{d}u_i, \qquad y_i = 0, 1, \dots. \tag{40}$$

The gamma density is a two-parameter distribution; $g(u) = [\theta^\gamma/\Gamma(\gamma)]\exp(-\theta u) u^{\gamma-1}$. The mean is γ/θ, so to impose the restriction that the mean is equal to one, we set $\gamma = \theta$. With this assumption, we find the unconditional distribution as

$$f(y_i|\mathbf{x}_i) = \int_0^\infty \frac{\exp(-\lambda_i u_i)(\lambda_i u_i)^{y_i}}{\Gamma(y_i + 1)} \frac{\theta^\theta}{\Gamma(\theta)}\exp(-\theta u_i)u_i^{\theta-1}\,\mathrm{d}u_i, \quad y_i =, 0, 1, \dots. \tag{41}$$

The variance of the gamma distribution is $\gamma/\theta^2 = 1/\theta$, so the smaller is θ, the larger is the amount of overdispersion in the distribution. (Note we have used the identity $y_i! = \Gamma(y_i + 1)$.) Using properties of the gamma integral and a bit of manipulation, we can write this as.

$$f(y_i|\mathbf{x}_i) = \frac{\Gamma(y_i + \theta)}{\Gamma(y_i + 1)\Gamma(\theta)} \left(\frac{\theta}{\lambda_i + \theta}\right)^\theta \left(\frac{\lambda_i}{\lambda_i + \theta}\right)^{y_i}, \qquad y_i = 0, 1, \dots. \tag{42}$$

By dividing all terms by θ, we obtain another convenient form,

$$f(y_i|\mathbf{x}_i) = \frac{\Gamma(y_i + \theta)}{\Gamma(y_i + 1)\Gamma(\theta)} \left(\frac{1}{1 + (\lambda_i/\theta)}\right)^\theta \left(1 - \frac{1}{1 + (\lambda_i/\theta)}\right)^{y_i}, \quad y = 0, 1, \dots. \tag{43}$$

By defining the dispersion parameter $\alpha = 1/\theta$ so that there will be a direct relationship between the model mean and α, we can obtain another convenient form of the density,

$$f(y_i|\mathbf{x}_i) = \frac{\Gamma(y_i + 1/\alpha)}{\Gamma(y_i + 1)\Gamma(1/\alpha)} \left(\frac{1}{1 + \alpha\lambda_i}\right)^{1/\alpha} \left(\frac{\alpha\lambda_i}{1 + \alpha\lambda_i}\right)^{y_i}, \qquad y = 0, 1, \dots. \tag{44}$$

One of the important features of the NB model is that the conditional mean function is the same as in the Poisson model,

$$E[y_i|x_i] = \lambda_i. \tag{45}$$

The implication is that the partial effects are computed the same way.

3.2. Estimation of the negative binomial model

Direct estimation of the NB model parameters (β,α) can be done easily with a few modern software packages including *LIMDEP*, *Stata*, and *SAS*. The likelihood equations for the algorithm are revealing

$$\frac{\partial \log L}{\partial \beta} = \sum_{i=1}^{N}\left(\frac{(y_i - \lambda_i)}{1 + \alpha\lambda_i}\right)\mathbf{x}_i = \mathbf{0}. \tag{46}$$

We can see immediately, as might be expected, that these are not the same as for the Poisson model, so the estimates will differ. On the other hand, note that as α approaches zero, the condition approaches that for the Poisson model – a point that will become important below. The other necessary condition for estimation is the derivative with respect to α,

$$\frac{\partial \log L}{\partial \alpha} = \sum_{i=1}^{N}\left\{\frac{1}{\alpha^2}\left[\log(1 + \alpha\lambda_i) - \log\left(\frac{\Gamma(y_i + 1/\alpha)}{\Gamma(1/\alpha)}\right)\right] - \left(\frac{y_i - \lambda_i}{\alpha(1 + \alpha\lambda_i)}\right)\right\}. \tag{47}$$

Second derivatives or outer products of the first derivatives can be used to estimate the asymptotic covariance matrix of the estimated parameters. An example appears below.

3.3. Robust estimation of count models

The conditional mean in the mixture model is $E[y_i|\mathbf{x}_i,u_i] = \lambda_i u_i$. By a simple application of the law of iterated expectations, we find $E[y_i|\mathbf{x}_i] = E_u[\lambda_i u_i|u_i] = \lambda_i E[u_i] = \lambda_i$. (Since the terms are independent, the mean is just the product of the means.) The fact that the conditional mean function in the NB model is the same as in the Poisson model has an important and intriguing implication. It follows from the result that the Poisson MLE is a generalized mixed models (GMM) estimator for the NB model. In particular, the conditional mean result for the NB model implies that the score function for the Poisson model,

$$\mathbf{g} = \sum_i (y_i - \lambda_i)\mathbf{x}_i \tag{48}$$

has mean zero even in the presence of the the overdispersion. The useful result for current purposes is that as a consequence, the Poisson MLE of β is consistent even in the presence of the overdispersion. (The result is akin to the consistency of ordinary least squares in the presence of heteroskedastic errors in the linear model for panel data.) The Poisson MLE is robust to this kind of model misspecification. The asymptotic covariance matrix for the Poisson model is not appropriate, however. This is one of those rare instances in which the increasingly popular 'robust' covariance matrix (see (35)) is actually robust to something specific that we can identify. The upshot of this is that one can estimate the parameters, an appropriate asymptotic covariance matrix, and appropriate partial effects for the slope parameters of the NB model just by fitting the Poisson model and using (32). Why then would one want to go the extra distance and effort to fit the NB model? One answer is that the NB estimator will be more efficient. Less obvious is that we do not have a test with demonstrable power against the equidispersion hypothesis in the Poisson model. With the NB model, we can begin to construct a test statistic, though as shown below, new problems do arise.

3.4. Application and generalizations

Table 3 presents both Poisson and negative binomial estimates of the count model for doctor visits. As anticipated, the estimates do differ noticeably. On the other hand, we are using quite a large sample, and both sets of estimates are consistent. The large differences might make one suspect that something else is amiss with the model; perhaps a different specification is called for, and neither estimator is consistent. Unfortunately, this cannot be discerned internally based on just these estimates, and a more detailed analysis would be needed. In fact, the differences persist in the partial effects – in some cases, these are quite large as well. We might add here that there is an efficacy gain from the NB2 model since the standard errors are roughly 25% less than the heteroskedasticity-robust standard errors for the Poisson.

Testing for the specification of the NB model against that of the Poisson model has a long and wide history in the relevant literature (see Anscombe, 1949; Blom, 1954). Unfortunately, none of the tests suggested, save for the Cameron and Trivedi tests used earlier, are appropriate in this setting. These tests include the LM tests against the negative binomial for overdispersed data, and against the Katz system for underdispersed data. Hilbe (2007) discusses a generalized Poisson which can also be used for underdispersed data. Regardless, the problem is that the relevant parameter, α, is on the edge of the parameter space, not in its interior. The test is directly analogous to a test for a zero variance. In practical terms, the LM test cannot be computed because the covariance matrix of the derivatives is singular at $\alpha = 0$. The Wald and likelihood-ratio tests can be computed, but again, there is the issue of the appropriate distribution for the test statistic. It is not $\chi^2(1)$. For better or worse, practitioners routinely compute these statistics in spite of the ambiguity.[6] It is certainly obvious that the hypothesis $\alpha = 0$ would be rejected by either of these tests.

Table 3 also presents robust standard errors for the NB model. For the pooled data case, these differ only slightly from the uncorrected standard errors. This is to be expected, since the NB model already accounts for the specification failure (heterogeneity) that would be accommodated by the robust standard errors. This does call into question why one would compute a robust covariance matrix for the NB model. Any remaining violation of the model assumptions is likely to produce inconsistent parameter estimates, for which robust standard errors provide dubious virtue.

The literature, mostly associating the result with Cameron and Trivedi's (1986) early work, defines two familiar forms of the NB model. Where

$$\lambda_i = \exp(\boldsymbol{\beta}'\mathbf{x}_i), \tag{49}$$

---

[6] Stata reports one half the standard $\chi^2[1]$ statistic. While this surely is not the appropriate test statistic, one might surmise that it is a conservative result. If the hypothesis that $\alpha = 0$ is rejected by this test, it seems extremely that it would not be rejected by the appropriate χ^2 test, whatever that is.

Table 3
Poisson and negative binomial models

	Poisson			Negative Binomial Model (NB-2)			Robust Standard Errors	
	Coeff.	Std. Err.	Part. Eff.	Coeff.	Std. Err.	Part. Eff.	Robust SE	Cluster SE
Constant	2.48612758	.06626647	0.	2.93815327	.14544040	0.	.14550426	.17427529
FEMALE	.28187106	.00774175	.89734351	.35108438	.01643537	1.14442153	.01680855	.02128039
AGE	-.01835519	.00277022	-.05843420	-.03604169	.00610034	-.11748426	.00616981	.00737181
AGESQ	.26778487	.03096216	.85249979	.46466762	.07006707	1.51466615	.07108961	.08528665
HSAT	-.21345503	.00141482	-.67953940	-.22320535	.00339028	-.72757725	.00344216	.00387560
HANDDUM	.09041129	.00963870	.28782659	.03863554	.02154854	.12593935	.02155752	.02070723
HANDPER	.00300153	.00017626	.00955544	-.00598082	.00050291	.01949555	.00050309	.00064984
MARRIED	.0387812	.00881265	.12332377	.05048344	.01856803	.16455967	.01857855	.02249464
EDUC	-.00342252	.00187631	-.01089568	-.01126970	.00390703	-.03673558	.00393156	.00495663
HHNINC	-.16498398	.02291240	-.52523061	-.01356497	.00472261	-.04421742	.00489946	.00556370
HHKIDS	-.09762798	.00862042	-.31080111	-.09439713	.01724797	-.30770411	.01781272	.02144006
SELF	-.23243199	.01806908	-.73995303	-.24001686	.03042783	-.78237732	.03128019	.03727414
BEAMT	.03640374	.01921475	.11589220	.04321571	.03494549	.14086922	.03531910	.04368996
BLUEC	-.01916882	.01006783	-.06102440	-.00355440	.02073448	-.01158621	.02083167	.02530838
WORKING	.00041819	.00941149	.00133132	.02487987	.02060004	.08110034	.02086701	.02435497
PUBLIC	.14122076	.01565581	.44957981	.11074510	.03041037	.36099319	.03066638	.03558399
ADDON	.0258454	.02544319	.08227672	.03713781	.06968404	.12105726	.07002987	.07939311
α	0.			1.46273783	.01654079	0.	.04080414	.04893952
log L	-89,431.01			-57,982.79				

NB Model Form	α	P	log L
Negbin – 0	0.0000 (.00000)	0.0000 (.0000)	-89,431.01
Negbin – 1	4.8372 (.05306)	1.0000 (.00000)	-57,861.96
Negbin – 2	1.4627 (.01654)	2.0000 (.00000)	-57,982.79
Negbin – P	2.6380 (.05891)	1.4627 (.01663)	-57,652.60

the *Negbin 2* or NB-2 form of the probability is the one we have examined thus far

$$\text{Prob}(Y = y_i|\mathbf{x}_i) = \frac{\Gamma(\theta + y_i)}{\Gamma(\theta)\Gamma(y_i + 1)} u_i^\theta (1 - u_i)^{y_i}, \tag{50}$$

where $u_i = \theta/(\theta + \lambda_i)$ and $\theta = 1/\alpha$. This is the default form of the model in most (if not all) of the received statistics packages that provide an estimator for this model. The signature feature of the model is the relationship between the mean and the variance of the model,

$$\text{Var}[y_i|\mathbf{x}_i] = \lambda_i[1 + \alpha\lambda_i^{P-1}]. \tag{51}$$

Thus, when $\alpha = 0$, we revert to the Poisson model. The model considered thus far has $P = 2$, hence the name NB-2. The *Negbin 1* form of the model results if θ in the preceding is replaced with $\theta_i = \theta\lambda_i$. Then, u_i becomes $u = \theta/(1+\theta)$, and the density becomes

$$\text{Prob}(Y = y_i|\mathbf{x}_i) = \frac{\Gamma(\theta\lambda_i + y_i)}{\Gamma(\theta\lambda_i)\Gamma(y_i + 1)} w^{\theta\lambda_i}(1 - w)^{y_i}, \tag{52}$$

where $w = \theta/(\theta + 1)$. In this instance, $P = 1$, and the model is one of a more pure form of overdispersion,

$$\text{Var}[y_i|\mathbf{x}_i] = \lambda_i[1 + \alpha]. \tag{53}$$

Note that this is not a simple reparameterization of the model – it is a NB model of a different form. The general Negbin P or NB-P model is obtained by allowing P in (51) to be a free parameter. This can be accomplished by replacing θ in (50) with $\theta\lambda^{2-P}$. For convenience, let $Q = 2 - P$. Then, the density is

$$\text{Prob}(Y = y_i|\mathbf{x}_i) = \frac{\Gamma(\theta\lambda_i^Q + y_i)}{\Gamma(\theta\lambda_i^Q)\Gamma(y_i + 1)} \left(\frac{\theta\lambda_i^Q}{\theta\lambda_i^Q + \lambda_i}\right)^{\theta\lambda_i^Q} \left(\frac{\lambda}{\theta\lambda_i^Q + \lambda_i}\right)^{y_i}. \tag{54}$$

(As of this writing, this model is only available in *LIMDEP*.) The table following the parameter estimates shows this specification analysis for our application. Though the NB-1 and NB-2 specifications cannot be tested against each other, both are restricted cases of the NB-P model. The likelihood-ratio test is valid in this instance, and it decisively rejects both models (see Hilbe, 1993; Hilbe, 1994; Lawless, 1987; Long and Freese, 2006).

4. Important extensions of the models for counts

The accommodation of overdispersion, perhaps induced by latent unobserved heterogeneity, is arguably the most important extension of the Poisson model for the applied researcher. But, other practicalities of 'real' data have motivated analysts to consider many other varieties of the count models. We will consider four broad areas here that are often encountered in received data: censoring and truncation, zero inflation, two part models, and panel data applications. In this section, we will turn to a sample of more exotic formulations that are part of the (very large) ongoing frontier research.

4.1. Censoring and truncation

Censoring and truncation are generally features of data sets that are modified as part of the sampling process. Data are censored when values in certain ranges of the distribution of outcomes are collapsed into one (or fewer) values. For example, we can see in Fig. 1 for the doctor visits data that the distribution of outcomes has an extremely long (perhaps implausibly so) right tail. Perhaps if one were skeptical of the data gathering process, or even if just to restrict the influence of outliers, they might recode all values above a certain value, say 15 in those data, down to some upper limit (such as 8). Values in a data set may be censored at either or both tails, or even in ranges within the distribution (see, e.g., Greene's (2003, pp. 774–780) analysis of Fair's (1978) data on extramarital affairs). The most common applications of censoring in counts will, however, involve recoding the upper tail of the distribution, as suggested in our example.

Truncation, in contrast, involves not masking a part of the distribution of outcomes, but discarding it. Our health care data suggest two possibilities. The number of zeros in our data is extremely large, perhaps larger than a Poisson model could hope to predict. One (perhaps not very advisable, but we are speaking theoretically here) modeling strategy might be simply to discard those zeros, as not representative. The distribution that describes the remaining data is truncated – by construction, only values greater than zero will be observed. In fact, in many quite reasonable applications, this is how data are gathered. In environmental and recreation applications, researchers are often interested in numbers of visits to sites. Data are gathered on site, so, again, by construction, it is not possible to observe a zero. The model, however, constructed, applies only to value 1,2, ... One might, as well truncate a distribution at its upper tail. Thus, in our data set, again referring to the histogram in Fig. 1, rather than censor the values larger than 15, we might just discard them. The resulting distribution then applies to the values 0,1, ..., 15, which is a truncated distribution.

Estimation of count models for censored or truncated distributions requires a straightforward extension of the base model. We illustrate for the Poisson case, but by a simple change of the function, the results can be extended to negative binomial or, in fact, any other specification.

The applicable distribution for the random variable that is censored is formed by using the laws of probability to produce a density that sums to one. For example, suppose the data are censored at an upper value, U. Thus, any actual value that is U or larger is recorded as U. The probability distribution for this set of outcomes is

$$f(Y|\mathbf{x}_i) = Prob[Y = y|\mathbf{x}_i] = \frac{\exp(-\lambda_i)\lambda_i^y}{y!}, \quad y = 0, 1, \ldots, U-1,$$

$$Prob[Y = U|\mathbf{x}_i] = \sum_{u=U}^{\infty} \frac{\exp(-\lambda_i)\lambda_i^u}{u!}, \quad \lambda_i = \exp(\boldsymbol{\beta}'\mathbf{x}_i) > 0. \tag{55}$$

The log-likelihood is formulated by using these probabilities for the observed outcomes. Note that the upper tail involves an infinite number of terms. This is transformed to a finite sum by noting that

$$\text{Prob}[Y = U|\mathbf{x}_i] = 1 - \text{Prob}[Y < U|\mathbf{x}_i]. \tag{56}$$

(For a detailed development of this result, see Econometric Software, Inc., 2007, Chapter 25). There are three important implications of this specification:

- Estimation of the model ignoring the censoring produces an inconsistent estimator of β. The result is precisely analogous to ignoring censoring in the linear regression model (see Greene, 2003, Chapter 22)
- Under this specification, the mean of Y is no longer λ_i. It is easy to see based on how the model is constructed that the mean must be less than λ_i. Intuitively, large values are being converted into small ones, so this must shrink the mean. (The opposite would be true if the censoring were in the lower tail.)
- Because the conditional mean is affected by the censoring, the partial effects are also. A full development of the appropriate partial effects is fairly complicated (see, again, Econometric Software, Inc. (ESI), 2007). The end result is that the censoring dampens the partial effects as well.

The analysis here parallels the development of the censored regression (Tobit) model for continuous data. See Terza (1985) for extensive details. (An alternative representation of censoring in count models in terms of discrete survival models can be found in Hilbe (2007).)

The truncation case is handled similarly. In this case, the probability distribution must be scaled so that the terms sum to one over the specified outcomes. Suppose, for example, that the distribution is truncated at lower value L. This means that only values $L+1, L+2, \dots$ appear in an observed sample. The appropriate probability model would be

$$f(Y|\mathbf{x}_i) = Prob[Y = y|\mathbf{x}_i] = \frac{\left[\exp(-\lambda_i)\lambda_i^y\right]/y!}{Prob[Y > L]}, \qquad y = L+1, L+2, \dots,$$
$$\lambda_i = \exp(\boldsymbol{\beta}'\mathbf{x}_i) > 0. \tag{57}$$

Once again, we use complementary probabilities to turn infinite sums into finite ones. For example, consider the common case of truncation at zero. The applicable distribution for the observed counts will be

$$\begin{aligned}
f(Y|\mathbf{x}_i) = \text{Prob}[Y = y|\mathbf{x}_i] &= \frac{\left[\exp(-\lambda_i)\lambda_i^y\right]/y!}{\text{Prob}[Y > 0]} \\
&= \frac{\left[\exp(-\lambda_i)\lambda_i^y\right]/y!}{1 - \text{Prob}[Y = 0]} \\
&= \frac{\left[\exp(-\lambda_i)\lambda_i^y\right]/y!}{1 - \exp(-\lambda_i)}, \qquad Y = 1, 2, \dots. \tag{58}
\end{aligned}$$

As in the censoring case, truncation affects both the conditional mean and the partial effects. (A detailed analysis appears in ESI, 2007.) Note, finally, these (and the cases below) are among those noted earlier in which computing a 'robust' covariance matrix does not solve the problem of nonrobustness. The basic MLE that ignores the censoring or truncation is inconsistent, so it is not helpful to compute a robust covariance matrix.

To demonstrate these effects, we continue the earlier application of the Poisson model. Table 4 shows the impact of censoring at 8 in the distribution. This masks about 10% of the observations, which is fairly mild censoring. The first set of results in the table at the left is based on the original uncensored data. The center set of results is based on the censored data, but ignore the censoring. Thus, the comparison to the first set shows the impact of ignoring the censoring. There is no clear generality to be drawn in the table, because it is clear that some of the changes in the coefficients are quite large, while others are quite small. The partial effects, however, tell a somewhat different story. These change quite substantially. Note, for example, that the estimated partial effect of income (HHNINC) falls by 80% while that of children (HHKIDS) falls by half. The third set of results in Table 4 is based on the corrected likelihood function. In principle, these should replicate the first set. We see, however, that for these data, the full MLEs for the censored data model actually more closely resemble those for the estimator that ignored the censoring. One might expect this when the censoring is only a small part of the distribution. The impact of the censoring is likely to be more severe when a larger proportion of the observations are censored.

Table 5 repeats the calculations for the truncation at zero case. The zeros are 37% of the sample (about 10,200), so we would expect a more noticeable impact. Indeed, the effect of ignoring the truncation is quite substantial. Comparing the left to the center set of estimates in Table 5, we see that some coefficients change sign, while others change considerably. The third should replicate the first. However, truncating 37% of the distribution quite substantively changes the distribution, and the replication is not particularly good. One might suspect, as we explore below, that the data process that is producing the zeros actually differs from that underlying the rest of the distribution.

Hilbe (2007) developed a survival parameterization of the censored Poisson and NB models. Rather than having cut points below or above which censored observations fall, and observation in the data may be censored. Characterized after traditional survival models such as the Cox proportional hazards model and parametric survival models such as exponential, Weibull, gamma, log-logistic, and so forth, the censored Poisson and censored NB response is parameterized in terms of a discrete count. For example, a typical count response in health care analysis is hospital length of stay data. The response we have been using for our examples, number of patient visits to the hospital, is also appropriate for modeling censored count models. If various counts are lost to a length of stay study after reaching a certain time in the hospital, these counts may be considered as right censored. In modeling LOS data, it is important to take into account the days that were counted for particular patients, even though records are lost thereafter.

Survival parameterized censored count models will differ from what has been termed (Hilbe, 2007) the econometric parameterization as earlier discussed in that the values of censored responses are not recast to the cut level. This method

Table 4
The effect of censoring on the Poisson model

	Poisson Based on Uncensored Data			Poisson Model Ignoring Censoring			Censored Data (at 8) Poisson Model		
	Coeff.	Std. Err.	Part. Eff.	Coeff.	Std. Err.	Part. Eff.	Coeff.	Std. Err.	Part. Eff.
Constant	2.48612758	.06626647	0.	2.14986800	.07524413	0.	2.25968677	.07596690	0.
FEMALE	.28187106	.00774175	.89734351	.27709347	.00894003	.66233310	.29202937	.00904040	.66106102
AGE	-.01835519	.00277022	-.05843420	-.03211408	.00318455	-.07676189	-.03403051	.00322451	-.07703417
AGESQ	.26778487	.03096216	.85249979	.42280492	.03578592	1.01062538	.44605854	.03627228	1.00973377
HSAT	-.21345503	.00141482	-.67953940	-.15716683	.00166910	-.37567393	-.16927552	.00171922	-.38318561
HANDDUM	.09041129	.00963870	.28782659	.03913318	.01132602	.09353955	.04291882	.01147955	.09715448
HANDPER	.00300153	.00017626	.00955544	.00308629	.00021489	.00737711	.00353402	.00022065	.00799989
MARRIED	.03873812	.00881265	.12332377	.05122800	.01024523	.12244965	.05587384	.01038134	.12648049
EDUC	-.00342252	.00187631	-.01089568	-.00021599	.00211001	-.00051628	.00072296	.00212106	.00163656
HHNINC	-.16498398	.02291240	-.52523061	-.02645213	.02544113	-.06322820	-.03024873	.02566863	-.06847344
HHKIDS	-.09762798	.00862042	-.31080111	-.06493632	.00985764	-.15521648	-.06795371	.00994926	-.15382544
SELF	-.23243199	.01806908	-.73995303	-.24973460	.02038677	-.59693753	-.25682829	.02045212	-.58137705
BEAMT	.03640374	.01921475	.11589220	-.00855232	.02140198	-.02044250	-.00464199	.02148378	-.01050797
BLUEC	-.01916882	.01006783	-.06102440	-.03340251	.01151415	-.07984161	-.03558453	.01159109	-.08055198
WORKING	.00041819	.00941149	.00133132	.03061167	.01080953	.07317070	.02669552	.01090431	.06043012
PUBLIC	.14122076	.01565581	.44957981	.06153310	.01722210	.14708182	.06893203	.01729248	.15604004
ADDON	.02584454	.02544319	.08227672	.08361017	.02824989	.19985236	.08126672	.02852185	.18396185

Table 5
The effect of truncation on the Poisson model

	Poisson Based on Original Data			Poisson Model Ignoring Truncation			Truncated (at 0) Poisson Model		
	Coeff.	Std. Err.	Part. Eff.	Coeff.	Std. Err.	Part. Eff.	Coeff.	Std. Err.	Part. Eff.
Constant	2.48612758	.06626647	0.	2.25206660	.06654230	0.	2.24409704	.06888683	0.
FEMALE	.28187106	.00774175	.89734351	.12026803	.00772833	.60860197	.12711629	.00795253	.54174405
AGE	-.01835519	.00277022	-.05843420	.00595941	.00278220	.03015687	.00668132	.00286642	.02847444
AGESQ	.26778487	.03096216	.85249979	-.04163927	.03115181	-.21071054	-.04695040	.03201880	-.20009316
HSAT	-.21345503	.00141482	-.67953940	-.14637618	.00144060	-.74071918	-.15271640	.00148358	-.65084657
HANDDUM	.09041129	.00963870	.28782659	.10255607	.00969572	.51897271	.10904012	.00990456	.46470706
HANDPER	.00300153	.00017626	.00955544	.00153298	.00017760	.00775747	.00145161	.00017977	.00618647
MARRIED	.03873812	.00881265	.12332377	-.01292896	.00882816	-.06542545	-.01233626	.00906142	-.05257467
EDUC	-.00342252	.00187631	-.01089568	-.00555201	.00189701	-.02809531	-.00598173	.00197010	-.02549295
HHNINC	-.16498398	.02291240	-.52523061	-.20206192	.02308216	-1.0225102	-.21657724	.02408796	-.92300865
HHKIDS	-.09762798	.00862042	-.31080111	-.05706609	.00865236	-.28877613	-.06100208	.00893594	-.25997858
SELF	-.23243199	.01806908	-.73995303	-.08128493	.01803489	-.41133269	-.08960050	.01886738	-.38185930
BEAMT	.03640374	.01921475	.11589220	.06077767	.01916495	.30755811	.06449740	.01999381	.27487497
BLUEC	-.01916882	.01006783	-.06102440	.00182451	.01002870	.00923271	.00230018	.01034645	.00980291
WORKING	.00041819	.00941149	.00133132	-.02881502	.00936256	-.14581498	-.02827975	.00963105	-.12052261
PUBLIC	.14122076	.01565581	.44957981	.11278164	.01557239	.57071800	.12294551	.01629795	.52396906
ADDON	.02584454	.02544319	.08227672	-.09224023	.02542136	-.46677065	-.09827798	.02645306	-.41884099

Note: Where Q is the regime probability and P(0) the Poisson, negative binomial, or other probability.

changes the values of censored data. Table 6 shows the results of survival censored Poisson and NB models using the same data as in Tables 4 and 5. Note the much better fit using the censored negative binomial. The AIC and BIC statistics have significantly lower values than the Poisson. Derivation of the respective likelihoods as well as a discussion of both methods can be found in Hilbe (2007). Supporting software is at http://ideas.repec.org/s/boc/bocode.html or at http://econpapers.repec.org/software/bocbocode/.

4.2. Zero inflation

The pattern in Fig. 1 might suggest that there are more zeros in the data on DOCVIS than would be predicted by a Poisson model. Behind the data, one might, in turn, surmise that the data contain two kinds of respondents, those who would never visit a doctor save for extreme circumstances, and those who regularly (or even more often) visit the doctor. This produces a kind of 'mixture' process generating the data. The data contain two kinds of zeros: a certain zero from individuals who never visit the physician and an occasional zero from individuals who for whatever reason, did not visit the doctor that period, but might in some other. (The pioneering study of this kind of process is Lambert's (1992) analysis of process control in manufacturing – the sampling mechanism concerned the number of defective items produced by a process that was either under control (y always zero) or not under control (y sometimes zero).)

The probability distribution that describes the outcome variable in a zero-inflated Poisson (ZIP) or zero-inflated negative binomial (ZINB) model is built up from first principles: The probability of observing a zero is equal to the probability that the individual is in the always zero group plus the probability that the individual is not in that group times the probability that the count process produces a zero anyway. This would be

$$\text{Prob}[y = 0] = Q + [1 - Q] \times P(0), \tag{59}$$

where Q is the regime probability and $P(0)$ the Poisson, negative binomial, or other probability for the zero outcome in the count process. The probability of a nonzero observation is, then

$$\text{Prob}[y = j > 0] = [1 - Q] \times P(j). \tag{60}$$

It remains to specify Q, then we can construct the log-likelihood function. Various candidates have been suggested (see ESI, 2007, Chapter 25); the most common is the logistic binary choice model,

$$
\begin{aligned}
Q_i &= \text{Prob[Regime 0]} \\
&= \frac{\exp(\gamma' \mathbf{z}_i)}{1 + \exp(\gamma' \mathbf{z}_i)},
\end{aligned} \tag{61}
$$

where $\mathbf{z}_i$ is a set of covariates – possibly the same as $\mathbf{x}_i$ that is believed to influence the probability of the regime choice and γ is a set of parameters to be estimated with $\boldsymbol{\beta}$.

Table 6
Survival parameterization of censored Poisson and negative binomial

Docvis Censored at Value of 8				Number of obs = 27,326	
Censored Poisson Regression				Wald $\chi^2(16)$ = 41,967.07	
Log-likelihood = −87,520.01				Prob > χ^2 = 0.0000	

docvis	Coeff.	Std. Err.	z	P>|z|	[95% CI]	
female	.2962892	.0078474	37.76	0.000	.2809086	.3116699
age	−.0201931	.0028097	−7.19	0.000	−.0257001	−.0146861
agesq	.2893301	.0314347	9.20	0.000	.2277191	.350941
hsat	−.2245135	.0014598	−153.80	0.000	−.2273746	−.2216523
handdum	.0935722	.0097864	9.56	0.000	.0743912	.1127532
handper	.0034529	.000181	19.08	0.000	.0030981	.0038076
married	.0464825	.0089499	5.19	0.000	.0289411	.0640239
educ	−.0022596	.0018888	−1.20	0.232	−.0059617	.0014425
hhninc	−.0163339	.0023175	−7.05	0.000	−.0208761	−.0117917
hhkids	−.1008135	.008725	−11.55	0.000	−.1179143	−.0837128
self	−.240174	.0181211	−13.25	0.000	−.2756908	−.2046572
beamt	.0402636	.0192906	2.09	0.037	.0024547	.0780725
bluec	−.0210752	.0101502	−2.08	0.038	−.0409693	−.0011812
working	−.0064606	.0095068	−0.68	0.497	−.0250937	.0121725
public	.1480981	.0157224	9.42	0.000	.1172827	.1789134
addon	.0189115	.0256716	0.74	0.461	−.0314039	.0692269
_cons	2.578406	.0670071	38.48	0.000	2.447075	2.709738

AIC statistic = 6.407 6	BIC statistic = −103,937.
LM value = 17,2762.665	LM $\chi^2(1)$ = 0.000
Score test OD = 428,288.802	Score $\chi(1)$ = 0.000

Censored Negative Binomial Regression

Log-likelihood = −55,066.082

Number of obs = 27,326
Wald $\chi^2(16)$ = 3472.65
Prob > χ^2 = 0.0000

docvis	Coeff.	Std. Err.	z	P>|z|	[95% CI]	
xb						
female	.2918081	.0244625	11.93	0.000	.2438626	.3397537
age	.0037857	.0089505	0.42	0.672	−.0137569	.0213284
agesq	−.0294051	.1015427	−0.29	0.772	−.2284252	.169615
hsat	−.252314	.0052074	−48.45	0.000	−.2625204	−.2421077
handdum	.0752106	.032167	2.34	0.019	.0121645	.1382567
handper	.0065435	.0007127	9.18	0.000	.0051466	.0079404
married	.0236717	.0276851	0.86	0.393	−.0305901	.0779335
educ	−.0375634	.0058873	−6.38	0.000	−.0491023	−.0260244
hhninc	−.0628296	.0066091	−9.51	0.000	−.0757832	−.049876
hhkids	−.2249677	.0260514	−8.64	0.000	−.2760276	−.1739078
self	−.0766637	.0518638	−1.48	0.139	−.1783148	.0249875
beamt	.2819248	.0579536	4.86	0.000	.1683378	.3955118
bluec	.1135119	.0302827	3.75	0.000	.0541589	.1728649
working	−.1079542	.0284011	−3.80	0.000	−.1636193	−.052289
public	.3378024	.0452985	7.46	0.000	.249019	.4265858
addon	−.2807842	.0797627	−3.52	0.000	−.4371163	−.1244522
_cons	4.62027	.2161169	21.38	0.000	4.196689	5.043851
lnalpha						
_cons	1.574162	.0117548	133.92	0.000	1.551123	1.597201
alpha	4.826693	.0567366	4.716763	4.939186		

AIC statistic = 4.032

BIC statistic = −168,835.3

The log-likelihood for this model based on the Poisson probabilities is

$$\log L = \sum_{y_i=0} \log \left[\frac{\exp(\gamma' z_i)}{1 + \exp(\gamma' z_i)} + \frac{\exp(-\lambda_i)}{1 + \exp(\gamma' z_i)} \right]$$

$$+ \sum_{y_i>0} \log \left[\frac{\exp(-\lambda_i)\lambda_i^{y_i}}{[1 + \exp(\gamma' z_i)]y_i!} \right]. \tag{62}$$

This formulation implies several new complications. First, its greater complexity is apparent. This log-likelihood function is much more difficult to maximize than that for the Poisson model. Second, the conditional mean function in this model is now

$$E[y|\mathbf{x}, \mathbf{z}] = Q_i \lambda_i = \frac{\exp(\gamma' z_i)\exp(\boldsymbol{\beta}' x_i)}{1 + \exp(\gamma' z_i)}, \tag{63}$$

which is much more involved than before, and involves both the original covariates and the variables in the regime model. Partial effects are correspondingly more involved;

$$\frac{\partial E[y|\mathbf{x}, \mathbf{z}]}{\partial \begin{pmatrix} \mathbf{x} \\ \mathbf{z} \end{pmatrix}} = \lambda_i Q_i \begin{pmatrix} \boldsymbol{\beta} \\ Q_i(1 - Q_i)\gamma \end{pmatrix}. \tag{64}$$

If there is any overlap between $\mathbf{x}$ and $\mathbf{z}$, the partial effect of that variable is the sum of the two effects shown.

The zero inflation model produces a substantial change in the specification of the model. As such, one would want to test the specification if possible. There is no counterpart to the LM test that would allow one to test the model without actually estimating it. Moreover, the basic model is not a simple restricted version of the ZIP (ZINB) model. Restricting γ to equal zero in the model above, for example produces $Q = 1/2$, not $Q = 0$, which is what one would hope for. Common practice is to use the Vuong (1989) test for these nonnested models. The statistic is computed as follows, based on the log-likelihood functions for the two models. Let $\log L_{i0}$ be an individual contribution (observation) in the log-likelihood for the basic Poisson model, and let $\log L_{i1}$ denote an individual contribution to the log-likelihood function for the zero inflation model. Let $m_i = (\log L_{i1} - \log L_{i0})$. The statistic is

$$Z = \frac{\sqrt{N}\bar{m}}{s_m} \tag{65}$$

where $\bar{m} = (1/N)\Sigma_i m_i$ and $s_m = (1/N)\Sigma_i(m_i - \bar{m})^2$. In large samples, the statistic converges to standard normal. Under the assumption of the base model, Z will be large and negative, while under the assumption of the zero inflation model, Z will be large and positive. Thus, large positive values (greater than 2.0) reject the Poisson model in favor of the zero inflation model.

To illustrate the ZIP model, we extend the Poisson model estimated earlier with a regime splitting equation

$$Q_i = \Lambda(\gamma_1 + \gamma_2 \text{FEMALE} + \gamma_3 \text{HHNINC} + \gamma_4 \text{EDUC} + \gamma_5 \text{ADDON}), \tag{66}$$

where $\Lambda(t)$ is the logistic probability shown in (60). The estimated model is shown in Table 7.

Table 7
Estimated zero-inflated Poisson model

	Base Poisson Model			Poisson Count Model		Zero Regime Equation		Partial Effect
	Coeff.	Std. Err.	Part. Eff.	Coeff.	Std. Err.	Coeff.	Std. Err.	
Constant	2.48612758	.06626647	0.	2.27389204	.02824420	-.86356818	.07269384	0.
FEMALE	.28187106	.00774175	.89734351	.14264681	.00289141	-.58033790	.02817964	.97216018
AGE	-.01835519	.00277022	-.05843420	.00194385	.00110859			.0056986
AGESQ	.26778487	.03096216	.85249979	.01169342	.01220742			.03428056
HSAT	-.21345503	.00141482	-.67953940	-.15791310	.00053102			-.46293957
HANDDUM	.09041129	.00963870	.28782659	.10648551	.00358290			.31217396
HANDPER	.00300153	.00017626	.00955544	.00158480	.597360D-04			.00464603
MARRIED	.03873812	.00881265	.12332377	-.00596092	.00334023			-.01747509
EDUC	-.00342252	.00187631	-.01089568	-.00335247	.00084300	.04090428	.00614014	-.04887430
HHNINC	-.16498398	.02291240	-.52523061	-.17752186	.01001860	.04894552	.08141084	-.56714692
HHKIDS	-.09762798	.00862042	-.31080111	-.05709710	.00342170			-.16738641
SELF	-.23243199	.01806908	-.73995303	-.12653617	.00764267			-.37095465
BEAMT	.03640374	.01921475	.11589220	.06028953	.00831117			.17674537
BLUEC	-.01916882	.01006783	-.06102440	.00195719	.00396727			.00573772
WORKING	.00041819	.00941149	.00133132	-.01322419	.00359116			-.03876818
PUBLIC	.14122076	.01565581	.44957981	.12484058	.00712261			.36598386
ADDON	.02584454	.02544319	.08227672	-.09812657	.01187915	-.51567053	.11710229	.20457682

The log-likelihood for the ZIP model is $-77{,}073.779$ compared to $-89{,}431.005$ for the Poisson model, which implies a difference of well over 12,000. On this basis, we would reject the Poisson model. However, as noted earlier, since the models are not nested, this is not a valid test. The Vuong statistic is $+39.08$, which does decisively reject the Poisson model. One can see some quite large changes in the results, particularly in the marginal effects. These are different models. On the specific point of the specification, the estimation results (using LIMDEP) indicate that the data contain 10,135 zero observations. The Poisson model predicts 2013.6 zeros. This is computed by multiplying the average predicted probability of a zero across all observations times the sample size. The zero inflation model predicts 9581.9 zeros, which is, as might be expected, much closer to the sample proportion.

4.3. Two part models

Two models that are related to the zero inflation model, hurdle models and sample selection models play important roles in the contemporary literature. A hurdle model (Mullahy, 1986) specifies the observed outcome as the result of two decisions, a participation equation and a usage equation. This is a natural variant of the ZIP model considered above, but its main difference is that the regime split is not latent. The participation equation determines whether the count will be zero or positive. The usage equation applies to the positive count outcomes. Thus, the formal model determining the observed outcomes is

$$\text{Prob}(y = 0) = R_i,$$
$$\text{Prob}(y > 0) = 1 - R_i, \tag{67}$$
$$\text{Prob}[y = j | y > 0][1 - R_i]P_i(j)/[1 - P_i(0)].$$

The participation equation is a binary choice model, like the logit model used in the previous section. The count equation is precisely the truncated at zero model detailed in Section 4.1. This model uses components that have already appeared. The log-likelihood function separates the probabilities into two simple parts:

$$\log L = \sum_{y=0} \log R_i$$
$$+ \sum_{y>0} \log[1 - R_i] - \log[1 - P_i(0)] + \log P_i(j). \tag{68}$$

The four terms of the log-likelihood partition into two log-likelihoods,

$$\log L = \sum_{d=0} \log R_i + \sum_{d=1} \log[1 - R_i]$$
$$+ \sum_{d=1} \log P_i(j) - \log[1 - P_i(0)], \tag{69}$$

where the binary variable d_i equals zero if y_i equals zero and one if y_i is greater than zero. Notice that the two equations can be estimated separately: a binary choice model for d_i and a truncated at zero Poisson (or negative binomial) model for the positive values of y_i.

We shall illustrate this model with the same specification as the ZIP model. The hurdle equation determines whether the individual will make any visits to the doctor. Then, the usage equation is, as before, a count model for the number of visits. This model differs from the ZIP model in that the main equation applies only to the positive counts of doctor visits. Not surprisingly, the model results are quite similar. The hurdle model and the zero inflation model are quite similar both in the formulation and in how the models are interpreted (Table 8).

Models for sample selection differ considerably from the frameworks we have considered so far. Loosely, while the two part models considered so far concern the utilization decision, the sample selection models can be viewed as a two part model in which the first involves a decision whether or not to be in the observed sample. A second crucial aspect of the model is that the effects of the first step are taken to operate on the unmeasured aspects of the usage equation, not directly in the specified equations.

To put this in a context, suppose we hypothesize that in our health care data, individuals who have insurance make their utilization decisions differently from those who do not, in ways that are not completely accounted for in the observed covariates. An appropriate model might appear as follows:

$$\text{Insurance decision } (0/1) = F(\boldsymbol{\alpha}'\mathbf{w}_i + u_i), \tag{70}$$

where $\mathbf{w}_i$ is the set of measured covariates and u_i is the unmeasured element of the individual's decision to have insurance. Then, the usage equation holds that

$$\text{Doctor visits (count)} = G(\boldsymbol{\beta}'\mathbf{x}_i + \varepsilon_i), \tag{71}$$

where ε_i accounts for those elements of the usage decision that are not directly measured by the analyst. The second equation is motivated by the same considerations that underlie the overdispersion models, such as the NB model. There can be unmeasured, latent elements in the usage equation that influence the outcome, but are not observable by the analyst. In our earlier application, this induced overdispersion, which was easily accommodated by extending the Poisson model to the NB framework. The effect is more pernicious here. If our estimation sample for the count variable contained only those individuals who have insurance, and if the unmeasured effects in the two equations are correlated, then the sampling mechanism becomes nonrandom. In effect, under these assumptions, the variables $\mathbf{w}_i$ will be acting in the background to influence the usage variable, and will distort our estimates of $\boldsymbol{\beta}$ in that equation.[7]

It is a bit ambiguous how the unmeasured aspects of the usage decision should enter the model for the count outcome. Note there is no 'disturbance' in (7)–(9). On the other hand, the presence of the latent heterogeneity in the overdispersion models in Section 3 provides a suitable approach. The following two part model for a count variable embodies these ideas:

$$z_i^* = \boldsymbol{\alpha}'\mathbf{w}_i + u_i,$$
$$z_i = 1 \text{ if } z_i^* > 0, \text{ 0 otherwise (a standard binary choice model)} \tag{72}$$

---

[7] In Greene (1994), this method is used to model counts of derogatory reports in credit files for a sample of individuals who have, in an earlier screening, applied for a specific credit card. The second step of the analysis is applied only to those individuals whose credit card application was approved.

Table 8
Estimated hurdle Poisson model

	Base Poisson Model			Poisson Count Model		Participation Equation		Partial Effect
	Coeff.	Std. Err.	Part. Eff.	Coeff.	Std. Err.	Coeff.	Std. Err.	
Constant	2.48612758	.06626647	0.	2.24409689	.02803268	.80374458	.06710834	0.
FEMALE	.28187106	.00774175	.89734351	.12711631	.00274746	.5919506	.02599107	.95763200
AGE	-.01835519	.00277022	-.05843420	.00668133	.00108985			.01821318
AGESQ	.26778487	.03096216	.85249979	-.04695053	.01195589			-.12798632
HSAT	-.21345503	.00141482	-.67953940	-.15271640	.00052262			-.41630224
HANDDUM	.09041129	.00963870	.28782659	.10904010	.00345227			.29724142
HANDPER	.00300153	.00017626	.00955544	.00145161	.586338D-04			.00395706
MARRIED	.03873812	.00881265	.12332377	-.01233627	.00316579			-.03362846
EDUC	-.00342252	.00187631	-.01089568	-.00598172	.00081933	-.04518713	.00566753	-.06295579
HHNINC	-.16498398	.02291240	-.52523061	-.21657725	.00981680	-.11523583	.07381806	-.70935153
HHKIDS	-.09762798	.00862042	-.31080111	-.06100214	.00326811			-.16629077
SELF	-.23243199	.01806908	-.73995303	-.08960050	.00698770			-.24424941
BEAMT	.03640374	.01921475	.11589220	.06449742	.00833036			.17581884
BLUEC	-.01916882	.01006783	-.06102440	.00230015	.00387887			.00627017
WORKING	.00041819	.00941149	.00133132	-.02827977	.00354930			-.07709015
PUBLIC	.14122076	.01565581	.44957981	.12294552	.00715542			.33514735
ADDON	.02584454	.02544319	.08227672	-.09827801	.01187417	.43208724	.10043663	.17816867

$$\text{Prob}[y_i = j|z_i = 1, \mathbf{x}_i, \varepsilon_i] = P(\boldsymbol{\beta}'\mathbf{x}_i + \sigma\varepsilon_i) \text{ (Poisson count model)}, \qquad (73)$$

where the data for the count model are only observed when $z_i = 1$, e.g., only for the insured individuals in the larger sample. The first equation is the participation equation. The second is the usage equation. The model is made operational by formal distributional assumptions for the unobserved components; (u_i, ε_i) are assumed to be distributed as joint standard normal with correlation ρ. It is the nonzero ρ that ultimately induces the complication of the selection effect.

Estimation of this model is considerably more involved than those considered so far. The presence of the unobserved variable makes familiar maximum likelihood methods infeasible. The model can be estimated by maximum simulated likelihood. (Development of the method is beyond the scope of our presentation here. Readers may refer to Greene (1994, 2003 or 2006) or ESI (2007) for details.) To illustrate the selection model, we have estimated a restricted version of the count model used earlier for doctor visits; the participation equation for whether or not the individual has PUBLIC health insurance is based on

$$\mathbf{w} = (\text{Constant, AGE, HHNINC, HHKIDS, EDUC}). \qquad (74)$$

The usage equation includes

$$\mathbf{x} = (\text{Constant, AGE, FEMALE, HHNINC, HHKIDS,}$$
$$\text{WORKING, BLUEC, SELF, BEAMT}). \qquad (75)$$

The estimates are given in Table 9. The leftmost estimates are obtained by the Poisson regression model ignoring the selection issue. The point of comparison is the second set of results for the Poisson model. (These are computed jointly with the probit equation at the far right of the table.) It can be seen that the effect of the selection correction is quite substantial; the apparently significant income effect in the first equation disappears; the effect of kids in the household becomes considerably greater; the positive and significant effect of BLUEC becomes negative and significant; and the insignificant BEAMT coefficient changes sign and becomes significant in the modified equation. Apparently, the latent effect of the insurance decision is quite important in these data. The estimate of ρ is $-.3928$, with a standard error of .0282. Based on a simple t-test, we would decisively reject the hypothesis of no correlation, which reinforces our impression that the selection effect in these data is indeed substantial. The fairly large negative estimate suggests that the latent effects that act to increase the likelihood that the individual will have insurance act in turn to reduce the number of doctor visits. A theory based on moral hazard effects of insurance would have predicted a positive coefficient, instead.

4.4. Panel data

The health care data we have been using are a panel. Data sets such as this one are becoming increasingly common in applications of count models. The main virtues of panel data are that they allow a richer specification of the model that we have been using so far, and they allow, under suitable assumptions, the researcher to learn more about the latent sources of heterogeneity that are not captured by the measured covariates already in the model. We shall examine the

Table 9
Estimated sample selection model

	Poisson Model; Subsample		Poisson Model; Maximum Likelihood		Probit Insurance Equation		Reestimated Probit Insurance Equation	
	Coeff.	Std. Err.	Coeff.	Std. Err.	Coeff.	Std. Err.	Coeff.	Std. Err.
Constant	.62950929	.02172139	-.25578895	.03277438	3.62691256	.07326231	3.60039973	.07232337
AGE	.01649406	.00035426	.01861389	.00052927	.00079753	.00104823	.00074654	.00108170
FEMALE	.23541478	.00783352	.33195368	.01057008				
HHNINC	-.35832703	.02330320	.01529087	.03513743	-.98823990	.05500769	-.98247429	.04954413
HHKIDS	-.16894816	.00843149	-.21559300	.01213431	-.07928466	.02276865	-.07028879	.02238365
WORKING	-.19400071	.00918292	-.22010784	.01272314				
BLUEC	.02209633	.00974552	-.03595214	.01371389				
SELF	-.26437394	.01978391	-.36281283	.02770759				
BEAMT	.03168950	.02771184	-.12155827	.04288937				
EDUC					-.17148226	.00403598	-.16970876	.00402272
σ	0.						1.31093146	.00494213
ρ	0.						-.39283049	.02820212
log L	-94,322.56		-62,584.14		-8320.77794			
N	24,203		27,326		27,326			

two most familiar approaches here, fixed effects and random effects. A wider variety of panel models is presented in Stata and ESI (2007). As suggested by the application, we assume that the sample contains N individuals, indexed by $i = 1, ..., N$. The number of observations available for each individual is denoted T_i; this may vary across individuals, as it does in our data set. [Note that T_i is used here differently than in Section 2.1.]

In general terms, the availability of panel data allows the analyst to incorporate individual heterogeneity in the model. For the fixed effects case, this takes the form of an individual-specific intercept term.

$$\log \lambda_{it} = \alpha_i + \boldsymbol{\beta}' \mathbf{x}_{it} (+\varepsilon_{it} \text{ for the negative binomial model}). \tag{76}$$

where α_i can be interpreted as the coefficient on a binary variable, d_i, which indicates membership in the ith group. A major difference between this and the linear regression model is that this model cannot be fit by least squares using deviations from group means – the transformation of the data to group mean form in this context brings no benefits at all. Two approaches are used instead. One possibility is to use a conditional maximum likelihood approach – the model conditioned on the sum of the observations is free of the fixed effects and has a closed form that is a function of $\boldsymbol{\beta}$ alone. This is provided for both Poisson and negative binomial (see Hausman et al., 1984). A second approach is direct, brute force estimation of the full model including the fixed effects. The *unconditional* estimator is obtained by a direct maximization of the full log-likelihood function and estimating all parameters including the group-specific constants. A result that is quite rare in this setting is that for the Poisson model (and few others), the conditional and unconditional estimators are numerically identical. The choice of approach can be based on what feature is available in the computer package one is using. The matter is more complicated in the NB case. The conditional estimator derived in HHG is not the same as the brute force estimator. Moreover, the underlying specifications are different. In HHGs specification, the fixed effect (dummy variable) coefficients appear directly in the distribution of the latent heterogeneity variable, not in the regression function as shown above. Overall, the fixed effects, negative binomial (FENB) appears relatively infrequently in the count data literature. Where it does occur, current practice appears to favor the HHG approach.

We note before turning to random effects models two important aspects of fitting FE models. First, as in the linear regression case, variables in the equation that do not differ across time become collinear with the individual-specific dummy variables. Thus, FE models cannot be fit with time invariant variables. (There is one surprising exception to this. The HHG FENB models can be fit with a full set of individual dummy variable and an overall constant – a result which collides with familiar wisdom. The result occurs because of the aforementioned peculiarity of the specification of the latent heterogeneity.) The second aspect of this model is relatively lightly documented phenomenon known as the incidental parameters problem (see Greene, 1995). The full unconditional maximum likelihood estimator of models that contain fixed effects is usually inconsistent – the estimator is consistent in T (or T_i), but T is usually taken to be fixed and small. The Poisson model is an exception to this rule, however. It is consistent even in the presence of the fixed effects. (One could deduce this from the discussion already. The brute force estimator would normally suffer from the incidental parameter problem. But, since it is numerically identical to the conditional estimator, which does not, the brute force estimator must be consistent as well.)

The random effects model is

$$\log \lambda_{it} = \boldsymbol{\beta}'\mathbf{x}_{it} + u_i. \tag{77}$$

Once again, the approach used for the linear model, in this case, two-step generalized least squares, is not usable. The approach is to integrate out the random effect and estimate by maximum likelihood the parameters of the resulting distribution (which, it turns out, is the NB model when the kernel is Poisson and the effect is log-gamma). The bulk of the received literature on random effects is based on the Poisson model, though HHG and modern software (e.g., LIMDEP and Stata) do provide estimators for NB models with random effects.

The random effects model for the count data framework is

$$\log \lambda_{it} = \boldsymbol{\beta}'\mathbf{x}_{it} + u_i, \quad i = 1,\ldots,N, \quad t = 1,\ldots,T_i, \tag{78}$$

where u_i is a random effect for the ith group such that $\exp(u_i)$ has a gamma distribution with parameters (θ,θ). Thus, $E[\exp(u_i)]$ has mean 1 and variance $1/\theta = \alpha$. This is the framework, which gave rise to the NB model earlier, so that, with minor modifications, this is the estimating framework for the Poisson model with random effects.

For the NB model, Hausman et al. proposed the following approach: We begin with the Poisson model with the random effects specification shown above. The random term, u_i is distributed as gamma with parameters (θ_i,θ_i), which produces the NB model with a parameter that varies across groups. Then, it is assumed that $\theta_i/(1 + \theta_i)$ is distributed as beta (a_n,b_n), which layers the random group effect onto the NB model. The random effect is added to the NB model by assuming that the overdispersion parameter is randomly distributed across groups. The two random effects models discussed above may be modified to use the normal distribution for the random effect instead of the gamma, with $u_i \sim N[0,\sigma^2]$. For the Poisson model, this is an alternative to the log-gamma model which gives rise to the negative binomial.

Table 10 displays estimates for fixed and random effects versions of the Poisson model, with the original model based on the pooled data. Both effects models lead to large changes in the coefficients and the partial effects. As usually occurs, the FE model brings the larger impact. In most cases, the fit of the model will improve dramatically – this occurs in linear models as well. The pooled model is a restriction on either of the panel models. Note that the log-likelihood function has risen from −89,431 in the pooled case to −45,480 for the FE model. The χ^2 statistic for testing for the presence of the fixed effects is about 87,900 with 7292 degrees of freedom. The 95% critical value is about 7500, so there is little question about rejecting the null hypothesis of the pooled model. The same result applies to the random effects model. The fixed effects and random effects are not nested, so one cannot use a likelihood-ratio test to test for which model is preferred. However, the Poisson model is an unusual nonlinear model in that the FE estimator is consistent – there is no incidental parameters problem. As such, in the same fashion

Table 10
Poisson models with fixed and random effects

	Pooled Poisson Model with No Effects			Fixed Effects Poisson Model			Random Effects Poisson Model		
	Coeff.	Std. Err.	Part. Eff.	Coeff.	Std. Err.	Part. Eff.	Coeff.	Std. Err.	Part. Eff.
Constant	2.48612758	.06626647	0.				2.24392235	.07371198	
FEMALE	.28187106	.00774175	.89734351	.51658559	.11586172	1.64456306	.30603129	.02119303	.97425823
AGE	-.01835519	.00277022	-.05843420	-.00645204	.00660632	-.02054024	-.02242192	.00240763	-.07138075
AGESQ	.26778487	.03096216	.85249979	.31095952	.06972973	.98994735	.39324433	.02574887	1.25190310
HSAT	-.21345503	.00141482	-.67953940	-.14713933	.00222146	-.46842172	-.16059023	.00074867	-.51124299
HANDDUM	.09041129	.00963870	.28782659	.05697301	.01101687	.18137500	.04903557	.00442617	.15610595
HANDPER	.00300153	.00017626	.00955544	-.00123990	.00034541	-.00394724	.00058881	.00011537	.00187449
MARRIED	.03873812	.00881265	.12332377	-.02568156	.02186501	-.08175789	-.02623233	.00773198	-.08351126
EDUC	-.00342252	.00187631	-.01089568	-.03829432	.01670290	-.12191093	-.01343872	.00427488	-.04278251
HHNINC	-.16498398	.02291240	-.52523061	-.12296257	.04266832	-.39145439	-.07074651	.01754451	-.22522326
HHKIDS	-.09762798	.00862042	-.31080111	.00275859	.01602765	.00878203	-.02970393	.00580292	-.09456319
SELF	-.23243199	.01806908	-.73995303	-.11580970	.03538353	-.36868304	-.16546368	.01330546	-.52675775
BEAMT	.03640374	.01921475	.11589220	-.07260535	.05533064	-.23114092	-.01814889	.02270099	-.05777745
BLUEC	-.01916882	.01006783	-.06102440	-.01636891	.01947144	-.05211084	-.01456716	.00775266	-.04637491
WORKING	.00041819	.00941149	.00133132	-.05009017	.01635782	-.15946331	-.04212169	.00711048	-.13409546
PUBLIC	.14122076	.01565581	.44957981	.09352915	.03072334	.29775238	.10688932	.01320990	.34028480
ADDON	.02584454	.02544319	.08227672	-.07453049	.03631482	-.23726967	-.05483927	.01859563	-.17458217
α							.87573201	.01570144	
log L	-89,431.01			-45,480.27			-68,720.91		

as in the linear model, one can use a Hausman (1978) (see also Greene, 2003, Chapter 13) test to test for fixed vs. random effects. The appropriate statistic is

$$H = (\hat{\boldsymbol{\beta}}_{FE} - \hat{\boldsymbol{\beta}}_{RE})'[\text{Est.Var}(\hat{\boldsymbol{\beta}}_{FE}) - \text{Est.Var}(\hat{\boldsymbol{\beta}}_{RE})]^{-1}(\hat{\boldsymbol{\beta}}_{FE} - \hat{\boldsymbol{\beta}}_{RE}). \qquad (79)$$

(Note the constant term is removed from the random effects results.) Applying this computation to the models in Table 10 produces a χ^2 statistic of 114.1628. The critical value from the table, with 16 degrees of freedom is 26.296, so the hypothesis of the random effects model is rejected in favor of the FE model.

Texts providing a thorough discussion of fixed and random effects models and generalized estimating equations (GEE) with an emphasis in health analysis include Zeger et al. (1988), Hardin and Hilbe (2003), Twist (2003), and Hilbe (2007). Texts discussing multilevel count models include Skrondal and Rabe-Hesketh (2005). Hilbe (2007) is the only source discussing multilevel NB models.

5. Software

Count response regression models include Poisson and NB regression, and all of the enhancements to each that are aimed to accommodate some violation in the distributional assumptions of the respective models. The most commonly used extended Poisson and NB models include zero-truncated, zero-inflated, and panel data models. Hurdle, sample selection, and censored models are used less frequently, and thus find less support in commercial software. The heterogeneous NB regression is a commonly used extension that has no Poisson counterpart. Other count model extensions that have been crafted have found support in *LIMDEP*, which has far more count response models available to its users than other commercial software.

LIMDEP and Stata are the only commercial statistical packages that provide their respective users with the ability to model Poisson, negative binomial, as well as their extensions. *LIMDEP* offers all of the enhanced models mentioned in this chapter, while Stata offers most of the models, including both base models, NB-1, zero-truncated and zero-inflated Poisson and negative binomial, a full suite of count panel data models, mixed models, and heterogeneous negative binomial. Stata users have written hurdle, censored, sample selection, and Poisson mixed model procedures. Both software packages provide excellent free technical support, have exceptional reference manual support with numerous interpreted examples, and have frequent incremental upgrades.

Unfortunately, other commercial programs provide limited support for count response models. *SAS* has Poisson and negative binomial as families within its *SAS/STAT GENMOD* procedure, *SAS*'s generalized linear models (GLM) and GEE facility. *SAS* also supports Poisson panel data models. *SPSS* provides no support for count response regression models, but is expected to release a GLM program in its next release, thereby providing the capability for Poisson regression. *GENSTAT* supports Poisson and NB regression, together with a variety of Poisson panel and mixed models.

R is a higher language statistical software environment that can be freely downloaded from the web. It enjoys worldwide developmental and technical support from members of academia as well as from statisticians at major research institutions or agencies. R statistical procedures are authored by users; thus its statistical capabilities depend entirely on the statistical procedures written and filed in user-supported R libraries. Although R has a rather complete suite of statistical procedures, it is at present rather weak in its support of count response models. R has software support for Poisson and NB regression, but not for any of the extensions we have discussed. A basic NB-2 model in R is provided as part of the *MASS* software package, based on the work of Venables and Ripley (2002). We expect, though, that this paucity of count response model offerings is only temporary and that most if not all of the extensions mentioned in this chapter will be available to users in the near future.

Other commercial statistical software either fails to support count response models, or provides only the basic models, and perhaps a GEE or fixed/random effects Poisson panel data module.

When evaluating software for its ability to model counts, care must be taken to check if the model offered has associated goodness-of-fit statistics and if it allows the user to generate appropriate residuals for model evaluation. Several of the software packages referenced in the previous paragraph may offer Poisson or NB regression, yet fail to provide appropriate fit statistics in their output. A model without fit analysis is statistically useless, and fosters poor statistical practice.

A caveat should be given regarding NB regression capability from within the framework of GLM. Since GLMs are one-parameter models, and the negative binomial has two parameters to estimate, the heterogeneity parameter, α, must be entered into the GLM algorithm as a constant. If the software also has a full maximum likelihood NB procedure, one may use it to obtain an estimate of α, and then insert it into the GLM negative binomial algorithm as the heterogeneity parameter constant. The value of adopting this two-stage procedure is that GLM procedures typically have a variety of goodness-of-fit output and residual analysis support associated with the procedure. Model evaluation may be enhanced. On the other hand, software such as *LIMDEP* provides extensive fit and residual support for all of its count regression models, thereby making the two-stage modeling task unnecessary. We advise the user of statistical software to be aware of the capability, as well as the limitations, of any software being used for modeling purposes.

With the increased speed of computer chips and the availability of cheap RAMs has made available the ability of statistical software to estimate highly complex models based on permutations. Cytel Corp has recently offered users of its *LogXact* program, the ability to model Poisson regression based on exact statistics. That is, the procedure calculates parameter estimate standard errors, and hence confidence intervals, based on exact calculations, not on traditional asymptotics. This is a particularly valuable tool when modeling small or ill-defined data sets. Software such as *SAS*, *SPSS*, *Stata*, and *StatXact* have exact statistical capabilities for tables, but only *LogXact* and *Stata* (version 10) provide exact statistical support for logistic and Poisson models. Cytel intends to extend *LogXact* to provide exact NB regression, but as of this writing the research has not yet been done to develop the requisite algorithms.

We have provided an overview of the count response regression capabilities currently available in commercial statistical software. *LIMDEP* and *Stata* stand far above other packages in the number of count models available, but also in their quality; i.e., providing a full range of goodness-of-fit statistics and residuals. As the years pass, other software vendors will likely expand their offerings to include most of the count models discussed in this chapter. As we mentioned before though, before using statistical software to model count responses, be certain to evaluate its fit analysis capability as well as its range of offerings.

6. Summary and conclusions

We have surveyed the most commonly used models related to the regression of count response data. The foundation for this class of models is Poisson regression. Though it has provided the fundamental underpinning for modeling counts, the equidispersion assumption of the Poisson model is a severe limitation. This shortcoming is generally overcome by the NB model, which can be construed as the unconditional result of conditioning the Poisson regression on unobservable heterogeneity, or simply as a more general model for counts that is not limited by the Poisson assumption on the variance of the response variable. We also considered the most common extensions of these two basic count models: zero inflation models, sample selection, two part (hurdle) models, and the most familiar panel data applications. The applications presented above focused on the Poisson model, though all of them have been extended to the NB model as well. The basic models are available in most commercial software packages, such as Stata, LIMDEP, GENSTAT, and SAS. The more involved extensions tend to be in more limited availability, with the most complex count response models only supported in LIMDEP and Stata.

The literature, both applied and theoretical, on this subject is vast. We have omitted many of the useful extensions and theoretical frontiers on modeling counts. (See, e.g., Winkelmann (2003), which documents these models in over 300 pages, Hilbe (2007), which provides detailed examples, most related to health data, for each major count response model, particularly all of the varieties of NB regression, or Cameron and Trivedi (1998), which has been a standard text on count response models, but emphasizes economic application.) Recent developments include many models for panel data, mixed models, latent class models, and a variety of other approaches. Models for counts have provided a proving ground for development of an array of new techniques as well, such as random parameters models and Bayesian estimation methods.

References

Anscombe, F.J. (1949). The statistical analysis of insect counts based on the negative binomial distribution. *Biometrics* **5**, 165–173.

Blom, G. (1954). Transformations of the binomial, negative binomial, Poisson, and χ^2 distributions. *Biometrika* **41**, 302–316.

Cameron, A., Trivedi, P. (1986). Econometric models based on count data: Comparisons and applications of some estimators and tests. *Journal of Applied Econometrics* **1**, 29–54.

Cameron, A., Trivedi, P. (1990). Regression based tests for overdispersion in the Poisson model. *Journal of Econometrics* **46**, 347–364.

Cameron, C., Trivedi, P. (1998). *Regression Analysis of Count Data*. Cambridge University Press, New York.

Econometric Software, Inc (1987). *LIMDEP*, version 4, Plainview, NY.

Econometric Software, Inc (2007). *LIMDEP and NLOGIT*. Plainview, New York.

Fair, R. (1978). A theory of extramarital affairs. *Journal of Political Economy* **86**, 45–61.

Greene, W. (1994). Accounting for excess zeros and sample selection in Poisson and negative binomial regression models. Working Paper No. EC-94-10, Department of Economics, Stern School of Business, New York University.

Greene, W. (1995). Sample selection in the Poisson regression model. Working Paper No. EC-95-6, Department of Economics, Stern School of Business, New York University.

Greene, W. (2003). *Econometric Analysis*, 5th ed. Prentice-Hall, Englewood Cliffs.

Greene, W. (2006). A general approach to incorporating selectivity in a model. Working Paper No. EC-06-10, Stern School of Business, Department of Economics.

Hardin, J., Hilbe, J. (2003). *Generalized Estimating Equations*. Chapman & Hall/CRC, London, UK.

Hardin, J., Hilbe, J. (2007). *Generalized Linear Models and Extensions*, 2nd ed. Stata Press, College Station, TX.

Hausman, J. (1978). Specification tests in econometrics. *Econometrica* **46**, 1251–1271.

Hausman, J., Hall, B., Griliches, Z. (1984). Economic models for count data with an application to the patents–R&D relationship. *Econometrica* **52**, 909–938.

Hilbe, J. (1994). Negative binomial regression., *Stata Technical Bulletin* **STB-18**, sg16.5.

Hilbe, J. (2007). *Negative binomial regression*. Cambridge University Press, Cambridge, UK.

Hilbe, J.M. (1993). Log negative binomial regression as a generalized linear model. Technical Report COS 93/94-5-26, Department of Sociology, Arizona State University.

Hilbe, J.M. (1994). Generalized linear models. *The American Statistician* **48**(3), 255–265.

Krinsky, I., Robb, A.L. (1986). On approximating the statistical properties of elasticities. *Review of Economics and Statistics* **68**, 715–719.

Lambert, D. (1992). Zero-inflated Poisson regression, with an application to defects in manufacturing. *Technometrics* **34**(1), 1–14.

Lawless, J.F. (1987). Negative binomial and mixed Poisson regression. *The Canadian Journal of Statistics* **15**(3), 209–225.

Long, J.S., Freese, J. (2006). *Regression Models for Categorical Dependent Variables using Stata*, 2nd ed. Stata Press, College Station, TX.

McCullagh, P., Nelder, J. (1983). *Generalized Linear Models*. Chapman & Hall, New York.

McCullagh, P., Nelder, J.A. (1989). *Generalized Linear Models*, 2nd ed. Chapman & Hall, New York.

Mullahy, J. (1986). Specification and testing of some modified count data models. *Journal of Econometrics* **33**, 341–365.

Rabe-Hesketh, S., Skrondal, A. (2005). *Multilevel and Longitudinal Modeling Using Stata*. Stata Press, College Station, TX.

Ripahn, R., Wambach, A., Million, A. (2003). Incentive effects in the demand for health care: A bivariate panel count data estimation. *Journal of Applied Econometrics* **18**(4), 387–405.

SAS Institute (1998). *SAS*. SAS Institute, Cary, NC.

Skrondal, A., Rabe-Hesketh, S. (2004). *Generalized Latent Variable Modeling*. Chapman & Hall/ CRC, Boca Raton, FL.

Stata Corp., (1993, 2006). *Stata*. Stata Corp., College Station, TX.

Terza, J. (1985). A Tobit type estimator for the censored Poisson regression model. *Economics Letters* **18**, 361–365.

Twist, J. (2003). *Applied Longitudinal Data Analysis for Epidemiology*. Cambridge University Press, Cambridge, UK.

Vuong, Q. (1989). Likelihood ratio tests for model selection and non-nested hypotheses. *Econometrica* **57**, 307–334.

Venables, W., Ripley, B. (2002). *Modern Applied Statistics with S*, 4th ed. Springer, New York.

Winkelmann, R. (2003). *Econometric Analysis of Count Data*, 4th ed. Springer, Heidelberg, Germany.

Zeger, S.L., Liang, K-Y., Albert, P.S. (1988). Models for longitudinal data: A generalized equation approach. *Biometrics* **44**, 1049–1060.

Handbook of Statistics, Vol. 27
ISSN: 0169-7161
DOI: 10.1016/S0169-7161(07)27008-7

5

Mixed Models

Matthew J. Gurka and Lloyd J. Edwards

Abstract

This paper provides a general overview of the mixed model, a powerful tool for analyzing correlated data. Numerous books and other sources exist that cover the mixed model comprehensively. However, we aimed to provide a relatively concise introduction to the mixed model and describe the primary motivations behind its use. Recent developments of various aspects of this topic are discussed, including estimation and inference, model selection, diagnostics, missing data, and power and sample size. We focus on describing the mixed model as it is used for modeling normal outcome data linearly, but we also discuss its use in other situations, such as with discrete outcome data. We point out various software packages with the capability of fitting mixed models, and most importantly, we highlight many important articles and books for those who wish to pursue this topic further.

1. Introduction

1.1. The importance of mixed models

Why mixed models? Simply put, mixed models allow one to effectively model data that are not independent. Of course, such a statement is quite general, and the actual use of mixed models varies widely across fields of study. Data suited for analysis via mixed models usually have some multilevel or hierarchical organization (hence mixed models are often times referred to as multilevel or hierarchical models). This usually means that this kind of data can be organized into different levels, or clusters. Observations made within a cluster are usually assumed to be dependent, whereas clusters themselves are assumed to be independent of one another.

One may wonder what kind of data lend themselves to such a cluster arrangement. The most convenient and common example of this sort of hierarchical organization is longitudinal data, in which observations are collected over time on a subject. Obviously characteristics unique to that subject or individual dictate that multiple observations collected over time on that individual will be correlated. Because of this, mixed models have become one common method for analyzing many types of longitudinal data, particularly from medical research.

But, mixed model analysis is by no means limited to longitudinal studies. Mixed models are often used in settings in which data are collected on families, schools, or hospitals. In using the individuals that comprise those groups, it is recommended that one take into account the natural correlation of those individuals from the same family, school, or hospital, depending on the motivation of the analysis. Mixed models can accommodate data from such studies easily and in a straightforward fashion that is easy to interpret.

Our aim for this chapter was to generally introduce the mixed model for the reader who is not an expert on such an analysis tool. In doing so, we describe the main aspects of the model, such as estimation and inference. We also discuss areas of research within the mixed model that are ongoing, such as model selection and power analysis. Our main goal was to provide a fairly comprehensive and current reference to textbooks, journal articles, and other sources of information that give details on more specific topics related to the mixed model for the reader who wishes to learn more about this popular method of analyzing data.

1.2. "Mixed" models

In introducing mixed models, one should discuss what makes a model "mixed." A model is "mixed" because it contains different types of effects to be estimated: namely, "fixed" effects and "random" effects. What sets apart a mixed model from a typical univariate or multivariate model is the addition of the random effects. While introducing the concept of linear mixed models, it is most straightforward to discuss with reference to linear models. However, mixed models can be applied to nonlinear models as well, and this concept will be introduced later.

In the case of the univariate linear model, the following form is typically observed:

$$y = X\beta + \varepsilon. \tag{1}$$

Here, we are fitting a model to data from N sampling units (subjects), considered to be independent of one another. In model (1), y is the $(N \times 1)$ vector of responses from the N subjects, X the $(N \times p)$ design matrix of known variables, β a $(p \times 1)$ vector of fixed, unknown parameters, and ε the $(N \times 1)$ vector whose rows represent unobservable random variables that capture the subject-specific deviation from the expected value. So, each row of y, X, and ε correspond to a subject. Typically, the rows of ε are assumed to be normally distributed with mean 0 and common variance σ^2; i.e., $\varepsilon \sim \mathcal{N}(0, \sigma^2 \mathcal{I})$.

Now, the linear mixed model, in the common form developed by Laird and Ware (1982) for longitudinal data analysis, is as follows:

$$y_i = X_i\beta + Z_ib_i + e_i. \tag{2}$$

Here, $i \in \{1, \ldots, m\}$, where m is the number of independent sampling units (subjects), y_i an $n_i \times 1$ vector of observations on the ith subject; X_i an $n_i \times p$ known, constant design matrix for the ith subject with rank p; β a $p \times 1$ vector of unknown, constant population parameters; Z_i an $n_i \times q$ known, constant design matrix for the ith subject with rank q corresponding to b_i, a $q \times 1$ vector of unknown, random individual-specific parameters (the "random effects"); and e_i an $n_i \times 1$ vector of random "within-subject," or "pure," error terms.

Additionally, let $\varepsilon_I = Z_i b_i + e_i$ be the "total" error term of model (2). The following distributional assumptions are usually held: b_i is normally distributed with mean vector 0 and covariance matrix D and b_i independent of b_j, $i \neq j$. Also, e_i is distributed normally with mean vector 0 and covariance matrix R_i, independent of b_i. The covariance matrices D and R_i are typically assumed to be characterized by unique parameters contained in the $k \times 1$ vector θ. Often, a "conditionally independent" model is assumed; i.e., $R_i = \sigma^2 I_{n_i}$. The total variance for the response vector in (2) is $\text{var}(y_i) = \text{var}(\varepsilon_i) = \Sigma_i(\theta) = Z_i D(\theta) Z_i' + R_i(\theta)$. It is common to write $\Sigma_i = \Sigma_i(\theta)$, $D = D\ (\theta)$, and $R_i = R_i(\theta)$ so that $\Sigma_i = Z_i D Z_i' + R_i$.

As alluded to in Section 1.1, the utility of the mixed model is primarily in its applicability to non-independent data. So, the standard univariate linear model (1) is valid when one observation each is collected on numerous "subjects" that are independent of one another.

A subject here can be a person, a family, a hospital, or so on. When multiple observations are collected on each person/family/hospital, independence of observations, at least taken from the same subject, can no longer be assumed. The mixed model (2), then, with its additional source of variation represented by the random effects (b_i) can accommodate such data.

1.3. An example

The mixed model is especially useful when fitting longitudinal data. It allows an analyst to not only make inferences about the population, but it also accommodates estimation and inference about subject-specific level deviation from the population estimates of typical interest. An especially useful property for the mixed model, particularly in longitudinal data analysis, is the fact that it can accommodate missing data. Missing data, usually in the form of withdrawals or drop outs, are a common characteristic of most studies collecting information on individuals over time. To be discussed later, depending on the nature of the missingness, mixed models can allow for missing data.

To exemplify the use of the mixed model in a repeated measures setting, we introduce an application to obesity research. In the United States, the prevalence of obesity has reached epidemic levels (Flegal et al., 2002). Additionally, obesity is a major risk factor for type 2 diabetes (Mokdad et al., 2001). Lifestyle treatment with modest weight loss has been shown to prevent type 2 diabetes (Knowler et al., 2002), and can thus be seen as a crucial element for diabetes control in obese individuals.

Improving Control with Activity and Nutrition (ICAN) was a randomized control trial designed to assess the efficacy of a modestly priced, registered dietician (RD)-led case management (CM) approach to lifestyle change in patients with type 2 diabetes (Wolf et al., 2004). The primary goal of the study was to compare the intervention to usual medical care with respect to weight loss for obese patients with type 2 diabetes. Weight in kilograms and waist circumference (cm) were recorded on 124 individuals at the beginning of the study, and then at 4, 6, 8, and 12 months following baseline. A significant overall difference was found in weight loss over the period of the trial favoring lifestyle CM over usual care (UC).

The primary focus of the study and the subsequent analysis of the data were in differences between the two groups, the lifestyle CM group and the UC group, with respect to weight loss over time. To do this, one would estimate and make inferences about the "fixed effects" portion of the model. One could with such a model fit a linear trend over time for each group and then compare groups, or one could examine polynomial effects over time.

It would also prove interesting to study the variation observed in the data as well. Namely, we could examine whether the variability in weight loss over time was different between the two groups. Such an examination would allow investigators to make decisions on the overall effectiveness of the CM intervention in facilitating consistent weight loss. The mixed model allows for separate models of the variation for the two intervention groups, and one could then make conclusions based on the resulting estimates. Similarly, examination of outliers in both groups using random effect estimates (i.e., subject-specific deviations from the average trend over time for the group) could also be useful in helping to identify underlying individual factors that may influence the response to such an intervention.

In order to achieve such goals, a linear mixed model was fitted to the data. Previous experience with the data coupled with careful model fitting strategies resulted in the following model of interest:

$$y_{ij} = \beta_1(\text{BASELINE WEIGHT})_i + \beta_2(\text{BASELINE AGE})_i + \beta_3(\text{UC}_i)$$
$$+ \beta_4(\text{CM}_i) + (\beta_5 \text{UC}_i + \beta_6 \text{CM}_i)t_{ij} + b_{1i}(\text{UC}_i) + b_{2i}(\text{CM}_i) + e_{ij}. \quad (3)$$

Here, y_{ij} is the change from baseline weight (kg) observed for individual i at month t_{ij} ($t_{ij} = 4,6,8,12$). CM_i and UC_i are indicator variables for those subjects in the CM and UC groups, respectively. The among-unit variation was modeled separately for each group; i.e., $\text{var}(b_{1i}) = \sigma_{b,\text{UC}}^2$ for those individuals in the UC group and $\text{var}(b_{2i}) = \sigma_{b,\text{CM}}^2$ for those individuals in the CM group. This variation, stemming from the random intercept included in the model (b_{1i} and b_{2i}, depending on the group assignment for subject i), represents the variation of the deviations of each subject's estimated intercept from the population intercepts (β_3 and β_4). In this instance, we assumed a constant within-unit variation between the two groups. Thus, $\text{var}(e_{ij}) = \sigma_e^2$.

In the majority of applications, as is the case here, primary interest lies in inference about the fixed effects; namely, we wish to know if there is a difference between the two groups with respect to weight loss over time. So, we wish to make inferences about the intercept and time parameters for the two groups. With this particular mixed model, we assume a linear change in weight loss over time for both groups, on average. But, the mixed model allows for individual deviations from these population estimates. Here, we only allow for deviation from the intercept; each individual has a random intercept estimate that will represent that person's deviation from the estimate of the average initial weight loss (intercept) for that particular group. However, one could add a number of random effects to account for multiple sources of variation that one believes can be modeled in such a fashion. In this particular case, we could have included a random slope term that represented the subject's deviation from the population slope estimate. As we will discuss later, there are methods to assess the necessity for including such random effects. In doing so, we decided that a random intercept term was only required, but we allowed for the random intercept's variation to differ between the two groups.

Figure 1 displays model-predicted weight loss at the mean values of age and weight (50 years old and 105 kg, respectively) for both groups, as well as a random sampling of individual profiles. These individual observations over time allow for estimation of average changes over time per group as well as estimation of variation from those average changes. The figure displays that in the UC group, there is no discernable pattern of weight change over the span of the study, as to be expected since this group of subjects did not receive any intervention more than what is considered "usual care." However, the subjects in the CM group on average lost more weight than those in the UC group. The figure of the individual profiles is extremely helpful in determining the appropriate model of the data. As one can see, there is considerable variation of the measurements for both groups over time, both among subjects as well as within-subjects.

Table 1 includes the estimates of the parameters in model (3). After using inference techniques described later, we can conclude from this model that there

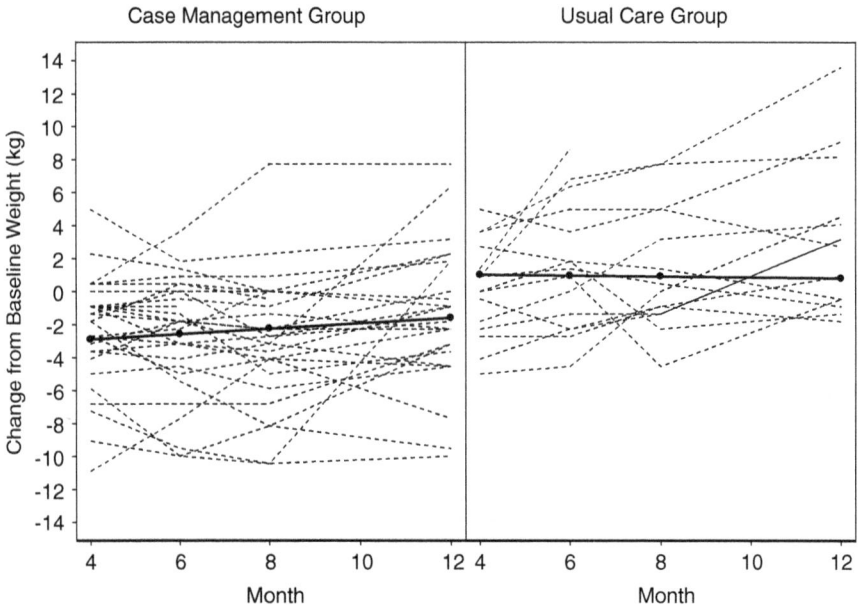

Fig. 1. Random sample of individual profiles of weight change from ICAN study along with estimated average weight loss (based on mixed model (3), using the mean values of age and weight (50 years old and 105 kg, respectively)).

Dashed lines represent observed weights for each individual over the span of the study. Solid lines represent the model-estimated weight change from baseline for each group. The individual profiles seen here represent only a random sampling of the entire set of subjects used to estimate the parameters of model (3).

Table 1
ICAN mixed model (3) parameter estimates

Effect	Parameter	Estimate	Standard Error
Baseline weight	β_1	−0.008	0.013
Baseline age	β_2	−0.084	0.042
Intercepts			
UC group	β_3	6.121	3.042
CM group	β_4	1.458	3.054
Month effect			
UC group	β_5	−0.025	0.069
CM group	β_6	0.164	0.076
Var(b_{1i})	σ_b^2,UC	8.626	2.035
Var(b_{2i})	σ_b^2,CM	10.404	2.477
Var(e_{ij})	σ_e^2	10.573	0.798

is a significantly greater initial amount of weight loss at four months in the CM group, compared to the UC group. However, there is no significant difference in the two population slopes, signifying that the two groups do not differ in weight loss/gain over time after the initial weight change at four months. In fact, the subjects in the CM group actually gained weight throughout the rest of the study on average, while the patients in the UC group remained relatively stable in terms of weight change throughout the year. Thus, we can conclude based on the fixed effect estimates that the intervention to be tested is effective at initial weight loss on average, but that those who received this intervention could not maintain this weight loss over the span of the study. Additionally, we observe that the subjects in the CM group experienced greater variation in their initial weight loss than those in the UC group. We could then look at actual random intercept estimates (not displayed) to determine those subjects who experienced the most weight loss.

1.4. Marginal versus hierarchical

To begin, it is worth writing the linear mixed model (2) again:

$$y_i = X_i\beta + Z_ib_i + e_i.$$

The motivation behind the analysis or scientific question of interest will drive the interpretation of the estimates resulting from fitting model (2) to the data. As alluded to in the discussion of the ICAN example, most often analysts are interested in estimation and inference about the fixed effects parameters, β, and possibly the "variance components," the variance parameters of θ. In this setting, model (2) with $\varepsilon_i = Z_ib_i + e_i$, i.e., $y_i = X_i\beta + \varepsilon_i$, is often referred to as the marginal model (Verbeke and Molenberghs, 2000), or the population-averaged model (Zeger et al., 1988). Here, the following distributional assumptions are all that are needed in making the conclusions necessary from the analysis of the data:

$$y_i \sim \mathcal{N}\left(X_i\beta, \Sigma_i = Z_iDZ_i' + R_i\right). \qquad (4)$$

Use of the marginal model does not imply that random effects are unnecessary for such an analysis. On the contrary, proper modeling of the random effects provides for a typically intuitive way of modeling variation of complex data that allows for accurate estimation and inference on the parameters of interest, β, and sometimes θ. Although not explicitly defined or needed in this case, random effects make it convenient in modeling the variation of multilevel data.

But, many times it is also important for one to focus on the random effects themselves. In this case, we should view (2) as a "hierarchical" model (Verbeke and Molenberghs, 2000), or a "subject-specific" model (Vonesh and Chinchilli, 1997). Rather than explicitly ignore the random effects in the model, b_i, we now define the distributional assumptions of the model conditional on b_i:

$$\mathbf{y}_i|\mathbf{b}_i \sim \mathcal{N}(\mathbf{X}_i\boldsymbol{\beta} + \mathbf{Z}_i\mathbf{b}_i, \; \mathbf{R}_i);$$
$$\mathbf{b}_i \sim \mathcal{N}(0, \mathbf{D}). \tag{5}$$

Notice that here, $\mathbf{y}_i \sim \mathcal{N}(\mathbf{X}_i\boldsymbol{\beta}, \Sigma_i)$, which is the same distributional assumption of the marginal model. However, the marginal model and the hierarchical model are not equivalent, at least in terms of interpretation and utility of the models. When we discuss the potential for using the mixed model, specifically the random effects portion of it, to focus on individual-specific deviation from the mean profiles (fixed effects), it is in the context of the hierarchical perspective. The hierarchical model then accommodates analyses to identify outlying individuals and to make predictions on the individual level.

Naturally, one may place certain restrictions on the structure and the number of parameters of both covariance matrices, $\mathbf{D}$ and $\mathbf{R}_i$. The structure of $\mathbf{D}$ is often dictated by the number of random effects included in the model. For example, in the context of longitudinal data, if one included only a random intercept, then one only needs to estimate the variance of this random intercept term. However, if one also includes a random slope as well, then one must decide whether or not to allow the two random effects to covary. Most software can accommodate many different specified parametric models of both covariance matrices of the mixed model. For more detailed information, see Verbeke and Molenberghs (2000).

2. Estimation for the linear mixed model

Seminal papers by Harville (1976, 1977) developed the linear mixed model as is written in (2), and Laird and Ware (1982) discussed its use for longitudinal data. Harville (1976) extended the Gauss–Markov theorem to cover the random effects, b_i, in estimating linear combinations of β and b_i. The prediction of b_i is also derived in an empirical Bayesian setting. Harville (1977) provided a review of the maximum likelihood (ML) approach to estimation in the linear mixed model. For model (2), the maximum log-likelihood is written as

$$l_{ML}(\boldsymbol{\theta}) = -\frac{N}{2}\log(2\pi) - \frac{1}{2}\sum_{i=1}^{m}\log|\Sigma_i|$$
$$-\frac{1}{2}\sum_{i=1}^{m}(\mathbf{y}_i - \mathbf{X}_i\boldsymbol{\beta})'\Sigma_i^{-1}(\mathbf{y}_i - \mathbf{X}_i\boldsymbol{\beta}). \tag{6}$$

Maximization of $l_{ML}(\boldsymbol{\theta})$ produces ML estimators (MLEs) of the unknown parameters $\boldsymbol{\beta}$ and $\boldsymbol{\theta}$. When $\boldsymbol{\theta}$ is known, the MLE of $\boldsymbol{\beta}$ is given by

$$\hat{\boldsymbol{\beta}} = \left(\sum_{i=1}^{m} X_i' \Sigma_i^{-1} X_i \right)^{-1} \sum_{i=1}^{m} X_i' \Sigma_i^{-1} y_i. \tag{7}$$

Kackar and Harville (1984) stated that the best linear unbiased estimators of the fixed and random effects are available when the true value of the variance parameter, $\boldsymbol{\theta}$, is known. In the usual case when $\boldsymbol{\theta}$ is unknown, Σ_i is simply replaced with its estimate, $\hat{\Sigma}_i$. Kackar and Harville (1984) concluded that if $\boldsymbol{\theta}$ needs to be estimated, the mean squared error of the estimates of $\boldsymbol{\beta}$ and $\boldsymbol{b}_i$ becomes larger. They also provided an approximation of this decrease in precision.

Harville (1974) also introduced the use of the restricted, or residual, maximum likelihood (REML) developed by Patterson and Thompson (1971) in estimating the covariance parameters of the linear mixed model. ML estimations of $\boldsymbol{\theta}$ are biased downward since the loss of degrees of freedom resulting from the estimation of the fixed effects is not taken into account. REML estimation acknowledges this loss of degrees of freedom and hence leads to less biased estimates. The REML estimator of $\boldsymbol{\theta}$ is calculated by maximizing the likelihood function of a set of error contrasts of y_i, $\boldsymbol{u}'y_i$, chosen so that $E(\boldsymbol{u}'y_i) = 0$. The resulting function, not dependent on $\boldsymbol{\beta}$, is based on a transformation of the original observations that lead to a new set of $N-p$ observations. Harville (1974) showed that the restricted log-likelihood function can be written in the following form based on the original observations:

$$l_{REML}(\boldsymbol{\theta}) = -\frac{N-p}{2}\log(2\pi) + \frac{1}{2}\log\left|\sum_{i=1}^{m} X_i' X_i\right| - \frac{1}{2}\sum_{i=1}^{m}\log|\Sigma_i|$$
$$- \frac{1}{2}\log\left|\sum_{i=1}^{m} X_i' \Sigma_i^{-1} X_i\right| - \frac{1}{2}\sum_{i=1}^{m}(y_i - X_i\hat{\boldsymbol{\beta}})'\Sigma_i^{-1}(y_i - X_i\hat{\boldsymbol{\beta}}), \tag{8}$$

where $\hat{\boldsymbol{\beta}}$ is of the form given above (7).

Laird and Ware (1982) introduced the linear mixed model in a general setting as it applies to longitudinal data, discussing how the model can be reduced to both growth curve models and repeated measures models. This two-stage random effects model is touted as being superior to ordinary multivariate models in its fitting of longitudinal data since it can handle unbalanced situations that typically arise when one gathers serial measurements on individuals. A unified approach to fitting the linear mixed model is the primary theme, comparing estimation of the model parameters using ML as well as empirical Bayes methods.

Harville (1977) noted that estimating the parameters of the linear mixed model via ML methods has computational disadvantages by requiring the solution of a nonlinear problem, an issue that is not as detrimental today with advances in computer technology that have dramatically increased the speed of estimation algorithms. Laird and Ware (1982) discussed the use of the Expectation-Maximization (EM) algorithm for estimation in the linear mixed model for longitudinal data. The EM algorithm was originally introduced by Dempster et al. (1977) as an iterative algorithm that can be used for computing ML estimates in the presence of incomplete data. Laird et al. (1987) attempted to improve the speed of convergence of the EM algorithm, noting the rate of convergence is dependent on the data and the specified forms of the covariance matrices, D and R_i.

Lindstrom and Bates (1988) proposed an efficient version of the Newton–Raphson (NR) algorithm for estimating the parameters in the linear mixed model via both ML and REML. They also developed computationally stable forms of both the NR and EM algorithms and compared the two in terms of speed and performance. While the NR algorithm is concluded to require fewer iterations to achieve convergence, it is not guaranteed to converge, whereas the EM algorithm will always converge to a local maximum of the likelihood. The faster convergence time of the NR algorithm has made it the preferred estimation method of choice for most mixed model fitting procedures.

3. Inference for the mixed model

3.1. Inference for the fixed effects

As stated previously, it is extremely common to be primarily interested in making conclusions regarding the fixed effects of the model. Not surprisingly, then, inference tools for the fixed effect parameters in the mixed model have received most of the attention methodologically. Likelihood ratio tests (LRTs) can compare two nested mixed models (Palta and Qu, 1995; Vonesh and Chinchilli, 1997; Verbeke and Molenberghs, 2000) with ML estimation and are assumed to exhibit a χ^2 distribution.

McCarroll and Helms (1987) evaluated a "conventional" LRT with a linear covariance structure via simulation studies. They showed that the LRT inflates Type I error rates. In addition, the LRT gave observed power values that were usually higher than the hypothesized values. McCarroll and Helms (1987) recommended using tests other than the LRT.

Use of the LRT based on the REML log-likelihood function is not valid when interest lies in the comparison of models with different sets of fixed effects. Welham and Thompson (1997) proposed adjusted LRTs for the fixed effects using REML, while Zucker et al. (2000) developed what they termed "refined likelihood ratio tests" in order to improve small sample inference. The adjusted tests of Welham and Thompson (1997) are reasonably well approximated by χ^2 variables. Zucker et al. (2000) found that an adjusted LRT based on the Cox–Reid adjusted likelihood produced Type I error rates lower than nominal. Consequently, a Bartlett correction greatly improved the Type I error rates of the adjusted LRT. Though the techniques appear promising, new and extensive analytic work seems required for each specific class of model.

Approximate Wald and F-statistics allow testing hypotheses regarding β. However, Wald tests can underestimate the true variability in the estimated fixed effects because they do not take into account the variability incurred by estimating θ (Dempster et al., 1981). The approximate F-test is more commonly used. The null hypothesis H_0: $C\beta = 0$, with C a $a \times p$ contrast matrix, can be tested with

$$T_F = a^{-1}(C\hat{\beta})' \left[C \left(\sum_{i=1}^{m} X_i' \hat{\Sigma}_i^{-1} X_i \right)^{-1} C' \right]^{-1} (C\hat{\beta}). \qquad (9)$$

Under the null hypothesis, it is assumed that T_F has an approximate F-distribution with a numerator degrees of freedom, and v denominator degrees of freedom, denoted $F(a,v)$. The denominator degrees of freedom, v, have to be estimated from the data. Determining the denominator degrees of freedom has been a source of research and debate for many years, with no clear consensus. However, in the analysis of longitudinal data, Verbeke and Molenberghs (2000, Section 6.2.2, p. 54) noted that "... different subjects contribute independent information, which results in numbers of degrees of freedom which are typically large enough, whatever estimation method is used, to lead to very similar p-values." Unfortunately, the approximate F-statistic is known to result in inflated Type I errors and poor power approximations in small samples, even for complete and balanced data (McCarroll and Helms, 1987; Catellier and Muller, 2000). Finally, Vonesh (2004) concluded that the denominator degrees of freedom of the F-test in the linear mixed model should be the number of independent sampling units minus "something" and we simply do not know what that "something" is.

Kenward and Roger (1997) presented a scaled Wald statistic with an approximate F-distribution for testing fixed effects with REML estimation that performs well, even in small samples. The Wald statistic uses an adjusted estimator of the covariance matrix to reduce the small sample bias. A drawback occurs when the variance components are constrained to be nonnegative and estimates fall on a boundary. In such cases the Taylor series expansions underlying the approximations may not be accurate. In addition, the procedure can fail to behave well with a nonlinear covariance structure. The technique has been implemented in popular mixed model fitting procedures such as SAS PROC MIXED (SAS Institute, 2003b). However, even this inference technique is not ideal, as documented performance of the Kenward–Roger F-statistic for some small sample cases has revealed inflated Type I error rates with various covariance model selection techniques (Gomez et al., 2005).

3.2. Inference for the random effects

When one is interested in the random effects themselves in the mixed model, then one needs to make inferences from the hierarchical model perspective. It is most convenient to estimate the random effects using Bayesian techniques, resulting in the following form of the estimates of b_i, assuming θ is known:

$$\hat{b}_i = DZ_i'\Sigma_i^{-1}(y_i - X_i\beta). \qquad (10)$$

The variance of $\hat{\boldsymbol{b}}_i$ is then approximated by

$$v(\hat{\boldsymbol{b}}_i) = \boldsymbol{D}\boldsymbol{Z}_i' \left\{ \boldsymbol{\Sigma}_i^{-1} - \boldsymbol{\Sigma}_i^{-1}\boldsymbol{X}_i \left(\sum_{i=1}^{m} \boldsymbol{X}_i'\boldsymbol{\Sigma}_i^{-1}\boldsymbol{X}_i \right)^{-1} \boldsymbol{X}_i'\boldsymbol{\Sigma}_i^{-1} \right\} \boldsymbol{Z}_i\boldsymbol{D}. \qquad (11)$$

As noted by Laird and Ware (1982), (11) underestimates the variability in $\hat{\boldsymbol{b}}_i - \boldsymbol{b}_i$ because it ignores the variation of $\boldsymbol{b}_i$. Consequently, inference about $\boldsymbol{b}_i$ is typically based on

$$v(\hat{\boldsymbol{b}}_i - \boldsymbol{b}_i) = \boldsymbol{D} - v(\hat{\boldsymbol{b}}_i). \qquad (12)$$

As with inference for the fixed effects, we typically do not know $\boldsymbol{\theta}$ beforehand. And, in this particular setting, we most often do not know $\boldsymbol{\beta}$. So, we usually replace $\boldsymbol{\theta}$ and $\boldsymbol{\beta}$ with their ML or REML estimates in the above equations. In this case, $\hat{\boldsymbol{b}}_i$ in (10) is known as the "empirical Bayes" estimate of $\boldsymbol{b}_i$. Again, as is the case when making inference about the fixed effects, when we use $\hat{\boldsymbol{\theta}}$ in place of $\boldsymbol{\theta}$, we then underestimate the variability of $\hat{\boldsymbol{b}}_i$. In this setting too, then, it is recommended that inference on the random effects be based on approximate F-tests with specific procedures for the estimation of the denominator degrees of freedom (Verbeke and Molenberghs, 2000).

3.3. Inference for the covariance parameters

Even though focus typically lies on the fixed effects, it is important to effectively model the variation of the data via the variance parameters in such a model. Making valid conclusions about the variability of the data are important information in itself, but it also leads to proper inference about the fixed effects as well. As discussed in Verbeke and Molenberghs (2000), likelihood theory allows for the distribution of both the ML and REML estimators of $\boldsymbol{\theta}$, $\hat{\boldsymbol{\theta}}$, to be approximated by a normal distribution with mean vector $\boldsymbol{\theta}$ and covariance matrix equaling the inverse of the Fisher information matrix. Thus, techniques such as LRTs and Wald tests can be used to make inferences about $\boldsymbol{\theta}$. Of course, there are restrictions to the possible values of the parameters contained in $\boldsymbol{\theta}$, most commonly that variance components be strictly positive. To demonstrate, in the example model (3), we assume $\mathrm{var}(b_{1i}) = \sigma_{b,\mathrm{UC}}^2 > 0$. Of course, in practice, when one fits the data using a mixed model procedure in a software package, if a value of a variance parameter is close to the boundary space (e.g., the variance is close to 0), this indicates that the source of variation may not need to be modeled. In the case when a negative value of the variance component parameter is not allowed, Verbeke and Molenberghs (2003) discuss the use of one-sided tests, in particular the score test.

In the context of a generalized nonlinear mixed model (to be discussed), Vonesh and Chinchilli (1997, Section 8.3.2) proposed a pseudo-likelihood ratio test (PLRT) used by Vonesh et al. (1996) to assess goodness-of-fit of the modeled covariance structure. The idea was to compare the robust "sandwich" estimator of the fixed effects covariance matrix to the usual estimated covariance matrix. The fixed effects covariance matrix is $\Omega = v(\hat{\boldsymbol{\beta}})$. The usual estimate and the robust "sandwich" estimator of the fixed effects covariance matrix for (2) are given by

$$\hat{\Omega} = \left(\sum_{i=1}^{m} X_i' \hat{\Sigma}_i^{-1} X_i \right)^{-1} \tag{13}$$

and

$$\hat{\Omega}_R = \hat{\Omega} \left[\sum_{i=1}^{m} X_i' \hat{\Sigma}_i^{-1} (y_i - X_i \hat{\beta})(y_i - X_i \hat{\beta})' \hat{\Sigma}_i^{-1} X_i \right] \hat{\Omega}. \tag{14}$$

By comparing the closeness of the estimators using a PLRT, one can evaluate the goodness-of-fit of the modeled covariance matrix Σ_i. Assuming that $m\hat{\Omega}_R$ has an approximate Wishart distribution, the PLRT is approximately distributed as a chi-square with $p(p+1)/2$ degrees of freedom. One advantage of the technique is that it does not require repeated fittings of models. The authors suggested that the PLRT should not be used when the outcomes exhibit a non-normal distribution. More work needs to be done to assess the performance of the PLRT for the mixed model in general. For more details of the technique, the reader is directed to Vonesh and Chinchilli (1997, Section 8.3.2).

4. Selecting the best mixed model

Discussion of estimation and inference on the parameters of the linear mixed model naturally falls under the discussion of model selection. Often, we usually perform hypothesis tests on model parameters to decide whether or not their inclusion in the model is necessary. Inference tools discussed previously are useful in linear mixed models when the parameters of note are nested. However, in the context of mixed models, it is common to want to compare models that are not nested, particularly when trying to determine the best model of the covariance.

4.1. Information criteria

Information theoretic criteria have played a prominent role in mixed model selection due to their relative validity in comparing non-nested models. Most practitioners use the Akaike Information Criterion (AIC, Akaike, 1974) and the Bayesian Information Criterion (BIC, Schwarz, 1978). Many variations have been introduced, including the corrected AIC, or AICC (Hurvich and Tsai, 1989), and the consistent AIC, or CAIC (Bozdogan, 1987). In their original forms, a larger value of the criteria for a given model indicates a better fit of the data. However, it is common to see them presented in a "smaller-is-better" form when they are calculated directly from the $-2 \times$ log-likelihood. Table 2 displays the formulas for the AIC, AICC, CAIC, and BIC from both angles, based on formulas familiar to readers of Vonesh and Chinchilli (1997).

Here, l is either $l_{REML}(\theta)$ or $l_{ML}(\theta)$, s refers to the number of parameters of the model, and N^* is a function of the number of observations. When using ML estimation, most often $s = p + k$, the total number of parameters in the model.

Table 2
General formulas for commonly used information criteria in mixed model selection

Criteria	Larger-is-Better Formula	Smaller-is-Better Formula
AIC	$l-s$	$-2l+2s$
AICC	$l-s(N^*/N^*-s-1)$	$-2l+2s(N^*/N^*-s-1)$
CAIC	$l-s(\log N^*+1)/2$	$-2l+s(\log N^*+1)$
BIC	$l-s(\log N^*)/2$	$-2l+s(\log N^*)$

Note: Here, l is either $l_{REML}(\theta)$ or $l_{ML}(\theta)$, s refers to the number of parameters of the model, and N^* a function of the number of observations.

The proper formulas and application of these formulas under REML is still debated; see Gurka (2006) for a summary of the various viewpoints and forms specific to REML model selection. The general consensus (Vonesh and Chinchilli, 1997) is that under ML, $N^* = N$, the total number of observations, and under REML, $N^* = N-p$, given that the restricted likelihood is based on $N-p$ observations. However, this recommendation has not been consistently employed and needs further investigation (see Gurka, 2006 for more discussion). Shi and Tsai (2002) noted that Akaike (1974) used the likelihood function as a basis for obtaining the AIC, but just like the variance estimates of a linear mixed model when using the unrestricted likelihood, the estimator used in the criterion is biased. They then proposed a "residual information criterion" (RIC) that uses REML, applying it to the classical regression setting. Extension of the RIC for use with the linear mixed model is an area of future research.

When discussing model selection criteria, one should introduce the large-sample notions of efficiency and consistency. Efficient criteria target the best model of finite dimension when the "true model" (which is unknown) is of infinite dimension. In contrast, consistent criteria choose the correct model with probability approaching 1 when a true model of finite dimension is assumed to exist. Selection criteria usually fall into one of the two categories; for instance, the AIC and AICC are efficient criteria, while the BIC and CAIC are considered to be consistent criteria. Debate has ensued as to which characteristic is preferred, as opinions are largely driven by the field of application in which one is interested in applying model selection techniques. For further discussion, see Burnham and Anderson (2002) or Shi and Tsai (2002).

In Hjort and Claeskens (2003) and Claeskens and Hjort (2003), the authors discuss model selection, inference after model selection, and both frequentist and Bayesian model averaging. Claeskens and Hjort (2003) noted that traditional information criteria aim to select a single model with overall good properties, but do not provide insight into the actual use of the selected model. Claeskens and Hjort (2003) proposed to focus on the parameter of interest to form the basis of their model selection criterion, and introduce a selection criteria for this purpose denoted as the focused information criterion (FIC). Discussions that follow the article describe limitations of the frequentist model averaging estimator and the FIC (Shen and Dougherty, 2003).

Jiang and Rao (2003) developed consistent procedures for selecting the fixed and random effects in a linear mixed model. Jiang and Rao (2003) focused on two types of linear mixed model selection problems: (a) selection of the fixed effects while assuming the random effects have already been correctly chosen and (b) selection of both the fixed effects and random effects. Their selection criteria are similar to the generalized information criterion (GIC), with the main idea centering on the appropriate selection of a penalty parameter to adjust squared residuals. Owing to the inability to provide an optimal way of choosing the best penalty parameter for a finite set of data, the methods require further investigation before recommending its widespread use.

It is very common to see values for information criteria in standard output of many mixed model fitting procedures, such as SAS PROC MIXED. The applicability of information criteria for mixed model selection is apparent. However, as one can observe by the above summary of this area of research, much more work needs to be performed to consolidate the utility of information criteria to mixed model selection. Thus, we must caution the analyst in using the values of computed information criteria from standard procedures without a through investigation of the research to date in this area.

4.2. Prediction

The introduction of cross-validation methods (Stone, 1974; Geisser, 1975) led to ensuing research in model selection focused on the predictive ability of models (Geisser and Eddy, 1979; Stone, 1977; Shao, 1993). The predictive approach generally involves two steps. For a given number of independent sampling units, m, the data are split into two parts, with $m = m_c + m_v$. Sample size m_c is used for model construction and sample size m_v is used for model validation.

For modeling repeated measures data with correlated errors, Liu et al. (1999) generalized a cross-validation model selection method, the Predicted Residual Sum of Squares (*PRESS*). Allen (1971) originally suggested *PRESS* as a model selection criterion in the univariate linear model. *PRESS* is a weighted sum of squared residuals in which the weights are related to the variance of the predicted values. Though Liu et al. (1999) presented various definitions of *PRESS*, only *PRESS* for the fixed effects was developed since it could be applied to unbalanced designs and the distribution of the statistic yielded useful results. As a result, the *PRESS* statistic should not be used for selecting random effects in the linear mixed model. No conclusive evidence exists of its performance against other model selection criteria. As with the LRT and information criteria, *PRESS* requires repeated fittings of mixed models and hence does not allow model adequacy to be assessed using only the chosen model of interest.

Vonesh et al. (1996) proposed a weighted concordance correlation coefficient as a measure of goodness-of-fit for repeated measurements. The concordance correlation coefficient for the linear and nonlinear mixed effects model (Vonesh and Chinchilli, 1997), denoted by r_c, is a function of the observed outcomes, y_i, and the model-predicted outcomes, $\hat{y}_i$. The r_c is a modification of Lin's (1989) proposed concordance correlation coefficient to assess the level of agreement between two bivariate measurements. In general, $-1 \leq r_c \leq 1$, with $r_c = 1$ being a perfect fit and $r_c \leq 0$ being significant lack of fit. Unlike the LRT, information criteria, or PRESS, r_c does not require repeated fittings of mixed models to evaluate adequacy of fit.

However, r_c can be used to differentiate between different hypothesized models by choosing the model with the largest r_c. It does not appear that r_c has been widely implemented in the literature for linear mixed models, and its performance has not been assessed via any large-scale simulation studies.

Vonesh and Chinchilli (1997) also presented a modification of the usual R^2-statistic from the univariate linear model that is interpreted as the explained residual variation, or proportional decrease in residual variation. Unlike r_c, the R^2-statistic requires specification of a hypothesized model and a null model (one that is simple but consistent with the application). As with the r_c, the lack of evidence describing the performance of R^2 strongly discourages its use in selecting a linear mixed model. Vonesh and Chinchilli (1997) noted that r_c may be preferred since it equals a concordance correlation between observed and predicted values.

Xu (2003) and Gelman and Pardoe (2005) investigated measures to estimate the proportion of explained variation under the linear mixed model. Xu (2003) considered three types of measures and generalized the familiar R^2-statistic from the univariate linear model to the linear mixed model for nested models. In order to measure explained variation, the method by Xu (2003) relies upon defining a "null" model such as a model with only a fixed effect and random effect intercept. Gelman and Pardoe (2005) presented a Bayesian method of defining R^2 for each level of a multilevel (hierarchical) linear model, which includes the linear mixed model. The method is based on comparing variances in a single-fitted model rather than comparing to a null model. Xu's (2003) simulation results demonstrated that the R^2 measure gives good estimates with reasonably large cluster sizes, but overestimates the proportion of variation in y explained by the covariates if the cluster sizes are too small. Gelman and Pardoe (2005) performed no simulations to assess the performance of their R^2 measure. More investigation must be done.

Weiss et al. (1997) presented a Bayesian approach to model selection for random effect models. In a data analysis example, Weiss et al. (1997) found conflicting results, showing that the selected model was dependent on the chosen priors and hyperparameter settings. In comparing their technique to the LRT, AIC, and BIC, the results were again mixed. There exists a lack of evidence that the Bayesian approach performs well in model selection for linear mixed models, since no in-depth simulation study or other additional comparative procedures have been conducted.

In the univariate linear model, Mallows' C_p criterion (Mallows, 1973) requires a pool of candidate models which are each separately nested within a single full model. It compares the mean square error (MSE) of each candidate model to the MSE of the full model, which then allows comparing one candidate to another. However, the MSE for the linear mixed model is not well defined since there are two independent sources of variation, one due to deviations about the population profile and one due to deviations about subject-specific profiles. Recently, Cantoni et al. (2005) suggested a generalized version of Mallows' C_p, denoted GC_p, for marginal longitudinal models. GC_p provides an estimate of a measure of adequacy of a model for prediction. Though the technique was developed for models fitted using generalized estimating equations (GEE), there is potential for considering the method in linear mixed model analysis.

The small sample characteristics of model selection methods based on predictive approaches require further investigation. Furthermore, in some cases the approach cannot be used. For example, in many small sample applications it is unacceptable to split the sample for determining model construction and model validation.

4.3. Graphical techniques

Graphical techniques have long been a component of model selection in both univariate and multivariate settings. Plotting the estimated response function or residuals against predicted values provides statisticians with visual aids that help in model selection. Similarly, graphical techniques can help select a linear mixed model. Plotting the estimated response function from the fixed effects and comparing it to a mean curve constructed using averages at selected time points provides one useful aid. For longitudinal data, plotting the collection of estimated individual response functions against the observed data can greatly help model selection.

For simple examples and some small sample applications, graphical techniques can work well, even though they are subjective aids. More complex scenarios make using graphical techniques either very challenging or render graphical techniques almost useless. In addition, due to the subjective nature of graphical procedures, perhaps the techniques can never be considered as a primary means of model selection. Grady and Helms (1995), Diggle et al. (2002) and Verbeke and Molenberghs (2000) gave expanded discussions of the use of graphical techniques.

5. Diagnostics for the mixed model

As is the case with ordinary linear regression, the linear mixed model has distributional assumptions that may or may not be valid when used with applied data. Unlike univariate linear regression, however, diagnostics to assess these assumptions, and consequent alternatives when violations of the assumptions are suspected have not been developed fully for the linear mixed model, primarily due to the relative youth of the analysis tool. An area that has received some attention is the assumed normality of the random effects, b_i. Lange and Ryan (1989) described a method for assessing the distribution assumption of the random effects that uses standardized empirical Bayes estimates of b_i. The assumed linearity of the covariance matrices of the observations, along with assuming $R_i = \sigma^2 I_{n_i}$, allows these standardized estimates to be independent across individuals. They then used classical goodness-of-fit procedures, in particular a weighted normal plot, to assess the normality of the random effects. Butler and Louis (1992) demonstrated that the normality assumption of the random effects has little effect on the estimates of the fixed effects; they did not investigate the effect on the estimates of the random effects themselves. Verbeke and Lesaffre (1996) investigated the impact of assuming a Gaussian distribution for the random effects on their estimates in the linear mixed model. They showed that if the distribution of the random effects is a finite mixture of normal distributions, then the estimates of b_i may be poor if normality is assumed. Consequently, they argued it is beneficial to assume a mixture of normal distributions and compare the fitted model to the model fit when assuming a Gaussian distribution.

Verbeke and Lesaffre (1997) showed that the ML estimates for the fixed effects as well as the variance parameters, θ, obtained when assuming normality of the random effects, are consistent and asymptotically normally distributed, even when the random effects distribution is not normal. But, they claimed that a sandwich-type correction to the inverse of the Fisher information matrix is needed in order to obtain the correct asymptotic covariance matrix. They showed through simulations that the obtained corrected standard errors are better than the uncorrected ones in moderate to large samples, especially for the parameters in D. Very little work has been done on the performance of the linear mixed model in small sample settings when normality of the random effects is assumed but not achieved.

Little attention has been given to the distribution assumption of the pure errors, e_i, in the linear mixed model. Often it is assumed that mixed models exhibit conditional independence, i.e., $R_i = \sigma^2 I_{n_i}$, as in some cases it is arguable that the correlation exhibited between observations within an individual can be accounted for fully by the random effects covariance structure. In certain instances this assumption is included simply for computational convenience. Chi and Reinsel (1989) developed a score test of the assumption of conditional independence compared to a model that assumes auto-correlation in the within-individual errors. They argued that assuming an auto-correlation structure for R_i can actually reduce the number of required random effects needed in the final model. One could note that not only does one assume independence when it is given that $R_i = \sigma^2 I_{n_i}$, but also that there is a constant within-unit error variance. Ahn (2000) proposed a score test for assessing this homoskedasticity of the within-unit errors.

Transformations have also been utilized in mixed model settings. Lipsitz et al. (2000) analyzed real longitudinal data by applying a Box–Cox transformation on the response of a marginal (population-averaged) model. Since the model did not explicitly contain random effects, the authors assumed the transformation achieved normality of the overall error term only. Gurka et al. (2006) discussed details that follow when extending the Box–Cox transformation to the linear mixed model. They showed that the success of a transformation may be judged solely in terms of how closely the total error, ε_i, follows a Gaussian distribution. Hence, the approach avoids the complexity of separately evaluating pure errors and random effects when one's primary interest lies in the marginal model. Oberg and Davidian (2000) extended the method for estimating transformations to nonlinear mixed effects models for repeated measurement data, employing the transform-both-sides model proposed by Carroll and Ruppert (1984).

6. Outliers

Of course, mixed models are sensitive to outlying observations. However, the multilevel structure of the mixed model allows for different definitions of outliers. When viewed as a marginal model, $y_i - X_i\hat{\beta}$ is one form of a residual that measures deviation from the overall population mean. Likewise, $y_i - X_i\hat{\beta} - Z_i\hat{b}_i$ measures the amount of difference from the observed value to a subject's predicted regression. As defined earlier, the random effect estimate itself, $\hat{b}_i$, is also an estimate of deviation; in the longitudinal setting, it is a measure of the subject-specific deviation. As one can imagine, then, due to the many definitions of residuals in the mixed model, diagnostic techniques regularly used for the univariate linear model (leverage, Cook's distance, etc.) do not extend to the mixed model in a straightforward fashion. For a more detailed discussion of influence for the linear mixed model, the reader is directed to Chapter 11 in Verbeke and Molenberghs (2000).

As is the case in the univariate linear model, some researchers have examined robust estimation and inference procedures that will not be greatly affected by such influential observations for mixed models. But, since mixed models are a relatively modern statistical technique, the literature on robust estimation for the linear mixed model is sparse. Fellner (1986) proposed a method for limiting the influence of outliers with respect to the random components in a simple variance components model. A robust modification of restricted ML estimation, Fellner's method uses influence functions attributed to Huber (1981) without explicitly using the likelihood function. Richardson and Welsh (1995) introduced the definitions of robust ML and robust restricted ML in the context of mixed models that are also based on bounding the influence. They applied the methods to data and performed simulation studies to show the advantages of these robust procedures.

7. Missing data

As introduced previously, one common characteristic of study data, particularly longitudinal data, is missing data. This is especially the case in biomedical studies of human beings over time, as it is impossible to ensure 100% compliance with the study protocol. Subjects drop out of studies for many reasons, or may simply miss a visit and continue the study.

The mixed model can accommodate missing data, thus making it an ideal tool to analyze longitudinal data. Unlike other multivariate models, such as the general linear multivariate model (Muller and Stewart, 2006), complete data are not required when fitting a mixed model as long as the missing data are of a certain type. However, the validity of the parameter estimates of the mixed model depends on the nature of the missingness.

Standard classifications of missing data exist. For a more comprehensive look at missing data, see Little and Rubin (1987). The "best" type of missing data is data that are missing completely at random (MCAR). Simply put, with MCAR the fact that the data are missing has nothing to do with any of the effects (e.g., the treatment to be studied) or outcomes of interest. Data in which MCAR is present will not lead to biased estimates of the parameters of the mixed model. The next classification of missingness, one that is also not "bad" from a validity standpoint for the mixed model, is missing at random (MAR). For MAR, the missingness depends on previous values of the outcome, but the missingness is still independent of the model covariates of interest. Handling MAR data is not as simple as MCAR, as careful strategies must be taken in order for valid conclusions to be made from the fitted mixed model.

The type of missingness that results in biased estimates of the parameters of the mixed model is generally referred to as non-ignorable missingness. Generally speaking, missingness that is non-ignorable results when the pattern of missingness is directly related to the covariates of interest. There is no way to accommodate this type of missingness while fitting standard mixed models.

It would be most helpful to give examples of each type of missingness in the context of the ICAN study, where we are comparing two intervention groups with respect to weight loss over time. If a few patients in each intervention group dropped out of the study because they moved out of the area, this most likely would be classified as MCAR. However, since the study participants were obese type 2 diabetes patients, it is quite possible that some of the subjects were so overweight and unhealthy that they could not continue to make their regularly scheduled visits. This pattern of missingness is not directly related to the intervention group in which they belong, but rather the outcome (their weight), and hence most likely this would be classified most likely as MAR. Finally, if many of the patients in the CM group, the intervention that was more intensive, dropped out due to the intensity of this intervention, this type of missingness would be non-ignorable.

To summarize, mixed models are extremely powerful in analyzing longitudinal data in particular due to its ability to accommodate missing data. However, the analyst must be careful in determining which pattern of missingness is present in the data they wish to model. Analytical tools exist to model the incompleteness, thus providing insight into the nature of the missingness. Additionally, imputation methods exist to "fill in the holes," so to speak. As alluded to earlier, missing data are an expansive area of research in itself, and the reader is referred to other articles and texts that deal exclusively with missing data issues. For an excellent overview of missing data in the context of linear mixed models for longitudinal data, see Verbeke and Molenberghs (2002). Also, Diggle et al. (2002) discuss missing data in the longitudinal data setting.

8. Power and sample size

The research on power analysis for mixed models is sparse. Exact power calculations are not available for the mixed model simply because the exact distributions of the tests used in the mixed model are not known. That being said, all hope is not lost in calculating power based on tests of the mixed model. To our knowledge, research on power analysis for the linear mixed model has been limited to calculations based on tests of the fixed effects of the model. As previously discussed, the test of the form (9) follows an approximate F-distribution under the null hypothesis. Simulation results in Helms (1992) support the notion that (9) follows an approximate non-central *F*-distribution under the alternative hypothesis. We must point out again the uncertainty regarding the denominator degrees of freedom of (9). We have no reason to believe that this uncertainty does not carry over to its use when considering the power of the test. For additional discussion regarding power and the mixed model in this setting, see Stroup (1999) and Littell et al. (2006, Chapter 12).

Power analyses in general require many assumptions. For simple analyses such as a *t*-test or a univariate linear model, one must have an estimate of the variability of the data, and some idea of what is considered a meaningful effect size before determining the appropriate sample size for a given power. As one can imagine, in settings where the mixed model is ideal (e.g., longitudinal studies), the amount of parameters to make assumptions is relatively large, and the required assumptions become more complicated. For instance, one must make assumptions about the structure of the correlation of the data, and then determine reasonable values to base the power analysis. Such a task is neither simple nor straightforward. Unfortunately, little has been done in terms of laying out sound strategies to perform power calculations for complicated settings such as repeated measures studies.

Calculating sample size for the linear mixed model is directly related to computing power analysis. As noted before, since little has been done to obtain sound strategies for power analysis, the same is then true for computing sample size. Sample size requirements for the linear mixed model, depending on the motivation behind the analysis, can be quite large. However, it is not clear what is sufficiently large with regard to sample size in order to make valid inferences about the model parameters. The primary application of mixed models, the analysis of clustered or longitudinal data, makes this question even more challenging. Should one focus on obtaining more subjects or clusters, or should one try to gather more measurements per subject, or individuals within a cluster? We mentioned earlier that it is generally recognized that for valid inference about the fixed effects, one should perhaps target a larger number of independent sampling units (Vonesh, 2004). However, this has not been proven definitively beyond simulation studies. One useful discussion regarding sample size calculations for repeated measures designs can be found in Overall and Doyle (1994).

9. Generalized linear mixed models

The linear mixed model discussed thus far is primarily used to analyze outcome data that are continuous in nature. One can see from the formulation of the model (2) that the linear mixed model assumes that the outcome is normally distributed. As mentioned previously, researchers have studied the utility of the linear mixed model when the continuous outcome does not follow a Gaussian distribution.

Often times, however, one is interested in modeling non-continuous outcome data, such as binary data or count data. The generalized linear model is appropriate for modeling such data. The generalized linear model encompasses many commonly used models, such as logistic regression, Poisson regression, and in fact linear regression. For an introduction to the generalized linear model, see McCullagh and Nelder (1989).

In the same way the linear mixed model builds on the capabilities of the linear model by allowing for clustered or longitudinal data, the generalized linear mixed model accommodates clustered or longitudinal data that are not continuous. Similar to the linear mixed model, the generalized linear mixed model can be viewed from a marginal or a hierarchical standpoint. Remember that in the hierarchical case of the linear mixed model,

$$E(y_i|b_i) = X_i\beta + Z_ib_i.$$

Now, for the generalized linear mixed model (McCulloch and Searle, 2001), again assuming $b_i \sim \mathcal{N}(0, D)$,

$$E(y_i|b_i) = f(X_i\beta + Z_ib_i), \tag{15}$$

where f is a function of the fixed and random effects of the model. The inverse of this function, say g, is typically called the "link" function. So, $g\{E(y_i|b_i)\} = X_i\beta + Z_ib_i$. There are many common link functions, each usually corresponding to an assumed distribution of $y_i|b_i$. The simplest function is $g\{E(y_i|b_i)\} = E(y_i|b_i)$, the identity link, where $y_i|b_i$ is assumed to be normally distributed. This simple case is the linear mixed model, a specific case of the generalized linear mixed model. For logistic regression, the link function is called the logit link, $g(x) = \log\{x/(1 - x)\}$, where x is assumed to follow a binary distribution. Logistic regression is popular in many epidemiological and other biomedical studies where the outcome has two options, e.g., disease or no disease, and interest lies in estimating the odds of developing the disease. For Poisson regression, the link function is the log link, $g(x) = \log(x)$, where x is assumed to follow a Poisson distribution. Poisson regression is often used to model count or rate data. There are many other link functions and corresponding distributions used in the case of generalized linear models, including generalized linear mixed models.

Again, the addition of the random effect term in this setting allows for clustered or repeated data. For instance, one may be interested in estimating the odds of developing a disease, but has data on multiple individuals from the same families. In this case, it may be unreasonable to assume that these individuals are independent of one another with respect to the risk of developing the disease. Here, then, the generalized linear mixed model allows the analyst to accommodate this dependence.

The above formulation applies to the hierarchical view of the mixed model, but the marginal view is applicable in this setting as well. In this case, we simply assume $E(y_i) = f(X_ib)$. If one is simply interested in population estimates (averages), then alternatives to the generalized linear mixed model exist, such as GEE. See Diggle et al. (2002) for a discussion of GEE. Thus, most often when generalized linear mixed models are used, the hierarchical standpoint is of interest; here the random effects included in the model are of importance and not just a nuisance.

Although at first glance the generalized linear mixed model, when using a link/distribution other than the identity/normal, does not seem to be much more complicated with respect to estimation and inference, the methodology involved for this model is actually quite a bit more complex. When using a link function other than the identity link, it is more difficult to express the likelihood of y_i, which now involves an integral with respect to b_i. The difficulty with expressing the likelihood, coupled with the lack of closed-form solutions, makes estimation much more computationally intensive. Sophisticated numerical techniques are necessary, and the body of literature in this area is relatively expansive. More in-depth introductions and discussions of generalized linear mixed models, along with estimation and inference about its parameters, can be found in many books (McCulloch and Searle, 2001; Diggle et al., 2002; Agresti, 2002; Demidenko, 2004; Molenberghs and Verbeke, 2005).

10. Nonlinear mixed models

Another version of the mixed model is the nonlinear mixed model. The nonlinear mixed model actually follows the same general form (15) as the generalized linear mixed model. However, the function f for a nonlinear mixed model is typically more complicated than the standard functions used for the generalized linear mixed model. It is common to see applications in which the data are best fitted by models that are nonlinear in the parameters of interest. As mentioned, generalized linear mixed models are one form of nonlinear mixed models. More complicated forms of nonlinear models are often used in pharmacokinetics and biological and agricultural growth models. In most of these cases, there is a known or suspected form, based on past experiences or theoretical knowledge, for how the parameters enter the model in a nonlinear fashion.

As an example of the applicability of the nonlinear mixed model in pharmacokinetic settings, Pinheiro and Bates (1995) fit what is referred to as a first-order compartment model to data on serum concentrations of the drug theophylline from 12 subjects observed over a 25-h period. The nonlinear mixed model in this case has the following form:

$$y_{it} = \left\{ \frac{Dk_{e_i} \cdot k_{a_i}}{Cl_i(k_{a_i} - k_{e_i})} \right\} \cdot \left\{ e^{(-k_{e_i}t)} - e^{(-k_{a_i}t)} \right\} + e_{it}. \tag{16}$$

Here, y_{it} is the observed serum concentration of the ith subject at time t, D the dose of theophylline, k_{e_i} the elimination rate constant, k_{a_i} the absorption rate constant, and Cl_i the clearance for subject i. Also, e_{it} represents the error term that is assumed to be normally distributed. The "mixed" model stems from the following assumed forms of k_{e_i}, k_{a_i}, and Cl_i:

$$Cl_i = e^{(\beta_1 + b_{i1})},$$
$$k_{e_i} = e^{(\beta_2 + b_{i2})},$$
$$k_{a_i} = e^{(\beta_3 + b_{i3})}. \tag{17}$$

Similar to the preceding treatment of linear mixed models, here β_1, β_2, and β_3 are fixed effect parameters representing population averages, and b_{i1}, b_{i2}, and b_{i3} are random effect parameters. As one can see, both the fixed effects and random effects of model (16) enter the model in a nonlinear fashion. Additionally, it is easy to imagine that estimating and inferring on the parameters of such a model is quite difficult from a computational perspective. Discussion of estimation and inference for the nonlinear mixed model is beyond the scope of this presentation on mixed models. However, the interested reader is referred to numerous texts that deal with the subject, including Davidian and Giltinan (1995), Vonesh and Chinchilli (1997) and Demidenko (2004). For demonstration of the analysis of data from this example, see Example 51.1 of the SAS online documentation (SAS OnlineDoc 9.1, SAS Institute Inc., 2003a, 2003b).

11. Mixed models for survival data

Random effects can also be included in models of time-to-event data as well. These types of models are often referred to as survival models, as one popular "event" of interest is death. The mixed model approach in estimating time to a certain event has two main uses, depending on the nature of the event to be modeled. When the event can only occur once, such as death, inclusion of random effects can be helpful when correlation among subjects may exist. For instance, subjects from the same hospital, nursing home, or even community may not be independent of one another, and this dependence might need to be taken into account depending on the motivation of the analysis. Mixed time-to-event models may also be useful when the event occurs repeatedly on the same individuals, and thus we have repeated durations that should be modeled accordingly. For a detailed discussion of what is often referred to as "multilevel" survival data models, see Goldstein (2003, Chapter 10).

12. Software

As alluded to often in this discussion, many computational techniques for fitting mixed models exist. We wish not to create an exhaustive list, but rather highlight some of the more popular tools.

Tools for fitting linear mixed models are the most readily available. PROC MIXED in SAS (2003b), lme in S-PLUS (MathSoft, 2002) and R (R Development Core Team, 2006), and xtmixed in STATA (StataCorp, 2005) are just a few of the linear mixed model fitting procedures. Additionally, SPSS (2006) has the ability to fit linear mixed models to data. Most of these procedures have similar capabilities, with many distinctions between them too detailed to list here. Rest assured that developers of most of these statistical software packages are kept abreast of the current mixed model research, and these procedures are continuously being updated and improved.

Tools exist for the analysis of generalized and nonlinear mixed models as well, although one must be warned that due to the complicated nature of these modeling scenarios, such procedures should not be used without substantial knowledge of both the modeling process as well as the procedure itself. PROC GLIMMIX and PROC NLMIXED are now available in SAS (2003) to fit generalized linear mixed models and nonlinear mixed models, respectively. S-PLUS (MathSoft, 2002) and R (R Development Core Team, 2006) have the nlme function for nonlinear mixed models. For an overview of fitting mixed models using S and S-PLUS, see Pinheiro and Bates (2000). Again, we simply wanted to cite some of the available options without trying to show favor to one particular software package. There are almost assuredly other options available in other software packages.

13. Conclusions

The powerful set of statistical analysis tools that collectively fit into the category "mixed models" is indeed quite large, and the capabilities of these tools continue to grow. It is impossible to write a comprehensive exposition of the topic of mixed models in a book, let alone a chapter of a book. We simply wished to introduce the mixed model in general, providing details regarding its applicability and utility. At the same time, we attempted to introduce some of the more recent areas of research that have been performed on the mixed model. More importantly, we aimed to provide references for areas of mixed model research for the reader interested in more details.

The theory behind the mixed model has existed for decades; however, advances in computing have made the mixed model a popular analytical tool only in the past 10–15 years. Consequently, the availability of this powerful method of analysis has led to more sophisticated study designs which in turn has allowed for answers to hypotheses previously too complicated to be addressed using standard statistical techniques. For example, more and more studies involve repeated measurements taken on subjects, as tools such as the mixed model can provide valid analyses of such data. For someone familiar with univariate linear models in a simple sense, mixed models are fairly intuitive and thus have great appeal to data analysts working with researchers without an extensive background in statistics.

The primary focus of this chapter is on the most straightforward form of the mixed model, the linear mixed model for continuous outcome data. We also introduce more general and complicated forms of the linear mixed model, the generalized, and the nonlinear mixed models. Owing to the computational intensity necessary for these more advanced types of mixed models, their use has become more commonplace only recently. The relatively recent expanded use of mixed models makes it necessary to continue methodological research on aspects of these models. For example, much more study is required on power analysis for the mixed model, and inference, particularly for small samples, needs to be further refined. Model selection and diagnostic tools also should be addressed in more detail. However, the practical utility of the mixed model in a variety of applications coupled with its complexity makes the mixed model a very exciting statistical analysis tool for future study.

References

Agresti, A. (2002). *Categorical Data Analysis*, 2nd ed. Wiley InterScience, New Jersey.

Ahn, C.H. (2000). Score tests for detecting non-constant variances in linear mixed models. *ASA Proceedings of the Biopharmaceutical Section* **0**, 33–38.

Akaike, H. (1974). A new look at the statistical model identification. *IEEE Transaction on Automatic Control* **AC-19**, 716–723.

Allen, D. M. (1971). The Prediction Sum of Squares as a Criterion for Selecting Predictor Variables, Technical Report 23, Department of Statistics, University of Kentucky.

Bozdogan, H. (1987). Model selection and Akaike's information criterion: The general theory and its analytical extensions. *Psychometrika* **52**, 345–370.

Burnham, K.P., Anderson, D.R. (2002). *Model selection and multimodel inference: A practical information-theoretic approach.* Springer, New York.

Butler, S.M., Louis, T.A. (1992). Random effects models with non-parametric priors. *Statistics in Medicine* **11**, 1981–2000.

Cantoni, E., Mills Flemming, J., Ronchetti, E. (2005). Variable selection for marginal longitudinal generalized linear models. *Biometrics* **61**, 507–514.

Carroll, R.J., Ruppert, D. (1984). Power transformations when fitting theoretical models to data. *Journal of the American Statistical Association* **79**, 321–328.

Catellier, D.J., Muller, K.E. (2000). Tests for Gaussian repeated measures with missing data in small samples. *Statistics in Medicine* **19**, 1101–1114.

Chi, E.M., Reinsel, G.C. (1989). Models for longitudinal data with random effects and AR(1) errors. *Journal of the American Statistical Association* **84**, 452–459.

Claeskens, G., Hjort, N.L. (2003). The focused information criterion. *Journal of the American Statistical Association* **98**, 900–916.

Davidian, M., Giltinan, D.M. (1995). *Nonlinear Models for Repeated Measures Data.* Chapman & Hall, London.

Demidenko, E. (2004). *Mixed Models: Theory and Application.* Wiley, New York.

Dempster, A.P., Laird, N.M., Rubin, R.B. (1977). Maximum likelihood with incomplete data via the E–M algorithm. *Journal of the Royal Statistical Society, Series B* **39**, 1–38.

Dempster, A.P., Rubin, R.B., Tsutakawa, R.K. (1981). Estimation in covariance components models. *Journal of the American Statistical Association* **76**, 341–353.

Diggle, P.J., Heagerty, P., Liang, K.Y., Zeger, S.L. (2002). *Analysis of Longitudinal Data.* Oxford University Press, Oxford.

Fellner, W.H. (1986). Robust estimation of variance components. *Technometrics* **28**, 51–60.

Flegal, K.M., Carroll, M.D., Ogden, C.L., Johnson, C.L. (2002). Prevalence and trends in obesity among US adults, 1999–2000. *Journal of the American Medical Association* **288**(14), 1723–1727.

Geisser, S. (1975). The predictive sample reuse method with applications. *Journal of the American Statistical Association* **70**, 320–328.

Geisser, S., Eddy, W.F. (1979). A predictive approach to model selection. *Journal of the American Statistical Association* **74**, 153–160.

Gelman, A., Pardoe, I. (2005). Bayesian measures of explained variance and pooling in multilevel (hierarchical) models. *Technometrics* **48**, 241–251.

Goldstein, H. (2003). *Multilevel Statistical Models*, 3rd ed. Arnold, London.

Gomez, E.V., Schaalje, G.B., Fellingham, G.W. (2005). Performance of the Kenward–Roger method when the covariance structure is selected using AIC and BIC. *Communications in Statistics-Simulation and Computation* **34**, 377–392.

Grady, J.J., Helms, R.W. (1995). Model selection techniques for the covariance matrix for incomplete longitudinal data. *Statistics in Medicine* **14**, 1397–1416.

Gurka, M.J. (2006). Selecting the best linear mixed model under REML. *The American Statistician* **60**, 19–26.

Gurka, M.J., Edwards, L.J., Muller, K.E., Kupper, L.L. (2006). Extending the Box–Cox transformation to the linear mixed model. *Journal of the Royal Statistical Society, Series A* **169**, 273–288.

Harville, D.A. (1974). Bayesian inference for variance components using only error contrasts. *Biometrika* **61**, 383–385.

Harville, D.A. (1976). Extension of the Gauss–Markov theorem to include the estimation of random effects. *Annals of Statistics* **4**, 384–395.

Harville, D.A. (1977). Maximum likelihood approaches to variance component estimation and to related problems. *Journal of the American Statistical Association* **72**, 320–338.

Helms, R.W. (1992). Intentionally incomplete longitudinal designs: I. Methodology and comparison of some full span designs. *Statistics in Medicine* **11**, 1889–1913.

Hjort, N.L., Claeskens, G. (2003). Frequentist model average estimator. *Journal of the American Statistical Association* **98**, 879–899.

Huber, P.J. (1981). *Robust Statistics*. John Wiley, New York.

Hurvich, C.M., Tsai, C.L. (1989). Regression and time series model selection in small samples. *Biometrika* **76**, 297–307.

Jiang, J., Rao, J.S. (2003). Consistent procedures for mixed linear model selection. *The Indian Journal of Statistics* **65**, 23–42.

Kackar, R.N., Harville, D.A. (1984). Approximations for standard errors of estimators of fixed and random effect in mixed linear models. *Journal of the American Statistical Association* **79**, 853–862.

Kenward, M.G., Roger, J.H. (1997). Small sample inference for fixed effects from restricted maximum likelihood. *Biometrics* **53**, 983–997.

Knowler, W.C., Barrett-Connor, E., Fowler, S.E., Hamman, R.F., Lachin, J.M., Walker, E.A., Nathan, D.M. (Diabetes Prevention Program Research Group) (2002). Reduction in the incidence of type 2 diabetes with lifestyle intervention or metformin. *New England Journal of Medicine* **346**(6), 393–403.

Laird, N.M., Ware, J.H. (1982). Random-effects models for longitudinal data. *Biometrics* **38**, 963–974.

Laird, N.M., Lange, N., Stram, D. (1987). Maximum likelihood computations with repeated measures: Application of the EM algorithm. *Journal of the American Statistical Association* **82**, 97–105.

Lange, N., Ryan, L. (1989). Assessing normality in random effects models. *Annals of Statistics* **17**, 624–642.

Lin, L.I. (1989). A concordance correlation coefficient to evaluate reproducibility. *Biometrics* **45**, 255–268.

Lindstrom, M.J., Bates, D.M. (1988). Newton-Raphson and EM algorithms for linear mixed-effects models for repeated-measures data. *Journal of the American Statistical Association* **83**, 1014–1022.

Lipsitz, S.R., Ibrahim, J., Molenberghs, G. (2000). Using a Box-Cox transformation in the analysis of longitudinal data with incomplete responses. *Applied Statistics* **49**, 287–296.

Littell, R., Milliken, G., Stroup, W., Wolfinger, R., Schabenberger, O. (2006). *SAS for Mixed Models*, 2nd ed. SAS Institute Inc., Cary, NC, Chapter 12.

Little, R.J.A., Rubin, D.B. (1987). *Statistical Analysis with Missing Data*. John Wiley and Sons, New York.

Liu, H., Weiss, R.E., Jennrich, R.I., Wenger, N.S. (1999). PRESS model selection in repeated measures data. *Computational Statistics and Data Analysis* **30**, 169–184.

Mallows, C.L. (1973). Some comments on C_p. *Technometrics* **15**, 661–675.

MathSoft, Inc. (2002). *S-Plus (Release 6)*. MathSoft Inc., Seattle.

McCarroll, K.A., Helms, R.W. (1987). An evaluation of some approximate F statistics and their small sample distributions for the mixed model with linear covariance structure. *The Institute of Statistics Mimeo Series*. Department of Biostatistics, University of North Carolina, Chapel Hill, NC.

McCullagh, P., Nelder, J.A. (1989). *Generalized Linear Models*, 2nd ed. Chapman & Hall, New York.

McCulloch, C.E., Searle, S.R. (2001). *Generalized, Linear and Mixed Models*. Wiley, New York.

Mokdad, A.H., Bowman, B.A., Ford, E.S., Vinicor, F., Marks, J.S., Koplan, J.P. (2001). The continuing epidemics of obesity and diabetes in the United States. *Journal of the American Medical Association* **286**(10), 1195–1200.

Molenberghs, G., Verbeke, G. (2005). *Models for Discrete Longitudinal Data*. Springer, New York.

Muller, K.E., Stewart, P.W. (2006). *Linear Model Theory: Univariate, Multivariate, and Mixed Models*. Wiley, New York.

Oberg, A., Davidian, M. (2000). Estimating data transformations in nonlinear mixed effects models. *Biometrics* **56**, 65–72.

Overall, J.E., Doyle, S.R. (1994). Estimating sample sizes for repeated measurement designs. *Controlled Clinical Trials* **15**, 100–123.

Palta, M., Qu, R.P. (1995). Testing lack of fit in mixed effect models for longitudinal data. In: Tiit, E.-M., Kollo, T., Niemi, H. (Eds.), *New Trends in Probability and Statistics Volume 3: Multivariate Statistics and Matrices in Statistics (Proceedings of the 5th Tartu Conference)*. VSP International Science Publishers, Zeist, The Netherlands, pp. 93–106.

Patterson, H.D., Thompson, R. (1971). Recovery of inter-block information when block sizes are equal. *Biometrika* **58**, 545–554.

Pinheiro, J.C., Bates, D.M. (1995). Approximations to the log-likelihood function in the nonlinear mixed-effects model. *Journal of Computational and Graphical Statistics* **4**, 12–35.

Pinheiro, J.C., Bates, D.M. (2000). *Mixed Effects Models in S and S-Plus*. Springer, New York.

R Development Core Team (2006). *R: A Language and Environment for Statistical Computing*. R Foundation for Statistical Computing, Vienna.

Richardson, A.M., Welsh, A.H. (1995). Robust restricted maximum likelihood in mixed linear models. *Biometrics* **51**, 1429–1439.

SAS Institute Inc (2003a). *SAS OnlineDoc® 9.1*. SAS Institute Inc., Cary, NC.

SAS Institute Inc (2003b). *SAS/Stat User's Guide, Version 9.1*. SAS Institute Inc, Cary, NC.

Schwarz, G. (1978). Estimating the dimension of a model. *Annuals of Statistics* **6**, 461–464.

Shao, J. (1993). Linear model selection by cross-validation. *Journal of the American Statistical Association* **88**, 486–494.

Shi, P., Tsai, C.L. (2002). Regression model selectiona residual likelihood approach. *Journal of the Royal Statistical Society B* **64**(2), 237–252.

Shen, X., Dougherty, D.P. (2003). Discussion: Inference and interpretability considerations in frequentist model averaging and selection. *Journal of the American Statistical Association* **98**, 917–919.

SPSS for Windows (2006). *Rel. 14.0.1*. SPSS Inc., Chicago.

StataCorp (2005). *Stata Statistical Software: Release 9*. StataCorp LP., College Station, TX.

Stone, M. (1974). Cross-validatory choice and assessment of statistical predictions (with discussion). *Journal of the Royal Statistical Society, Series B* **36**, 111–147.

Stone, M. (1977). An asymptotic equivalence of choice of model by cross-validation and Akaike's criterion. *Journal of the Royal Statistical Society, Series B* **39**, 44–47.

Stroup, W.W. (1999). *Mixed model procedures to assess power, precision, and sample size in the design of experiments*. American Statistical Association, Alexandria, VA, (pp. 15–24).

Verbeke, G., Lesaffre, E. (1996). A linear mixed-effects model with heterogeneity in the random-effects population. *Journal of the American Statistical Association* **91**, 217–221.

Verbeke, G., Lesaffre, E. (1997). The effect of misspecifying the random-effects distribution in linear mixed models for longitudinal data. *Computational Statistics and Data Analysis* **23**, 541–556.

Verbeke, G., Molenberghs, G. (2000). *Linear Mixed Models for Longitudinal Data*. Springer, New York.

Verbeke, G., Molenberghs, G. (2003). The use of score tests for inference on variance components. *Biometrics* **59**, 254–262.

Vonesh, E.F. (2004). Hypothesis testing in mixed-effects models. Presented in Session 12: Estimation and Inference in Mixed-Effects Models. 2004 International Biometric Society Eastern North American Region Meetings, Pittsburgh, PA.

Vonesh, E.F., Chinchilli, V.M. (1997). *Linear and Nonlinear Models for the Analysis of Repeated Measurements*. Marcel Dekker, New York.

Vonesh, E.F., Chinchilli, V.M., Pu, K. (1996). Goodness-of-fit in generalized nonlinear mixed-effects models. *Biometrics* **52**, 572–587.

Weiss, R.E., Wang, Y., Ibrahim, J.G. (1997). Predictive model selection for repeated measures random effects models using Bayes factors. *Biometrics* **53**, 592–602.

Welham, S.J., Thompson, R. (1997). A likelihood ratio test for fixed model terms using residual maximum likelihood. *Journal of the Royal Statistical Society, Series B* **59**, 701–714.

Wolf, A.M., Conaway, M.R., Crowther, J.Q., Hazen, K.Y., Nadler, J.L., Oneida, B., Bovbjerg, V.E. (2004). Translating lifestyle intervention to practice in obese patients with type 2 diabetes: Improving control with activity and nutrition (ICAN) study. *Diabetes Care* **27**(7), 1570–1576.

Xu, R. (2003). Measuring explained variation in linear mixed effects models. *Statistics in Medicine* **22**, 3527–3541.

Zeger, S.L., Liang., K-Y., Albert, P.S. (1988). Models for longitudinal data: A generalized estimating equation approach. *Biometrics* **44**(4), 1049–1060.

Zucker, D.M., Lieberman, O., Manor, O. (2000). Improved small sample inference in the mixed linear model. *Journal of the Royal Statistical Society, Series B* **62**, 827–838.

Handbook of Statistics, Vol. 27
ISSN: 0169-7161
© 2007 Elsevier B.V. All rights reserved
DOI: 10.1016/S0169-7161(07)27012-9

6

Factor Analysis and Related Methods

Carol M. Woods and Michael C. Edwards

Abstract

*This chapter introduces exploratory and confirmatory factor analysis (EFA
and CFA) with brief mention of the closely related procedures principle components analysis and multidimensional item response theory. For EFA, emphasis is on rotation, the principle factors criterion, and methods for selecting
the number of factors. CFA topics include identification, estimation of model
parameters, and evaluation of model fit. EFA and CFA are introduced for
continuous variables, and then extensions are described for non-normal continuous variables, and categorical variables. Study characteristics that influence sample size (for EFA or CFA) are discussed, and example analyses are
provided which illustrate the use of three popular software programs.*

1. Introduction

Factor analysis (FA) refers to a set of latent variable models and methods for
fitting them to data. Factors are latent variables: Unobservable constructs presumed to underlie manifest variables (MVs). The objective of FA is to identify
the number and nature of the factors that produce covariances or correlations
among MVs. The variance of each MV is partitioned into *common variance* which
is shared with other MVs, and *unique variance*, which is both random error and
systematic variance unshared with other MVs (called *specific variance*). Because
specific variance and random error are not modeled separately in FA, unique
variance is often considered "error" variance. *Common factors* represent common variance and *unique factors* represent unique variance.

The FA model is:

$$\sum_{xx} = \Lambda\Phi\Lambda^{\mathrm{T}} + \mathbf{D}_{\psi},\tag{1}$$

where Σ_{xx} is the $p \times p$ covariance matrix among MVs $x_1, x_2, \ldots, x_p$, Λ is a $p \times m$
matrix of regression coefficients called *factor loadings* that relate each factor to
each MV, Φ is an $m \times m$ matrix of correlations among m factors, and $\mathbf{D}_{\psi}$ is a
$p \times p$ diagonal matrix of unique variances (one for each MV). The model could

be fitted to a matrix of correlations instead of covariances; this standardizes the factor loadings and elements of $\mathbf{D}_{\psi}$. Standardized unique variances are referred to as *uniquenesses*. The sum of squared standardized factor loadings, incorporating the correlations among factors (i.e., $\mathbf{\Lambda\Phi\Lambda}^{\mathrm{T}}$) gives the *communalities* for the MVs. The communality for an MV is the proportion of total variance it shares with other MVs, or its reliability. Notice that the communality and the uniqueness sum to 1.

Classic FA is applicable to continuous MVs and is analogous to multivariate linear regression, except that the predictors are unobservable. Assumptions comparable to those made in linear regression are made in FA: Common and unique factors are presumed uncorrelated, unique factors are presumed uncorrelated with one another, and MVs are assumed to be linearly related to the (linear combination of) factors. Additional assumptions are needed to identify the model because latent variables have no inherent scale. The scale of the common factors is often identified by fixing the mean and variance to 0 and 1, respectively. The mean of the unique factors is also usually fixed to 0, but the variance is estimated. The variance of a unique factor is usually interpreted as the error variance of the MV.

FA can be exploratory or confirmatory depending on the degree to which investigators have prior hypotheses about the number and nature of the underlying constructs. Although some of the methods used in exploratory and confirmatory factor analysis (EFA and CFA) are distinct, the boundary between them is often blurred. Rather than imagining them as completely separate techniques, it is useful to think of EFA and CFA as opposite ends of the same continuum.

In EFA, a preliminary sense of the latent structure is obtained, often without significance testing. Additional research is needed to make definitive claims about the number and nature of the common factors. In CFA, a hypothesized model is tested, and sometimes compared to other hypothesized models. CFA is a special case of a structural equation model (SEM); thus many principles of SEM also apply to CFA. CFA models are evaluated using significance tests and other indices of fit. Though replication and cross-validation is important for both types of FA, results from CFA are more definitive because prior hypotheses are tested.

2. Exploratory factor analysis (EFA)

EFA is performed when investigators are unable or unwilling to specify the number and nature of the common factors. A key task is to select the number of common factors (m) that best accounts for the covariance among MVs. Several models with differing m are fitted to the same data and both statistical information and substantive interpretability are used to select a model. The goal is to identify the number of major common factors such that the solution is not only parsimonious, but also plausible and well matched to the data. Typically, all pm elements of $\mathbf{\Lambda}$ are estimated rather than constrained to a particular value. Unique variances and correlations among factors are also estimated.

Once the parameters of a model with a particular m are estimated, the solution is rotated to improve substantive interpretability. Rotated, not un-rotated, factor loadings aid in the selection of m. The term *factor rotation* was coined during an era when FA was carried out by hand. FA models were represented graphically in m-dimensional space with an axis for each factor and a point for each MV. Axes were literally rotated to a subjective, *simple structure* solution. Thurstone (1947) specified formal criteria for simple structure, but essentially, each factor should be represented by a distinct subset of MVs with large factor loadings, subsets of MVs defining different factors should overlap minimally, and each MV should be influenced by only a subset of common factors.

In contemporary FA, rotation is objective and automated by computer software. The matrix of rotated loadings is produced by multiplying $\boldsymbol{\Lambda}$ by an $m \times p$ *transformation matrix*, $\mathbf{T}$. The elements of $\mathbf{T}$ are chosen to either maximize a *simplicity* function or minimize a *complexity* function. These functions mathematically specify simple structure, or its opposite (complexity) in the pattern of loadings.

The EFA model is *rotationally indeterminate*, meaning that if a single $\boldsymbol{\Lambda}$ can be found that satisfies the model for a particular $\boldsymbol{\Sigma}_{xx}$, then infinitely many other $\boldsymbol{\Lambda}$s exist that satisfy the model equally well. Procedures used to estimate EFA model parameters (discussed in a subsequent section) impose criteria to obtain unique values; however, an infinite number of alternative $\boldsymbol{\Lambda}$s could replace the initial solution.

Numerous rotation methods have been developed (see Browne, 2001). One major distinction among them is whether factors are permitted to correlate. *Orthogonal* rotations force factors to be uncorrelated whereas *oblique* rotations permit nonzero correlations among factors. Orthogonal rotations are primarily of didactic or historical interest; they are easier and were developed first. It is usually best to use an oblique rotation because factors are typically correlated to some degree, and correlation estimates will be 0 if they are not. A few of the most popular oblique rotation procedures are described next.

2.1. Rotation

The two-stage *oblique Promax rotation* procedure (Hendrikson and White, 1964) is frequently used and widely implemented in software. Orthogonal rotation is carried out first, followed by a procedure that permits correlations among factors. The first stage consists of rotating loadings to an orthogonal criterion called "Varimax" (Kaiser, 1958). The transformation matrix for *orthogonal Varimax rotation* maximizes the sum of the variances of the squared factor loadings on each factor. The simplicity criterion is:

$$V = \sum_{k=1}^{m} \frac{1}{p} \sum_{j=1}^{p} (\lambda_{jk}^2 - \bar{\lambda}_{.k}^2)^2, \quad \text{where } \bar{\lambda}_{.k}^2 = \frac{1}{p} \sum_{k=1}^{m} \lambda_{jk}^2 \tag{2}$$

and λ_{jk} is an element of $\boldsymbol{\Lambda}$ for the jth MV and the kth factor. Greater variability in the magnitude of the squared loadings indicates better simple structure.

The second stage of the Promax procedure is to raise Varimax-rotated loadings to a power (often the 4th), restore the signs, and estimate new loadings that are as close as possible to the powered loadings. Least squares estimation is used to minimize the sum of squared differences between the Varimax-rotated loadings and the powered (target) loadings, t_{jk}, which is the complexity function:

$$P = \sum_{k=1}^{m} \sum_{j=1}^{p} (\lambda_{jk}^2 - t_{jk})^2. \tag{3}$$

Because variables with larger communalities have more influence on the rotated solution than variables with smaller communalities, each row of Λ is standardized before rotation and returned to the original scale after rotation. Loadings for each MV are divided by the square root of the communality (called a *Kaiser weight*) before rotation, and then multiplied by the Kaiser weight after rotation. This process of *row standardization* was originally introduced for orthogonal Varimax rotation, but is now commonly used with most rotations, both orthogonal and oblique.

Other popular oblique rotations are members of a family described by Crawford and Ferguson (1970). The general complexity function is:

$$CF = (1 - \kappa) \sum_{j=1}^{p} \sum_{k=1}^{m} \sum_{\substack{\ell=1 \\ k \neq \ell}}^{m} \lambda_{jk}^2 \lambda_{j\ell}^2 + \kappa \sum_{k=1}^{m} \sum_{j=1}^{p} \sum_{\substack{h=1 \\ j \neq h}}^{p} \lambda_{jk}^2 \lambda_{hk}^2, \tag{4}$$

where κ weights MV complexity (first term) and factor complexity (second term), and $0 \leq \kappa \leq 1$. MV complexity is minimized when there is a single nonzero loading in each row of Λ; factor complexity is minimized when there is a single nonzero loading in each column of Λ.

Researchers select κ and specify whether the rotation is orthogonal or oblique. When $\kappa = 1/p$, and orthogonal rotation is specified, the Crawford–Ferguson (CF) criterion is the same as the orthogonal Varimax criterion. Oblique Varimax rotation is also possible. When $\kappa = 0$, complexity in the MVs, but not the factors, is minimized. Oblique rotation renders the CF criterion equivalent to the oblique quartimax criterion (also called "quartimin" or "direct quartimin"), introduced by Jennrich and Sampson (1966).

Some FA experts prefer oblique quartimax rotation (e.g., Browne, 2001), but the best approach may depend on the particular data set and the goals of the FA. It is sometimes useful to use two or three different rotation criteria and then select the most substantively interpretable solution.

We turn now to methods for estimating the parameters of EFA models. The two most common methods are iterative principle factors and maximum likelihood (ML) estimation. Typically, correlations rather than covariances are analyzed because factor loadings are easier to interpret when standardized. Also, note that the columns of Λ (i.e., the factors) are always uncorrelated following initial estimation. In EFA, correlations among factors are introduced only by oblique rotation.

2.2. Principle factors

Because the EFA model is rotationally indeterminate, an additional criterion is imposed when the parameters are estimated so that initial factor loadings are unique. By the *criterion of principle factors*, each common factor should account for the maximum possible amount of variance in the MVs. Only one Λ satisfies the principle factors criterion. A principle factors solution uses eigenvalues and eigenvectors to estimate Λ. If S is a symmetric matrix and $Su = \ell u$, then ℓ is an eigenvalue of S and u is an eigenvector of S.

In EFA, eigenvalues and eigenvectors of the *reduced correlation matrix*, R_{xx}, are used to compute Λ. R_{xx} has communalities for each MV on the diagonal (rather than 1's). For a given m, Λ is constructed from the m largest eigenvalues and the corresponding eigenvectors: $\Lambda = UD_\ell^{1/2}$. U is a $p \times m$ orthogonal matrix with columns equal to eigenvectors, and $D_\ell^{1/2}$ is an $m \times m$ diagonal matrix with nonzero elements equal to square roots of eigenvalues. An eigenvalue is equal to the sum of squared loadings down each column of Λ, interpreted as the proportion of variance accounted for by each factor.

A complication inherent in the procedure just described is that communalities are needed prior to the computation of factor loadings. These so-called prior communalities must be estimated. Guttman (1940) showed that the squared multiple correlation (R^2) from the regression of an MV on the $p-1$ other MVs is a lower bound for the communality. Though somewhat conservative, R^2s from these regressions are usually used as estimates of prior communalities.

A newer way to estimate prior communalities is the *partitioning method* (Cudeck, 1991), which may be used only if $p \geq 2m+1$. For each MV, the remaining $p-1$ MVs are divided into two mutually exclusive subsets of m variables (because the method is contingent upon m, it must be repeated for every different m under consideration). The jth MV for which a communality is sought is subset 1, and the other mutually exclusive sets of MVs are subsets 2 and 3. The communality for the jth MV is given by $\rho_{13} P_{23}^{-1} \rho_{21}$, where ρ_{13} is the vector of correlations between subsets 1 and 3, ρ_{21} is the vector of correlations between subsets 1 and 2, and P_{23}^{-1} is the (inverse of) the $m \times m$ matrix of correlations between subsets 2 and 3.

The set of procedures described thus far is referred to as *principle factors conditional on prior communalities* (or simply, conditional principle factors). However, a closely related method, *iterative principle factors*, can provide better answers. Iterative principle factors minimizes the sum of squared residuals, which are discrepancies between sample correlations (or covariances) and a particular solution for the FA model:

$$\text{RSS} = \sum_{i=1}^{p} \sum_{j=1}^{p} [R_{xx} - (\Lambda \Phi \Lambda^T)]_{ij}^2, \tag{5}$$

where RSS is the residual sums of squares, Φ is diagonal (prior to rotation), and D_ψ is not shown because it has been subtracted from the full correlation matrix to create R_{xx}. A key feature of the iterative approach is that communalities placed on the diagonal of R_{xx} are estimated simultaneously with the factor loadings.

The iterative approach begins as conditional principle factors. Then the initial estimate of Λ is used to estimate new communalities as the sum of squared loadings across each row. These are placed on the diagonal of $\mathbf{R}_{xx}$, eigenvalues and eigenvectors are obtained as before, and Λ is re-estimated. This process continues until the communalities change minimally from one iteration to the next (i.e., converge).

2.3. Normal theory maximum likelihood (ML) estimation

One advantage of principle factors methods is that no distributional assumption about the MVs is needed. However, the disadvantage is that no standard errors (SEs), significance tests, or confidence intervals (CIs) are available. If MVs can be assumed to jointly follow a multivariate normal distribution, EFA parameters can be estimated as in conditional principle factors, with the additional requirement that they maximize a multivariate normal likelihood function. Normal theory ML estimation is the same as iterative principle factors except that loadings are chosen to maximize the likelihood function rather than to minimize RSS. The joint likelihood is

$$L = \prod_{i=1}^{N} \frac{|\Sigma_{xx}|^{.5}}{(2\pi)^{.5p}} \exp\left(-\frac{1}{2}(\mathbf{x}_i - \boldsymbol{\mu})^{\mathrm{T}}\Sigma_{xx}^{-1}(\mathbf{x}_i - \boldsymbol{\mu})\right), \tag{6}$$

where N is the total number of observations, $\mathbf{x}_i$ the vector of MV scores for observation i, and $\boldsymbol{\mu}$ is the vector of MV means.

When ML is used, a likelihood ratio (LR) test statistic and numerous descriptive indices may be used to evaluate global model fit. Two versions of the LR statistic are used. The classic LR statistic is $(N-1)(-2)[\log(L)]$, and Bartlett's (1950) corrected version is $(N - ((2p+11)/6) - (2m/3)) - (2)[\log(L)]$. L is (Eq. (6)) evaluated at the maximum. With sufficient N, the LR statistic is approximately χ^2-distributed with degrees of freedom:

$$df = \frac{1}{2}p(p+1) - \left\{p + pm - \frac{1}{2}m(m-1)\right\} = \frac{(p-m)^2 - (p+m)}{2} \tag{7}$$

Bartlett's correction may increase the degree to which the LR statistic is χ^2-distributed. The LR statistic may be used to test the null hypothesis (H_0) that the FA model with m factors holds. Rejection of H_o indicates that Σ_{xx} has no particular structure or that more factors are needed. Thus, failing to reject H_0 is desirable. However, this test of perfect fit is sensitive to N. Virtually any parsimonious model is rejected if N is large enough, and substantial misfit is missed if N is small.

Numerous descriptive indices of model fit have been developed that should be consulted along with, or instead of, the χ^2-test. These indices are usually studied or discussed in the context of CFA rather than EFA; thus it is more natural to review them when describing CFA. However, the indices are also useful for EFA, and are the primary method by which the number of factors is decided upon when ML is used. ML also provides SEs for the factor loadings and inter-factor correlations (following oblique rotation), which aids in the often subjective process of assigning MVs to factors in EFA.

2.4. Tools for choosing m

Three statistical tools used to choose m (which may be used with either principle factors or ML) are residuals, a scree plot, and parallel analysis. Smaller residuals indicate better model fit. A summary statistic, such as the root mean square residual or the maximum absolute residual, can be compared for models with different m. Examination of residuals for each correlation or covariance may help to identify specific areas of model misfit. The best model typically has many small residuals and no particularly large ones. Many software programs standardize residuals, which aid in the interpretation of their magnitude. Typically, a standardized residual greater than about 2 is considered large.

Another tool, the *scree plot* (Cattell, 1966), is a graph of the eigenvalues of R_{xx}. Figure 1 shows an example for 9 MVs. The vernacular definition of "scree" is an accumulation of loose stones or rocky debris lying on a slope or at the base of a hill or cliff. In a scree plot, it is desirable to find a sharp reduction in the size of the eigenvalues (like a cliff), with the rest of the smaller eigenvalues constituting rubble. When the eigenvalues drop dramatically in size, an additional factor would add relatively little to the information already extracted. Because scree plots can be subjective and arbitrary to interpret, their primary utility is in providing two or three reasonable values of m to consider. The plot in Fig. 1 suggests that a useful model for these data may have 3 or 4 factors.

Parallel analysis (Horn, 1965) helps to make the interpretation of scree plots more objective. The eigenvalues of R_{xx} are plotted with eigenvalues of the reduced correlation matrix for simulated variables with population correlations of 0 (i.e., no common factors). An example is displayed in Fig. 2. The number of eigenvalues above the point where the two lines intersect (3 for the example in

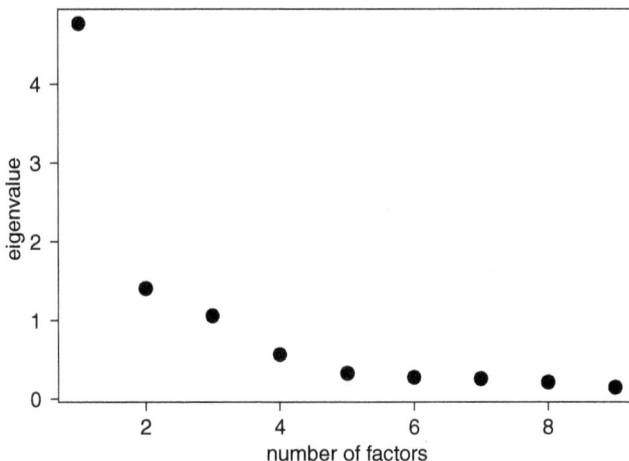

Fig. 1. Example scree plot.

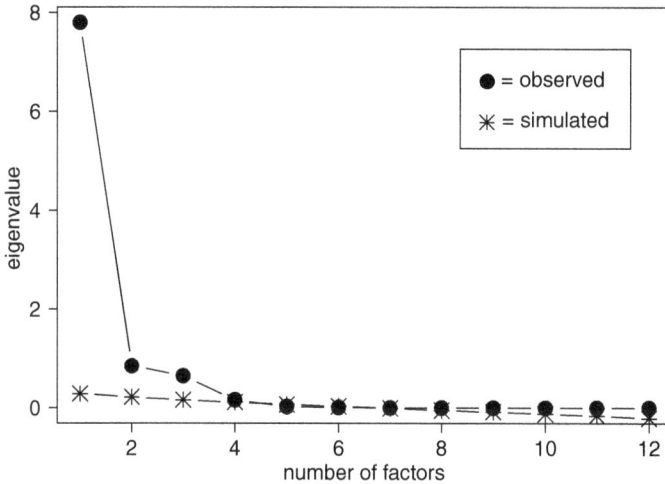

Fig. 2. Example of parallel analysis.

Fig. 2) is the suggested *m*. The rationale for parallel analysis is that useful factors account for more variance than could be expected by chance. Recall that an eigenvalue is the proportion of variance explained by each factor. Only factors with eigenvalues greater than those from uncorrelated data are useful.

We are not aware of a commercial computer program that implements parallel analysis, but any software that will simulate data from a normal distribution and compute eigenvalues may be used. To carry out parallel analysis, generate N observations from a normal distribution for p variables (N and p for the simulated data match those for the observed data). Then compute the reduced correlation matrix among simulated MVs and its eigenvalues, repeat this process approximately 100 times, and average the eigenvalues for each simulated MV. It is these mean eigenvalues that are plotted against the eigenvalues of $\mathbf{R}_{xx}$. Syntax for parallel analysis using SPSS (SPSS Incorporated, 2006), or SAS software (SAS Institute, 2006) was published by O'Connor (2000).

Additional tools are available to help select m when ML is used. Global indices of model fit may be compared among models with differing m. Increasing m improves model fit to some degree, but the goal is to identify m such that one fewer factor results in substantially poorer fit and one additional factor has little impact on the fit. Additionally, nested models can be statistically compared using a χ^2-difference test. The difference between the LR statistics for a model with k factors and a model with $k-1$ factors is approximately χ^2-distributed with degrees of freedom (*df*) equal to the difference between the *df* for the two models. A significant difference suggests that fit is better for the model with k factors. Otherwise, the more parsimonious model is preferred. The final model selected should fit in an absolute, as well as relative, sense.

We conclude this section with a warning about an approach commonly employed to select m, which is theoretically unjustifiable and likely to be misleading. The eigenvalue-greater-than-one rule (also called the Kaiser criterion or the Kaiser–Guttman rule) leads researchers to select m equal to the number of eigenvalues of $\mathbf{R}_{xx}$ that exceed 1. The number of eigenvalues greater than 1 is a lower bound for the number of *components* to extract in *principle components analysis* (discussed next), but it should never be used as the sole criterion to select *m* for EFA.

3. Principle components analysis (PCA)

PCA is a data reduction method sometimes confused with EFA. Conditional principle factors EFA is mathematically similar to PCA. For both, parameters interpreted as standardized regression coefficients are calculated from eigenvectors and eigenvalues of a correlation matrix. However, EFA analyzes the *reduced* correlation matrix, with prior communalities on the diagonal, whereas PCA analyzes the *full* correlation matrix, with 1's on the diagonal. Because a communality is the proportion of MV variance that is reliable, PCA treats MVs as error-free. Thus, what may seem like a small technical difference between PCA and EFA has important implications for interpretation.

The purpose of EFA and PCA differs, as does interpretation of the results. EFA seeks to explain covariation among MVs and is useful for understanding underlying structure in the data. Total MV variance is separated into common and unique elements, and common factors are constructs thought to give rise to MVs. In contrast, PCA is useful for reducing a large number of variables into a smaller set. Instead of separating common and unique variance, total MV variance is reorganized into linear combinations called *components*. A component is a linear combination of MVs, not a latent variable. Component loadings are standardized regression coefficients indicating the strength of relation between each MV and each component. However, a component has no particular interpretation beyond "linear combination of" MVs. When the goal of an analysis is to understand underlying dimensions implied by correlations (or covariances) among MVs, and interpret the dimensions as constructs, FA is applicable and PCA is not.

4. Confirmatory factor analysis (CFA)

CFA is used to test a hypothesized model. Investigators specify the number of factors, and typically constrain many factor loadings to 0. Thus, fewer loadings are estimated in CFA than in EFA because not all factors are hypothesized to underlie all MVs. MVs with nonzero loadings on a factor are *indicators* of the factor. Researchers decide when fitting the model to data which parameters are *free* (i.e., to be estimated) and which are *fixed* (i.e., constrained to some value).

Because more restrictions are placed on the parameters than in EFA, CFA models are not rotationally indeterminate. Thus, eigenvalues and eigenvectors are not used in CFA, and correlations among factors are not introduced by rotation. Instead, researchers specify whether correlations among factors are free or fixed. Typically, unique variances are estimated as in EFA and correlations among them can be estimated if relationships are hypothesized. An important consideration in CFA that influences how many parameters can be freed is model identification.

4.1. Identification

A CFA model is *identified* if parameter estimates are unique, otherwise the model is *unidentified* (also called *under-identified*) and the results are not trustworthy. At a minimum, there must be more known quantities (e.g., non-redundant elements of Σ_{xx}) than unknown quantities (i.e., parameters to estimate). This is a necessary but not sufficient condition for model identification. Bollen (1989) describes conditions that are sufficient but not necessary for identification that are useful for models matching these criteria. Models with $m > 1$ are identified if there are 3 or more indicators per factor, each indicator has a nonzero loading on only 1 factor, and unique variances are uncorrelated. Only 2 indicators per factor are acceptable if either all the factors are correlated (i.e., Φ has no zeros), or each row of Φ has at least one nonzero off-diagonal element.

Many possible models can be specified and identified which do not match Bollen's (1989) criteria above. Identification can be proven by matrix algebra, but this is tedious, error-prone, and unrealistic for some users. Most software programs detect some types of under-identification and warn users that re-specification may be needed. If identification is uncertain, Jöreskog and Sörbom (1986) suggest fitting the model to data, computing the model-implied covariance matrix, and then re-fitting the model treating the model-implied covariances as if they were observed. If parameter estimates from the two fittings differ, the model is not identified.

In addition to model identification, the scales of all latent variables must be identified in CFA. Typically, unique factors are handled as in EFA: Means are fixed to 0 and variances are free. The scales of common factors also may be identified as in EFA, by fixing the means and variances to 0 and 1, respectively. Alternatively, a common factor can be assigned the scale of one MV to which it is highly related by fixing that MV's loading to 1. This permits estimation of the common-factor variance which is sometimes of interest. Model fit is unaffected by the procedure used to identify the scales of the factors.

4.2. Estimation

A CFA model is usually fitted to data with ML under the assumption that MVs are continuous and multivariate normal. The likelihood is:

$$L_{CFA} = \log\left|\hat{\Sigma}_{xx}\right| + \mathrm{tr}(\Sigma_{xx}\hat{\Sigma}_{xx}^{-1}) - \log|\Sigma_{xx}| - p, \tag{8}$$

where Σ_{xx} is the observed covariance matrix, $\hat{\Sigma}_{xx}$ the model-implied covariance matrix, and "tr" refers to the trace (i.e., sum of diagonal elements). Thus, SEs for factor loadings and inter-factor correlations are available, as is an LR statistic for evaluating model fit that is χ^2-distributed in large samples. The LR statistic is $(N-1)L_{CFA}$ (where L_{CFA} is (Eq. (8)) evaluated at the maximum) with *df* equal to the number of nonredundant elements in Σ_{xx} less than the number of free parameters, t:

$$df = \frac{1}{2}p(p+1) - t \tag{9}$$

CFA models should be fitted to covariance, not correlation, matrices, unless one's software is known to handle correlation matrices correctly (Cudeck, 1989). The statistical theory that justifies CFA does not apply to correlation matrices without modification. Because the procedures are more complicated for correlation versus covariance matrices, many computer programs do not handle correlation matrices appropriately and will provide incorrect SEs (and possibly an incorrect LR statistic). The RAMONA program (Browne et al., 1994) and PROC CALIS in SAS (SAS Institute, 2006) handle correlation matrices appropriately, but with most software programs, it is best to fit a CFA model to a covariance matrix to ensure a proper analysis.

4.3. Evaluation of model fit

After a CFA model has been specified, identification has been addressed, and parameters have been estimated, a fundamental concern is how well the model fits the data. First, there should be no improper parameter estimates. If a correlation is outside the range -1 to 1, or a variance is negative (called a *Heywood case*), the solution should not be interpreted and causes of the problem should be explored. Improper estimates can occur when the population parameter is near the boundary, when outliers or influential observations are present in the data, when the model is poorly specified, or because of sampling variability.

If all parameter estimates are within permissible ranges, global model fit is evaluated. As in EFA, the χ^2-test of absolute fit is sensitive to sample size and could provide misleading results. However, the difference between LR statistics for two nested models provides a useful χ^2-difference test (for large samples) with df equal to the difference in dfs for the two models. A significant difference supports the larger model; otherwise, the more parsimonious model is preferred.

Absolute fit is evaluated using descriptive indices. Available options are abundant and sometimes contradict one another. However, Hu and Bentler (1998, 1999) extensively studied many indices and provide guidance for selecting and interpreting a manageable subset. They recommend reporting one residuals-based measure such as the standardized root mean square residual (SRMR; Bentler, 1995; Jöreskog and Sörbom, 1981), and one or more of the following: (a) the root mean square error of approximation (RMSEA; Browne and Cudeck, 1993; Steiger, 1990; Steiger and Lind, 1980), (b) the Tucker–Lewis (1973) incremental fit index (TLI; also known as the non-normed fit index due to Bentler and Bonett, 1980), (c) Bollen's (1988) non-normed index (Δ_2), and (d) Bentler's (1990) comparative fit index (CFI).

The SRMR summarizes the differences between the observed and model-implied covariance matrices:

$$\text{SRMR} = \sqrt{\frac{2}{p(p+1)} \left\{ \sum_{i=1}^{p} \sum_{j=1}^{i} \left[\frac{(\sigma_{ij} - \hat{\sigma}_{ij})}{\sigma_{ii}\sigma_{jj}} \right]^2 \right\}}, \tag{10}$$

where σ_{ij} is an element of $\boldsymbol{\Sigma}_{xx}$ and $\hat{\sigma}_{ij}$ is an element of $\hat{\boldsymbol{\Sigma}}_{xx}$. Values closer to 0 indicate better fit; Hu and Bentler (1999) suggested that fit is good if SRMR $\leq$ about .09.

The RMSEA indicates the degree of discrepancy between the model and the data per degree of freedom:

$$\text{RMSEA} = \sqrt{\frac{-2L_{\text{CFA}} - \frac{df}{N-1}}{df}}, \tag{11}$$

where L_{CFA} is (Eq. (8)) evaluated at the maximum. Values closer to 0 indicate better fit.

Roughly, model fit is quantified as close (RMSEA $<$ .05), reasonably good (.05 $<$ RMSEA $<$ .08), mediocre (.08 $<$ RMSEA $<$ .10), or unacceptable (RMSEA $>$ .10) (Browne and Cudeck, 1993). Hu and Bentler (1999) suggested that RMSEA $\leq$ about .06 indicates good fit. The RMSEA is unique because under certain assumptions, its sampling distribution is known; thus, CIs can be computed (Browne and Cudeck, 1993; Curran et al., 2003).

The TLI, CFI, and Δ_2 are the incremental fit indices that measure the proportionate improvement in fit by comparing our model to a more restricted, hypothetical baseline model. Usually the baseline model has independent MVs, thus 0 factors. The TLI and Δ_2 indicate where our model lies on a continuum between a hypothetical worst (baseline) model and a hypothetical perfect model, for which the LR statistic equals its df (thus, the ratio is 1):

$$\text{TLI} = \frac{\frac{\chi_b^2}{df_b} - \frac{\chi_m^2}{df_m}}{\frac{\chi_b^2}{df_b} - 1}, \tag{12}$$

and

$$\Delta_2 = \frac{\chi_b^2 - \chi_m^2}{\chi_b^2 - df_m}. \tag{13}$$

Subscripts "b" and "m" refer to the baseline model and the fitted model with m factors.

The CFI shows how much less misfit there is in our model than in the worst-fitting (baseline) model:

$$\text{CFI} = \frac{(\chi_b^2 - df_b) - (\chi_m^2 - df_m)}{\chi_b^2 - df_b}. \tag{14}$$

If our model fits perfectly, $\chi_m^2 = df_m$ and CFI $= 1$. The worst possible fit for our model is $\chi_m^2 = \chi_b^2$ with $df_m = df_b$; thus, CFI $= 0$. The TLI and Δ_2 are also typically between 0 and 1 with larger values indicating better fit, but values outside that range are possible. Hu and Bentler (1999) suggested that values of TLI, CFI, or Δ_2 equal to at least .95 indicate good fit.

It is possible for a model that fits well globally to fit poorly in a specific region; thus additional elements of model fit should be evaluated. Parameter estimates should make sense for the substantive problem, and most factor loadings should be statistically significant. It is useful to screen for extreme residuals, because specific misfit may not be reflected in the SRMR summary statistic. Models that are well matched to the data have moderate to large R^2s for each MV and reliable factors that explain substantial variance in the MVs.

The R^2 is the proportion of total variance in an MV that is accounted for by the common factors (i.e., the communality). Larger values are generally preferred. Fornell and Larcker (1981) recommend interpreting a reliability coefficient, ρ_η, for each factor:

$$\rho_\eta = \frac{\left(\sum_{j=1}^{p} \lambda_j\right)^2}{\left(\sum_{j=1}^{p} \lambda_j\right)^2 + \sum_{j=1}^{p} \sigma_{jj}^2}, \tag{15}$$

where σ_{jj}^2 is the (estimated) unique variance for the jth MV. A rule of thumb is that .7 or larger is good reliability (Hatcher, 1994). Fornell and Larcker (1981) suggest an additional coefficient, $\rho_{vc(\eta)}$, as a measure of the average variance explained by each factor in relation to the amount of variance due to measurement error:

$$\rho_{vc(\eta)} = \frac{\sum_{j=1}^{p} \lambda_j^2}{\sum_{j=1}^{p} \lambda_j^2 + \sum_{j=1}^{p} \sigma_{jj}^2}. \tag{16}$$

If $\rho_{vc(\eta)}$ is less than .50, the variance due to measurement error is larger than the variance measured by the factor; thus, the validity of both the factor and its indicators is questionable (Fornell and Larcker, 1981, p. 46).

5. FA with non-normal continuous variables

In practice, MVs are often not approximately multivariate normal. This should be evaluated before methods described in the previous sections are applied. If ML estimation is used to fit an FA model to non-normal (continuous) data, the LR statistic and SEs are likely to be incorrect (Curran et al., 1996; Yuan et al., 2005; West et al., 1995). Thus, significance tests, CIs, and indices of model fit are potentially misleading. Coefficients and tests of multivariate skewness and kurtosis (e.g., Mardia, 1970) are available in many computer programs and should be used routinely. Outliers can cause non-normality, so screening for outliers also should be common practice.

If non-normality is detected in CFA, one alternative is a weighted least squares estimator called asymptotically distribution free (ADF) (Browne, 1982, 1984). Parameter estimates minimize the sum of squared deviations between $\boldsymbol{\Sigma}_{xx}$ and $\hat{\boldsymbol{\Sigma}}_{xx}$, weighted by approximate covariances among elements of $\boldsymbol{\Sigma}_{xx}$. However, with large p, it becomes impractical to invert the $p \times p$ weight matrix, and it appears that large sample sizes (e.g., 1,000–5,000) are needed for the ADF method to perform well (Curran et al., 1996; West et al., 1995).

A more generally applicable alternative is to use ML with a correction to the LR statistic and SEs. The Satorra–Bentler correction (Satorra and Bentler, 1988; Satorra, 1990) has performed well with moderate sample sizes such as 200–500 (Chou et al., 1991; Curran et al., 1996; Hu et al., 1992; Satorra and Bentler, 1988). It is implemented in the EQS (Bentler, 1989) and Mplus (Muthén and Muthén, 2006) programs for CFA. ML with the Satorra–Bentler correction can also be used for EFA and is implemented in Mplus. If SEs and an LR statistic are not needed, conditional or iterative principle factors could be used for EFA because multivariate normality is not required.

6. FA with categorical variables

Both EFA and CFA are commonly used to assess the dimensionality of questionnaires and surveys. Typically, such items have binary or ordinal response scales; thus, classic FA is not appropriate for several reasons. For one, linear association is not meaningful because absolute distances between categories are unknown. Thus, the classic model of linear association among MVs, and between each MV and the factor(s), is inapplicable. Also, Pearson correlations are attenuated for categorical data, which can lead to underestimates of factor loadings if classic FA is applied. Strictly speaking, discrete variables cannot follow the continuous multivariate normal distribution. Serious biases can result when standard ML is used for FA with Pearson correlations computed from categorical data (DiStefano, 2002; West et al., 1995). An alternative to classic FA is needed for categorical data.

One solution is to posit that a continuous but unobserved distribution underlies the observed categories. In other words, in addition to an observed categorical MV, x, there is an unobserved continuous variable, x^*. It is assumed that the categorization occurs such that:

$$x_1 = \begin{cases} 1, & \text{if } x_1^* \leq \tau_1 \\ 2, & \text{if } \tau_1 < x_1^* \leq \tau_2 \\ \cdots & \cdots \\ c-1, & \text{if } \tau_{c-2} < x_1^* \leq \tau_{c-1} \\ c, & \text{if } \tau_{c-1} < x_1^* \end{cases} \tag{17}$$

where τ_j is the threshold separating category j from $j+1$ and $j = 1, 2, \ldots, c$. While a linear relationship between x and the latent construct(s) is untenable, linearity is reasonable for x^*.

If it can be assumed for a given research context that the observed categorical data arose through a categorization of unobserved continuous data, and that every pair of unobserved variables is bivariate normal, then the correlations among the underlying, continuous variables can be estimated by *polychoric correlations* (called *tetrachoric correlations* when both variables are binary). Typically, a polychoric correlation is computed in two stages (Olsson, 1979). First, τs are estimated for each MV based on the proportions of people responding in each category (and the normality assumption). Second, the correlation between each pair of underlying variables is estimated by ML. The likelihood is a function of the τs and the bivariate frequencies. The classic FA model is then fitted to the matrix of polychoric correlations. However, an alternate estimator is also needed.

Unweighted least squares requires no distributional assumptions about the MVs and produces consistent estimates of the factor loadings. However, SEs, significance tests, and most fit indices are not available; thus, it is only useful for EFA. Weighted least squares (WLS) is a popular alternative that may be used for EFA or CFA. When the asymptotic covariance matrix (i.e., the covariances among all the elements in the covariance matrix among MVs) is used as the weight matrix, WLS can provide accurate estimates of the SEs and the LR statistic. Unfortunately, inversion of the weight matrix (required for WLS) becomes increasingly difficult as the number of MVs increases, and very large sample sizes are needed for accurate estimation (West et al., 1995).

A compromise solution, called diagonally weighted least squares (DWLS; Jöreskog and Sörbom, 2001), uses only the diagonal elements of the asymptotic covariance matrix; thus, the weight matrix is much easier to invert. This results in a loss of statistical efficiency, but corrective procedures (e.g., the Satorra–Bentler correction) can be used to obtain accurate estimates of the SEs and the LR statistic. DWLS with these corrections is sometimes called *robust DWLS*. Recent simulations suggested that robust DWLS performs well, and better than WLS based on a full weight matrix (Flora and Curran, 2004). Robust DWLS is implemented in the LISREL (Jöreskog and Sörbom, 2005) and Mplus (Muthén and Muthén, 2006) programs.

Another way to evaluate the latent dimensionality of categorical MVs is with models and methods in the domain of item response theory (IRT; Embretson and Reise, 2000; Thissen and Wainer, 2001). Unlike FA, IRT models were originally developed for categorical data. As in FA, IRT models are based on the premise that latent variables give rise to observed data, and parameters provide information about relationships between MVs and factor(s). The exploratory–confirmatory continuum described for FA also applies in IRT. In certain circumstances, FA parameters may be converted by simple algebra to IRT parameters (McLeod, Swygert, and Thissen, 2001; Takane and de Leeuw, 1987). Multidimensional IRT (MIRT) methods (i.e., those involving more than one common factor) are sometimes referred to as full information item factor analysis (Bock et al., 1988; Muraki and Carlson, 1995) in acknowledgment of the similarities between classic FA and IRT. "Full information" reflects the fact that

IRT models are fitted to the raw data directly rather than to summary statistics such as polychoric correlations. An ML-based estimation scheme described by Bock and Aitkin (1981) is typically used to fit the models.

MIRT is not as widely used as categorical FA, probably because software development has lagged behind that for FA. At the time of this writing, the commercially available TESTFACT program (v.4; Bock et al., 2002) performs exploratory MIRT and fits one very specific type of hierarchical confirmatory model known as the bi-factor model (Holzinger and Swineford, 1937; Gibbons and Hedeker, 1992). However, the only models implemented are for binary MVs. The ltm package (Rizopoulos, 2006) for R offers slightly more flexibility in the factor structure, but is limited to dichotomous variables and a maximum of two latent factors. The POLYFACT program (Muraki, 1993) performs exploratory MIRT for ordinal MVs, but this program has not been as widely distributed. Software for general kinds of confirmatory MIRT models is not readily available.

MIRT methods are appealing because the model is fitted to the data directly, thus polychoric correlations need not be calculated. However, the disadvantage is that m-dimensional numerical integration is required (m = number of factors); thus, solutions are more difficult to obtain as m increases. Nevertheless, Markov chain Monte Carlo estimation methods may hold promise for use with MIRT models (Edwards, 2006), and we anticipate advancements in software for MIRT in future years.

7. Sample size in FA

For classic FA (without assumption violations), how many observations are needed for accurate estimation? Historically, minimum Ns have been suggested such as 100 (Gorsuch, 1983; Kline, 1979), 200 (Guilford, 1954), 250 (Cattell, 1978), or 300 (Comrey and Lee, 1992), or minimum ratios of N to p such as 3 (Cattell, 1978), or 5 (Gorsuch, 1983; Kline, 1979). More recently, MacCallum, Widaman, Zhang, and Hong (1999) astutely pointed out that such rules of thumb are meaningless because the optimal N depends on characteristics of the study. These authors showed that under certain conditions 60 observations can be adequate, whereas in other situations, more than 400 observations are needed. Results apply to both EFA and CFA.

The theoretical arguments presented by MacCallum et al., 1999 (see also MacCallum and Tucker, 1991) are based on the fact that nonzero correlations between common and unique factors, and among unique factors, are a major source of error in the estimation of factor loadings. The correlations tend to be farther from zero with smaller N. However, small uniquenesses (e.g., $\leq .3$), and highly *overdetermined* factors, having four or more indicators with large loadings, can offset the limitations of small samples. Uniquenesses act as weights on the matrices of correlations between unique and common factors and among unique factors. The less these correlations are weighted, the less impact they have on the FA results. Further, with the number of MVs held constant, increasing the number of indicators per factor reduces m, which reduces the number of correlations among common and unique factors and among unique factors, giving them less overall influence on results.

MacCallum et al. (1999) found that when uniquenesses were small (.2, .3, or .4), accurate recovery of Λ could be achieved with around 60 observations with highly overdetermined factors, and 100 observations with weakly determined factors having 2 or 3 indicators. When uniquenesses were large (.6, .7, or .8), 400 observations were inadequate for recovery of Λ unless the factors had 6 or 7 strong indicators each, in which case $N \geq 200$ was required. When uniquenesses varied over MVs (.2, .3, ..., .8), $N = 60$ provided pretty good recovery of Λ for factors with 6 or 7 strong indicators, but $N \geq 200$ was needed with weakly determined factors. These results were observed both with (MacCallum et al., 2001) and without (MacCallum et al., 1999) mis-specification of the model in the population.

The sample size question is perhaps even more crucial when analyzing categorical MVs. As mentioned above, WLS requires many observations (perhaps several thousand) for stable parameter estimates (Potthast, 1993), primarily because of the potentially massive number of parameters in the weight matrix. Robust DWLS has performed well with smaller samples. For example, Flora and Curran (2004) found that a sample size of 200 was adequate for relatively simple CFA models (e.g., 10 or 20 MVs and 1 or 2 factors), MVs with 2 or 5 categories, and communalities of .49.

With either WLS or robust DWLS, adequate sample size is needed for estimation of polychoric correlations because sparseness in the 2-way contingency tables used in their computation can cause serious instability in the correlation estimate. Sparseness is especially problematic for two dichotomous MVs, because a tetrachoric correlation is inestimable when there is a zero cell in the 2×2 contingency table. In addition, no easily implemented method exists to deal with missingness, and the common practice of listwise deletion can further exacerbate the problem. Robust DWLS is a relatively new procedure and additional research on the sample-size question is warranted.

8. Examples of EFA and CFA

In this section we present three example FAs. Many software packages are capable of estimating some (or all) of the FA models discussed in this chapter. We selected CEFA (Browne et al., 2004) because it is one of the most flexible EFA programs, and we chose LISREL (Jöreskog and Sörbom, 2005), and Mplus (Muthén and Muthén, 2006) to illustrate CFA because they are very popular, easy to use, and have many features. Other popular software programs that perform EFA and CFA include SAS (SAS Institute, 2006), Splus (Insightful Corporation, 2005), and R (R Development Core Team, 2005); all SEM programs carry out CFA. Our examples use only a fraction of currently available options in the selected programs and the software is always expanding and improving. Nevertheless, these examples should provide a valuable introduction to persons unfamiliar with the software or with FA.

8.1. EFA with continuous variables using CEFA

The first example is an EFA carried out using CEFA.[1] Continuous multivariate normal data were simulated using Mplus from a model with three correlated factors and 18 MVs ($N = 400$). For each factor, six different MVs had nonzero loadings, and all other MVs had zero loadings. The population factor loadings and communalities are given in Table 1. Population correlations among factors i and j (ρ_{ij}) were: $\rho_{12} = .3$, $\rho_{13} = .5$, and $\rho_{23} = .4$. The total sample of 400 was divided in half to provide one sample for EFA and another for a follow-up CFA (described in the next section).

For EFA, we analyzed a Pearson correlation matrix using ML (presuming multivariate normality). A scree plot of the eigenvalues, given in Fig. 3, suggests that no more than four factors should be extracted. Table 2 compares the fit of models with between one and four factors. The maximum absolute residual is in a correlation metric; thus, values of .33 and .29 are very large. The information in Table 2 indicates that fit is very poor for the one- and two-factor models. However, the three-factor model fits well, and is not significantly improved upon by the addition of a fourth factor. A χ^2-difference test comparing the three- and four-factor (nested) models is nonsignificant ($\chi^2(15) = 21.99$, $p = .108$). With real data, the substantive interpretability of the rotated factor loadings with different numbers of factors is as important as the fit and should be considered as part of model selection.

Estimated factor loadings, their SEs, and communalities for the three-factor model are given in Table 1. The loadings have been rotated using the oblique quartimax criterion. The estimated parameters match up well with the values used to generate the data. The estimated correlations among factors and their SEs were: $r_{12} = .37$ (.06), $r_{13} = .47$ (.07), and $r_{23} = .44$ (.07). These are also close to the population values.

CEFA is unusual among EFA programs because it provides SEs (and CIs) for the parameters which can be useful for assigning MVs to factors. Often, factor assignment is done using an arbitrary criterion such as "MVs with a loading of .30 or larger load on the factor". Arbitrary criteria are still needed when SEs are available, but sampling variability can be incorporated into the process. In Table 1, the MVs we assigned to each factor are highlighted in bold. In this case, loadings are either small or large so factor assignment is fairly straight-forward.

8.2. CFA with continuous variables using LISREL

Once a structure has been determined from an EFA, it is useful to cross-validate it with CFA using a new sample. Splitting the initial sample in half is often a practical way to cross-validate EFA results. In this section, the other half of the simulated data described in the previous section is analyzed with CFA using LISREL.

---

[1] The CEFA software and user's manual may be downloaded for free from http://faculty.psy.ohio state.edu/browne/software.php.

Table 1
Factor loadings and communalities for the EFA example

MV	Population Values				Sample Estimates ($N = 200$)			
	λ_{j1}	λ_{j2}	λ_{j3}	h_j^2	$\hat{\lambda}_{j1}(SE)$	$\hat{\lambda}_{j2}(SE)$	$\hat{\lambda}_{j3}(SE)$	$\hat{h}_j^2$
1	.6	0	0	.36	**.61** (.06)	−.02 (.07)	.07 (.07)	.41
2	.6	0	0	.36	**.63** (.06)	−.03 (.07)	.04 (.07)	.40
3	.6	0	0	.36	**.48** (.07)	−.12 (.08)	.23 (.08)	.33
4	.7	0	0	.49	**.71** (.06)	.05 (.06)	−.02 (.06)	.52
5	.7	0	0	.49	**.64** (.06)	.07 (.07)	−.05 (.07)	.42
6	.7	0	0	.49	**.71** (.06)	.04 (.06)	−.03 (.06)	.51
7	0	.7	0	.49	−.05 (.05)	**.70** (.06)	.05 (.06)	.50
8	0	.7	0	.49	−.08 (.04)	**.81** (.05)	−.01 (.05)	.60
9	0	.7	0	.49	.07 (.05)	**.65** (.07)	.10 (.06)	.53
10	0	.8	0	.64	.04 (.04)	**.81** (.05)	−.04 (.05)	.65
11	0	.8	0	.64	.05 (.04)	**.80** (.05)	−.03 (.05)	.65
12	0	.8	0	.64	.04 (.04)	**.76** (.05)	−.06 (.05)	.65
13	0	0	.6	.36	−.11 (.06)	.08 (.06)	**.72** (.06)	.50
14	0	0	.6	.36	−.02 (.06)	−.05 (.06)	**.67** (.07)	.41
15	0	0	.6	.36	.06 (.07)	.22 (.08)	**.42** (.08)	.34
16	0	0	.8	.64	.03 (.06)	.10 (.06)	**.65** (.06)	.50
17	0	0	.8	.64	.01 (.05)	.01 (.05)	**.80** (.05)	.66
18	0	0	.8	.64	.11 (.05)	−.06 (.05)	**.75** (.06)	.61

Note: MV, measured variable; λ_{jk}, true factor loading for MV j on factor k; h_j^2, true communality for MV j; $\hat{\lambda}_{jk}(SE)$, estimated factor loading for MV j on factor k, with its standard error; $\hat{h}_j^2$, estimated communality for MV j. The estimated loadings have been rotated using the oblique quartimax criterion.

   Performing CFA in LISREL is a two-stage process. In the first stage, a covariance matrix is estimated from the raw data using the PRELIS program, which is distributed with LISREL. The PRELIS syntax we used is given in Appendix A. The first two lines are the title, followed by a data format line (DA) that specifies the number of indicators (NI), the number of observations (NO), and where the data are stored (FI). The last line tells PRELIS to output (OU) a

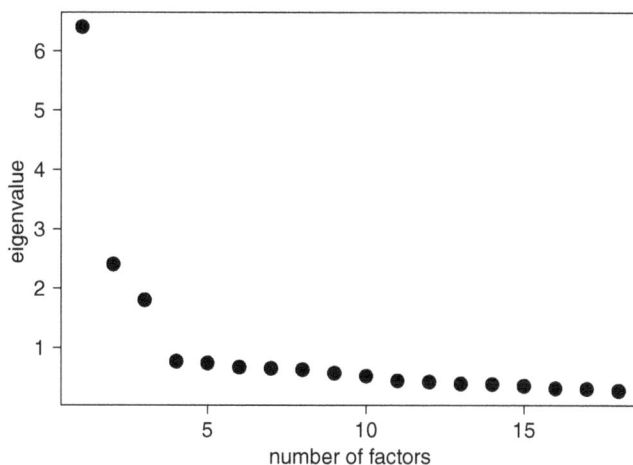

Fig. 3. Scree plot for EFA example.

Table 2
Comparisons among EFA models with differing numbers of factors

m	$\chi^2(df)$	Max. Residual	RMSEA (90% CI)
1	645.64	.33	.14
	(135)		(.13, .15)
2	300.69	.29	.09
	(118)		(.08, .10)
3	105.58	.08	.01
	(102)		(.00, .04)
4	83.59	.09	.00
	(87)		(.00, .04)

Note: m, number of factors; Max. Residual, maximum absolute correlation residual (range: 0–1); RMSEA (90% CI), root mean square error of approximation, with 90% confidence interval.

sample covariance matrix (CM) from the data described in the preceding line. The output file will be created in the same folder as the syntax file.

The second stage is to estimate the CFA model in LISREL. The syntax we used is given in Appendix A. The first line provides a title (TI) for the output file. The second line describes the data (DA) being used in terms of number of indicators (NI), number of observations (NO), number of groups (NG), and the kind of matrix (MA) that is to be analyzed. The third line specifies the file that contains the matrix to be analyzed. The next line contains a model statement (MO) that describes the CFA generally. In addition to indicating the number of MVs to be modeled (NX) and the number of factors (NK), this line indicates how the factor loading matrix (LX), error covariance matrix (TD), and the inter-factor correlation matrix (PH) should be structured. For this example, the error covariance matrix is diagonal (DI) and freely estimated (FR) and the inter-factor correlation matrix is standardized (i.e., it has 1's on the diagonal) and symmetric (ST). The factor-loading matrix is set to be full (FU) and fixed (FI) meaning there is a complete 18 by 3 loading matrix (Λ), but none of the loadings are to be estimated. This is not the model we are interested in, but this is remedied in the next three lines. These lines, each of which begins with FR, indicate to LISREL which elements of the factor loading matrix are to be estimated. For instance, LX 3 1 is the factor loading for the third measured variable on the first factor, found in row 3, column 1 of Λ. The last two lines indicate the output desired. The PD line produces a path diagram of the model being estimated, which is a convenient way to verify that the model being estimated is the desired model. The final line is an output line (OU), which defines the structure of the output file (RS prints residuals, ND $= 2$ sets the number of decimal places in the output file to two) and indicates which method of estimation (ME) should be used (ML indicates maximum likelihood).

There were no improper estimates such as negative variances, thus we proceed to evaluation of model fit. Though LISREL produces numerous global fit statistics, we followed Hu and Bentler's (1999) recommendations (described above) for selecting and evaluating a subset of them. The model fits very well (SRMR: .04; RMSEA: .00 with 90% CI: .00, .03; TLI: 1.00; CFI: 1.00). LISREL also provides a great deal of information about residuals which are differences between the sample covariance matrix and the model-implied covariance matrix (labeled the "fitted covariance matrix" in the output). Residuals are presented in both raw and standardized metrics, and plotted several ways. A model that fits the data well has mostly small residuals that do not show any particular pattern.

The estimated factor loadings, their SEs and the communalities (usually referred to as squared multiple correlations in a CFA context) are given in Table 3. Correlations among factors and their SEs were: $r_{12} = .43$ (.07), $r_{13} = .37$ (.07), and $r_{23} = .54$ (.06). The estimates match the true values reasonably well; accuracy improves with larger samples. LISREL provides t-statistics for testing whether each factor loading or inter-factor correlation is significantly different from 0. All the estimates were significant ($\alpha = .05$) for this example.

8.3. CFA with categorical MVs using Mplus

The data for this example were simulated using Mplus from a model with three correlated factors and 18 MVs ($N = 400$). As before, there were six indicators for each factor. The variables are binary (coded 0 or 1), thus each one has a single threshold parameter. The population thresholds, factor loadings and communalities are given in Table 4. Population correlations among factors were: $\rho_{12} = .3$, $\rho_{13} = .5$, and $\rho_{23} = .4$.

The Mplus syntax we used for the CFA is given in Appendix B. Following the title is the DATA line that specifies a path for the raw data file. The VARIABLE command specifies names for the variables. For the correct analysis, it is extremely important to indicate here that the MVs are categorical. The MODEL statement specifies the model. BY indicates a directional path and WITH requests estimation of a correlation or covariance. In the context of CFA, relationships between MVs and factors are directional paths; thus, "f1 BY y1-y6" indicates that factor 1 should load on MVs y1, y2, y3, y4, y5, and y6. An asterisk

Table 3
Factor loadings and communalities for the CFA example

MV	Sample Estimates ($N = 200$)			
	$\hat{\lambda}_{j1}(SE)$	$\hat{\lambda}_{j2}(SE)$	$\hat{\lambda}_{j3}(SE)$	R_j^2
1	.60 (.07)	–	–	.36
2	.58 (.07)	–	–	.32
3	.57 (.07)	–	–	.31
4	.65 (.07)	–	–	.45
5	.66 (.07)	–	–	.41
6	.79 (.07)	–	–	.59
7	–	.75 (.06)	–	.56
8	–	.73 (.06)	–	.53
9	–	.79 (.07)	–	.56
10	–	.78 (.06)	–	.61
11	–	.91 (.06)	–	.69
12	–	.91 (.06)	–	.72
13	–	–	.58 (.07)	.35
14	–	–	.61 (.07)	.36
15	–	–	.64 (.07)	.42
16	–	–	.75 (.06)	.59
17	–	–	.81 (.06)	.64
18	–	–	.83 (.06)	.67

Note: MV, measured variable; –, loading was fixed to 0 (not estimated); $\hat{\lambda}_{jk}(SE)$, estimated factor loading for MV j on factor k, with its standard error; R_j^2, squared multiple correlation for MV j.

is used to override the default method for setting the scale (fixing the first factor loading for each factor to one) and the last three lines of the MODEL statement fix the factor variances to 1. The ANALYSIS line specifies the estimation method; WLSMV is robust DWLS. Finally, the OUTPUT line controls elements of the output. For categorical MVs, thresholds are obtained by requesting sample statistics (SAMPSTAT).

Table 4
Population parameters for the CFA example with categorical MVs

MV	τ_j	λ_{j1}	λ_{j2}	λ_{j3}	h_j^2
1	−.5	.5	0	0	.25
2	0	.5	0	0	.25
3	.5	.5	0	0	.25
4	−.5	.6	0	0	.36
5	0	.6	0	0	.36
6	.5	.6	0	0	.36
7	−.5	0	.6	0	.36
8	0	0	.6	0	.36
9	.5	0	.6	0	.36
10	−.5	0	.7	0	.49
11	0	0	.7	0	.49
12	.5	0	.7	0	.49
13	−.5	0	0	.5	.25
14	0	0	0	.5	.25
15	.5	0	0	.5	.25
16	−.5	0	0	.7	.49
17	0	0	0	.7	.49
18	.5	0	0	.7	.49

Note: MV, measured variable; τ_j, true threshold for MV j; λ_{jk}, true factor loading for MV j on factor k; h_j^2, true communality for MV j.

There were no improper estimates such as negative variances and global model fit was very good (SRMR: .07; RMSEA: .02; TLI: .98; CFI: .98). The estimated thresholds, factor loadings, their SEs, and the squared multiple correlations are given in Table 5. Correlations among factors and their SEs were: $r_{12} = .48$ (.08), $r_{13} = .48$ (.08), and $r_{23} = .41$ (.07). The estimates are fairly close to the generating values. All of the loadings and inter-factor correlations were significantly ($\alpha = .05$) different from 0 for this example.

For comparison, the analysis was redone using classic WLS (with a full weight matrix). The only change needed in the Mplus input file is the name of the estimator in the ANALYSIS statement. There were no improper estimates or other estimation difficulties, but global model fit declined quite a bit (SRMR: .12; RMSEA: .05; TLI: 88; CFI: .90) compared to the robust DWLS solution. WLS estimates of the thresholds, factor loadings, and communalities are given in Table 5. Correlations among factors and their SEs were: $r_{12} = .49$ (.05), $r_{13} = .55$ (.05), and $r_{23} = .49$ (.04). Two-thirds of the robust DWLS factor loadings are closer to the true values than the WLS estimates. This is consistent with Flora and Curran's (2004) finding that robust DWLS performs better than WLS in smaller (realistic) sample sizes.

9. Additional resources

This has been an introduction to EFA and CFA, with brief mention of the closely related procedures PCA and MIRT. For additional information, readers are referred to several textbooks on FA and related methods (Bartholomew and

Table 5
Factor loadings, thresholds, and communalities for the CFA example with categorical MVs

MV	$\hat{\tau}_j$	Robust DWLS $\hat{\lambda}_{j1}(SE)$	$\hat{\lambda}_{j2}(SE)$	$\hat{\lambda}_{j3}(SE)$	R^2_j	WLS $\hat{\lambda}_{j1}(SE)$	$\hat{\lambda}_{j2}(SE)$	$\hat{\lambda}_{j3}(SE)$	R^2_j
1	−.52	.45 (.08)	–	–	.20	.48 (.06)	–	–	.23
2	−.03	.49 (.07)	–	–	.24	.50 (.05)	–	–	.25
3	.38	.42 (.08)	–	–	.17	.62 (.06)	–	–	.38
4	−.55	.52 (.08)	–	–	.27	.59 (.05)	–	–	.35
5	−.01	.55 (.07)	–	–	.31	.64 (.05)	–	–	.41
6	.43	.64 (.08)	–	–	.41	.66 (.06)	–	–	.44
7	−.44	–	.67 (.06)	–	.45	–	.74 (.04)	–	.54
8	.06	–	.59 (.06)	–	.35	–	.57 (.04)		.33
9	.43	–	.71 (.06)	–	.51	–	.82 (.04)	–	.67
10	−.62	–	.65 (.06)		.43	–	.79 (.04)	–	.62
11	.04	–	.77 (.05)	–	.59	–	.84 (.03)	–	.70
12	.52	–	.78 (.06)	–	.61	–	.74 (.04)	–	.54
13	−.46	–	–	.61 (.06)	.37	–	–	.66 (.04)	.43
14	−.01	–	–	.58 (.06)	.34	–	–	.73 (.04)	.53
15	.53	–	–	.53 (.08)	.28	–	–	.57 (.05)	.32
16	−.57	–	–	.59 (.06)	.35	–	–	.72 (.04)	.52
17	−.01	–	–	.73 (.05)	.54	–	–	.89 (.03)	.80
18	.53	–	–	.69 (.07)	.48	–	–	.86 (.04)	.74

Note: MV, measured variable; $\hat{\tau}_j$, estimated threshold for MV j; $\hat{\lambda}_{jk}(SE)$, estimated factor loading for MV j on factor k, with its standard error; R^2_j, squared multiple correlation for MV j.

Knott, 1999; Bollen, 1989; Brown, 2006; Comrey and Lee, 1992; Gorsuch, 1983; McDonald, 1985; Thissen and Wainer, 2001). Many special issues in FA were not mentioned here, such as multiple group analyses, hierarchical FA, and missing data. Some of these topics are covered in the texts listed above, but developments are ongoing and the methodological literature should be consulted for the most current developments in FA.

Appendix A:. PRELIS and LISREL code for the CFA example with continuous MVs

PRELIS Code

```
PRELIS code to get covariance matrix for
FA chapter continuous CFA example
DA NI = 18 NO = 200 FI = '***insert your directory here***/conFA-2.dat'
OU CM = conFA-2.cm
```

LISREL Code

```
TI FA chapter continuous CFA example
DA NI = 18 NO = 200 NG = 1 MA = CM
CM = conFA-2.cm
MO NX = 18 NK = 3 LX = FU,FI TD = DI,FR PH = ST
FR LX 1 1 LX 2 1 LX 3 1 LX 4 1 LX 5 1 LX 6 1
FR LX 7 2 LX 8 2 LX 9 2 LX 10 2 LX 11 2 LX 12 2
FR LX 13 3 LX 14 3 LX 15 3 LX 16 3 LX 17 3 LX 18 3
PD
OU RS ND = 2 ME = ML
```

Appendix B:. Mplus code for CFA example with categorical MVs

```
TITLE: CFA with categorial measured variables in Mplus
DATA: FILE IS catFA.dat;
VARIABLE: NAMES ARE y1-y18;
    CATEGORICAL ARE y1-y18;
MODEL: f1 BY y1-y6;
    f2 BY y7-y12;
    f3 BY y13-y18;
    f1 WITH f2 f3;
    f2 WITH f3;
    f1 BY y1*.5;
    f2 BY y7*.5;
    f3 BY y13*.5;
    f1@1;
    f2@1;
    f3@1;
!ANALYSIS: ESTIMATOR = WLS;
ANALYSIS: ESTIMATOR = WLSMV;
OUTPUT: SAMPSTAT;
```

References

Bartholomew, D.J., Knott, M. (1999). *Latent Variable Models and Factor Analysis*, 2nd ed. Oxford University Press, New York.

Bartlett, M.S. (1950). Tests of significance in factor analysis. *British Journal of Psychology: Statistical Section* **3**, 77–85.

Bentler, P.M. (1989). *EQS: Structural Equations Program Manual.* BMDP Statistical Software, Los Angeles.

Bentler, P.M. (1990). Comparative fit indices in structural models. *Psychological Bulletin* **107**, 238–246.

Bentler, P.M. (1995). *EQS Structural Equations Program Manual.* Multivariate Software, Encino, CA.

Bentler, P.M., Bonett, D.G. (1980). Significance tests and goodness-of-fit in the analysis of covariance structures. *Psychological Bulletin* **88**, 588–606.

Bock, R.D., Aitkin, M. (1981). Marginal maximum likelihood estimation of item parameters: An application of the EM algorithm. *Psychometrika* **46**, 443–459.

Bock, R.D., Gibbons, R., Muraki, E.J. (1988). Full information item factor analysis. *Applied Psychological Measurement* **12**, 261–280.

Bock, R.D., Gibbons, R., Schilling, S.G., Muraki, E., Wilson, D.T., Wood, R. (2002). *TESTFACT 4 [Computer Software].* Scientific Software International, Inc., Chicago, IL.

Bollen, K. (1988). *A new incremental fit index for general structural equation models.* Paper presented at Southern Sociological Society Meeting, Nashville, TN.

Bollen, K. (1989). *Structural Equations with Latent Variables.* Wiley, New York.

Brown, T.A. (2006). *Confirmatory Factor Analysis for Applied Research.* Guilford Press, New York.

Browne, M.W. (1982). Covariance structures. In: Hawkins, D.M. (Ed.), *Topics in Applied Multivariate Analysis.* Cambridge University Press, Cambridge, pp. 72–141.

Browne, M.W. (1984). Asymptotic distribution free methods in the analysis of covariance structures. *British Journal of Mathematical and Statistical Psychology* **37**, 127–141.

Browne, M.W. (2001). An overview of analytic rotation in exploratory factor analysis. *Multivariate Behavioral Research* **21**, 230–258.

Browne, M.W., Cudeck, R. (1993). Alternative ways of assessing model fit. In: Bollen, K.A., Long, J.S. (Eds.), *Testing Structural Equation Models.* Sage, Newbury Park, CA, pp. 136–162.

Browne, M.W., Cudeck, R., Tateneni, K., Mels, G. (2004). CEFA: Comprehensive Exploratory Factor Analysis, Version 2.00 [Computer software and manual]. Retreived from http://faculty.psy.ohio-state.edu/browne/software.php.

Browne, M.W., Mels, G., Coward, M. (1994). Path analysis: RAMONA. In: Wilkinson, L., Hill, M.A. (Eds.), *Systat: Advanced Applications.* SYSTAT, Evanston, IL, pp. 163–224.

Cattell, R.B. (1966). The scree test for the number of factors. *Multivariate Behavioral Research* **1**, 245–276.

Cattell, R.B. (1978). *The Scientific Use of Factor Analysis.* Plenum, New York.

Chou, C.P., Bentler, P.M., Satorra, A. (1991). Scaled test statistic and robust standard errors for nonnormal data in covariance structure analysis: A Monte Carlo study. *British Journal of Mathematical and Statistical Psychology* **44**, 347–357.

Comrey, A.L., Lee, H.B. (1992). *A First Course in Factor Analysis.* Erlbaum, Hillsdale, NJ.

Crawford, C.B., Ferguson, G.A. (1970). A general rotation criterion and its use in orthogonal rotation. *Psychometrika* **35**, 321–332.

Cudeck, R. (1989). Analysis of correlation matrices using covariance structure models. *Psychological Bulletin* **105**, 317–327.

Cudeck, R. (1991). Noniterative factor analysis estimators with algorithms for subset and instrumental variable selection. *Journal of Educational Statistics* **16**, 35–52.

Curran, P.J., Bollen, K.A., Chen, F., Paxton, P., Kirby, J.B. (2003). Finite sampling properties of the point estimators and confidence intervals of the RMSEA. *Sociological Methods and Research* **32**, 208–252.

Curran, P.J., West, S.G., Finch, J.F. (1996). The robustness of test statistics to nonnormality and specification error in confirmatory factor analysis. *Psychological Methods* **1**, 16–29.

DiStefano, C. (2002). The impact of categorization with confirmatory factor analysis. *Structural Equation Modeling* **9**, 327–346.

Embretson, S.E., Reise, S.P. (2000). *Item Response Theory for Psychologists.* Lawrence Erlbaum Associates, Mahwah, NJ.

Edwards, M.C. (2006). *A Markov chain Monte Carlo approach to confirmatory item factor analysis.* Unpublished doctoral dissertation, University of North Carolina at Chapel Hill, Chapel Hill, NC.

Flora, D.B., Curran, P.J. (2004). An empirical evaluation of alternative methods of estimation for confirmatory factor analysis with ordinal data. *Psychological Methods* **9**, 466–491.

Fornell, C., Larcker, D.F. (1981). Evaluating structural equation models with unobservable variables and measurement error. *Journal of Marketing Research* **18**, 39–50.

Gibbons, R.D., Hedeker, D.R. (1992). Full-information item bi-factor analysis. *Psychometrika* **57**, 423–436.

Gorsuch, R. (1983). *Factor Analysis*, 2nd ed. Erlbaum, Hillsdale, NJ.

Guilford, J.P. (1954). *Psychometric Methods*, 2nd ed. McGraw-Hill, New York.

Guttman, L. (1940). Multiple rectilinear prediction and the resolution into components. *Psychometrika* **5**, 75–99.

Hatcher, L. (1994). *A Step-by-Step Approach to Using SAS for Factor Analysis and Structural Equation Modeling*. SAS, Cary, NC.

Hendrikson, A.E., White, P.O. (1964). PROMAX: A quick method for rotation to oblique simple structure. *British Journal of Statistical Psychology* **17**, 65–70.

Holzinger, K.J., Swineford, F. (1937). The bi-factor model. *Psychometrika* **2**, 41–54.

Horn, J.L. (1965). A rationale and test for the number of factors in factor analysis. *Psychometrika* **30**, 179–185.

Hu, L., Bentler, P.M. (1998). Fit indices in covariance structure modeling: Sensitivity to underparameterized model misspecification. *Psychological Methods* **3**, 424–453.

Hu, L., Bentler, P.M. (1999). Cutoff criteria for fit indexes in covariance structure analysis: Conventional criteria versus new alternatives. *Structural Equation Modeling* **6**, 1–55.

Hu, L., Bentler, P.M., Kano, Y. (1992). Can test statistics in covariance structure analysis be trusted? *Psychological Bulletin* **112**, 351–362.

Insightful Corporation (2005). *S-PLUS Version 7.0 for Windows (Computer Software)*. Insightful Corporation, Seattle, Washington.

Jennrich, R.I., Sampson, P.F. (1966). Rotation for simple loadings. *Psychometrika* **31**, 313–323.

Jöreskog, K.G., Sörbom, D. (1981). *LISREL V: Analysis of linear structural relationships by the method of maximum likelihood*. National Educational Resources, Chicago.

Jöreskog, K.G., Sörbom, D. (1986). *LISREL VI: Analysis of linear structural relationships by maximum likelihood and least square methods*. Scientific Software International, Inc., Mooresville, IN.

Jöreskog, K.G., Sörbom, D. (2001). *LISREL 8: User's Reference Guide*. Scientific Software International, Inc., Lincolnwood, IL.

Jöreskog, K.G., Sörbom, D. (2005). *LISREL (Version 8.72) [Computer Software]*. Scientific Software International, Inc, Lincolnwood, IL.

Kaiser, H.F. (1958). The varimax criterion for analytic rotation in factor analysis. *Psychometrika* **23**, 187–200.

Kline, P. (1979). *Psychometrics and Psychology*. Academic Press, London.

MacCallum, R.C., Widaman, K.F., Zhang, S., Hong, S. (1999). Sample size in factor analysis. *Psychological Methods* **4**, 84–99.

MacCallum, R.C., Tucker, L.R. (1991). Representing sources of error in factor analysis: Implications for theory and practice. *Psychological Bulletin* **109**, 502–511.

MacCallum, R.C., Widaman, K.F., Preacher, K.J., Hong, S. (2001). Sample size in factor analysis: The role of model error. *Multivariate Behavioral Research* **36**, 611–637.

Mardia, K.V. (1970). Measures of multivariate skewness and kurtosis with applications. *Biometrika* **57**, 519–530.

McDonald, R.P. (1985). *Factor Analysis and Related Methods*. Erlbaum, Hillsdale, NJ.

McLeod, L.D., Swygert, K.A., Thissen, D. (2001). Factor analysis for items scored in two categories. In: Thissen, D., Wainer, H. (Eds.), *Test scoring*. Lawrence Erlbaum Associates, Inc., Mahwah, NH, pp. 189–216.

Muraki, E.J. (1993). *POLYFACT [Computer Program]*. Educational Testing Service, Princeton, NJ.

Muraki, E.J., Carlson, J.E. (1995). Full-information factor analysis for polytomous item responses. *Applied Psychological Measurement* **19**, 73–90.

Muthén, L.K., Muthén, B.O. (2006). *Mplus: Statistical Analysis with Latent Variables (Version 4.1) [Computer Software]*. Muthén & Muthén, Los Angeles, CA.

O'Connor, B.P. (2000). SPSS and SAS programs for determining the number of components using parallel analysis and Velicer's MAP test. *Behavior Research Methods, Instrumentation, and Computers* **32**, 396–402.

Olsson, U. (1979). Maximum likelihood estimation of the polychoric correlation coefficient. *Psychometrika* **44**, 443–460.

Potthast, M.J. (1993). Confirmatory factor analysis of ordered categorical variables with large models. *British Journal of Mathematical and Statistical Psychology* **46**, 273–286.

R Development Core Team. (2005). *R: A Language and Environment for Statistical Computing*. R Foundation for Statistical Computing, Vienna, Austria. ISBN 3-900051-07-0, URL http://www.R-project.org.

Rizopoulos, D. (2006). *ltm: Latent Trait Models under IRT, Version 0.5-1*. Retrieved from http://cran.r-project.org/src/contrib/Descriptions/ltm.html.

SAS Institute. (2006). *SAS/STAT Computer Software*. Cary, NC.

Satorra, A. (1990). Robustness issues in structural equation modeling: A review of recent developments. *Quality & Quantity* **24**, 367–386.

Satorra, A., Bentler, P.M. (1988). Scaling corrections for chi-square statistics in covariance structure analysis. *ASA Proceedings of the Business and Economics Section*, 308–313.

SPSS Incorporated. (2006). *SPSS Base 15.0 Computer Software*. Chicago, IL.

Steiger, J.H. (1990). Structural model evaluation and modification: An interval estimation approach. *Multivariate Behavioral Research* **25**, 173–180.

Steiger, J.H., Lind, J.M. (1980). *Statistically-based tests for the number of common factors*. Paper presented at the annual meeting of the Psychometric Society, May, Iowa City, IA.

Takane, Y., de Leeuw, J. (1987). On the relationship between item response theory and factor analysis of discretized variables. *Psychometrika* **52**, 393–408.

Thissen, D., Wainer, H. (eds.) (2001). Test Scoring. Lawrence Erlbaum Associates, Inc., Mahwah, NJ.

Thurstone, L.L. (1947). *Multiple Factor Analysis*. University of Chicago Press, Chicago.

Tucker, L.R., Lewis, C. (1973). A reliability coefficient for maximum likelihood factor analysis. *Psychometrika* **38**, 1–10.

West, S.G., Finch, J.F., Curran, P.J. (1995). Structural equation models with nonnormal variables: Problems and remedies. In: Hoyle, R.H. (Ed.), *Structural Equation Modeling: Concepts, Issues, and Applications*. Sage, Thousand Oaks, CA, pp. 56–75.

Yuan, K., Bentler, P.M., Zhang, W. (2005). The effect of skewness and kurtosis on mean and covariance structure analysis. *Sociological Methods and Research* **34**, 240–258.

Handbook of Statistics, Vol. 27
ISSN: 0169-7161
© 2007 Elsevier B.V. All rights reserved
DOI: 10.1016/S0169-7161(07)27013-0

7

Structural Equation Modeling

Kentaro Hayashi, Peter M. Bentler and Ke-Hai Yuan

Abstract

Structural equation modeling (SEM) is a multivariate statistical technique for testing hypotheses about the influences of sets of variables on other variables. Hypotheses can involve correlational and regression-like relations among observed variables as well as latent variables. The adequacy of such hypotheses is evaluated by modeling the mean and covariance structures of the observed variables. After an introduction, we present the statistical model. Then we discuss estimation methods and hypothesis tests with an emphasis on the maximum likelihood method based on the assumption of multivariate normal data, including the issues of model (parameter) identification and regularity conditions. We also discuss estimation and testing with non-normal data and with misspecified models, as well as power analysis. To supplement model testing, fit indices have been developed to measure the degree of fit for a SEM model. We describe the major ones. When an initial model does not fit well, Lagrange Multiplier (score) and Wald tests can be used to identify how an initial model might be modified. In addition to these standard topics, we discuss extensions of the model to multiple groups, to repeated observations (growth curve SEM), to data with a hierarchical structure (multi-level SEM), and to non-linear relationships between latent variables. We also discuss more practical topics such as treatment of missing data, categorical dependent variables, and software information.

1. Models and identification

1.1. Introduction

Structural equation modeling (SEM) is a multivariate statistical technique designed to model the structure of a covariance matrix (sometimes the structure of a mean vector as well) with a relatively few parameters, and to test the adequacy of such a hypothesized covariance (mean) structure in its ability to reproduce sample covariances (means). An interesting model would be well motivated substantively and provide a parsimonious and adequate representation of the data.

SEM emerged from several different modeling traditions, e.g., multiple regression, path analysis, exploratory factor analysis (Lawley and Maxwell, 1971), confirmatory factor analysis (Jöreskog, 1969), and simultaneous equation models in econometrics. It is meant to be a unifying methodology that can handle these various models as special cases, as well as generalized models that are hard or impossible to handle with earlier methods. Initially, SEM was developed in the social sciences, especially in psychology and sociology, where it is still popular (e.g., MacCallum and Austin, 2000). However, it has become employed as a useful research tool in a variety of other disciplines such as education and marketing to more medically oriented fields such as epidemiology, imaging, and other biological sciences (see e.g., Batista-Foguet et al., 2001; Bentler and Stein, 1992; Davis et al., 2000; Dishman et al., 2002; Duncan et al., 1998; Hays et al., 2005; Peek, 2000; Penny et al., 2004; Shipley, 2000; van den Oord, 2000).

Numerous texts have been written on SEM. Introductory-level textbooks include Byrne (2006), Dunn et al. (1993), Kline (2005), Loehlin (2004), Maruyama (1998), Raykov and Marcoulides (2006). The most well-known intermediate-level text is Bollen (1989). Two more advanced overviews are those of Bartholomew and Knott (1999) and Skrondal and Rabe-Hesketh (2004). Some collections of articles on a variety of topics related to SEM can be found in Berkane (1997), Marcoulides and Schumacker (1996, 2001), and Schumacker and Marcoulides (1998). The most complete and somewhat technical overview is given by the 18 chapters in Lee's (2007) *Handbook of Structural Equation Models*.

Structural models are often represented by a path diagram in which squares represent observed variables, ovals represent hypothesized latent variables, unidirectional arrows represent regression-type coefficients, and bidirectional arrows represent unanalyzed correlations or covariances. Any such diagram is precisely synonymous with a set of equations and variance and covariance specifications (see e.g., Raykov and Marcoulides, 2006 (Chapter 1) for more details). In this section we concentrate on the algebraic and statistical representation.

1.2. Structural equation models

By late 1970s, full SEM formulations were given by several authors. The earliest and most widely known is the factor analytic simultaneous equation model based on the work of Jöreskog, Keesling, and Wiley (see Bentler, 1986 for a history). It is widely known as the Lisrel model, after Jöreskog and Sörbom's (1979, 1981) computer program. Another approach is the Bentler–Weeks model (Bentler and Weeks, 1980). These models are formally equivalent, though differing in apparent mathematical structure. We start with the Bentler–Weeks structure. Let ξ be a vector of independent variables and η be a vector of dependent variables, where "independent" variables may be correlated but, unlike dependent variables, are not explicit functions of other variables. The structural equation that relates these variables is

$$\eta = L\eta + M\xi, \tag{1}$$

where L and M are coefficient matrices. Elements of these matrices are known as path coefficients, and would be shown as unidirectional arrows in a diagram.

Note that this allows dependent variables to be influenced not only by independent variables, as in regression and linear models in general, but also by other dependent variables. Let us denote $B = \begin{pmatrix} L & 0 \\ 0 & 0 \end{pmatrix}$, $\Gamma = \begin{pmatrix} M \\ I \end{pmatrix}$, and $v = \begin{pmatrix} \eta \\ \xi \end{pmatrix}$, where I is the identity matrix of an appropriate order. Then (1) can be expressed in an alternative form

$$v = Bv + \Gamma\xi. \tag{2}$$

Now assume that $I-B$ is non-singular so that the inverse of $I-B$ exists, then

$$v = (I - B)^{-1}\Gamma\xi. \tag{3}$$

This gives an expression of all the variables as a linear combination of the independent variables. For generality, we allow both independent and dependent variables to be observed variables, in the data file, as well as hypothesized latent variables such as factors, residuals, and so on. Thus, we introduce the matrix G whose components are either 1 or 0 which connects v to the observed variables x such that $x = Gv$. Let $\mu = E(x)$, $\mu_\xi = E(\xi)$, $\Sigma = Cov(x)$, and $\Phi = Cov(\xi)$. Various covariances ϕ_{ij} are shown as two-way arrows in path diagrams. The full mean and covariance structure analysis model (MCSA) follows as:

Mean structure : $\mu = G(I - B)^{-1}\Gamma\mu_\xi$ (4)

Covariance structure : $\Sigma = G(I - B)^{-1}\Gamma\Phi\Gamma'(I - B)^{-1'}G'.$ (5)

When the mean structure is saturated, i.e., μ does not have a structure as given by (4), then we may consider only the covariance structure (5). This explains the name covariance structure analysis (CSA) as another generic name for SEM in which means are ignored.

In the above, there is no obvious use of latent variables. Bollen (2002) provides a review of several definitions of such variables. Among these, Bentler's (1982) approach (see also Bentler and Weeks, 1980) is the clearest to differentiate a latent variable model from a measured variable model. In this approach, the ranks or dimensionality of Φ and Σ are compared. If $dim(\Phi) > dim(\Sigma)$, i.e., the dimensionality of the independent variables exceeds that of the data variables, the model is a latent variable model. This means that the measured variables x may be generated by the ξ, but the ξ cannot be generated by the x. This clarifies some traditional controversies in the field, e.g., it follows immediately that principal components analysis is not a latent variable model, since the principal components exist in the space of measured variables; and similarly that factor analysis, although typically talked about as a dimension-reducing method, actually is a dimension-inducing method since the space of factors is at least the number of variables plus one.

In a simple variant of the factor analytic simultaneous equation model, the measurement model, a factor analysis model, relates observed to latent variables via

$$x = \mu + \Lambda\xi + \varepsilon. \tag{6}$$

Here Λ is a matrix of factor loadings, ξ a vector of factors, and ε a vector of residuals often known as unique variates. The simultaneous equation model relates the latent variables to each other via

$$\xi = B\xi + \zeta, \tag{7}$$

where B is a coefficient matrix and ζ a vector of residuals. Equation (7) allows any factor ξ_i to be regressed on any other factor ξ_j. Assuming no correlations between ξ, ζ, ε, and a full rank $(I-B)$, we can rewrite

$$\xi = (I - B)^{-1}\zeta, \tag{8}$$

$$x = \mu + \Lambda(I - B)^{-1}\zeta + \varepsilon. \tag{9}$$

If the means are unstructured, $\mu = E(x)$. With a structure, we take $\mu = 0$ in (9) and let $\mu_\zeta = E(\zeta)$, and with the covariance matrix of the ζ and the ε given as Φ_ζ and Ψ, respectively, the mean and covariance structure of the model are given as:

$$\mu = \Lambda(I - B)^{-1}\mu_\zeta, \tag{10}$$

$$\Sigma = \Lambda(I - B)^{-1}\Phi_\zeta\{(I - B)^{-1}\}'\Lambda' + \Psi. \tag{11}$$

This representation makes it easy to show that the confirmatory factor analysis model

$$\Sigma = \Lambda\Phi_\zeta\Lambda' + \Psi \tag{12}$$

can be obtained as a special case by setting $B = 0$.

These two representation systems can also be made even more abstract. Considering the elements of the matrices in (4)–(5) or (10)–(11) as generic parameters arranged in the vector θ, we may write the SEM null hypothesis as $\mu = \mu(\theta)$ and $\Sigma = \Sigma(\theta)$. The statistical problem is one of estimating the unknown parameters in θ, and evaluating whether the population means μ and covariances Σ are consistent with the null hypothesis or whether $\mu \neq \mu(\theta)$ and/or $\Sigma \neq \Sigma(\theta)$. This notation can be made even more compact by arranging $\beta = \{\mu', vech(\Sigma)'\}'$, where $vech(A)$ vectorizes the lower or upper triangle of a symmetric matrix A, and writing $\beta = \beta(\theta)$. When only a covariance structure is of interest, we may write $\sigma = \sigma(\theta)$, where $\sigma = vech(\Sigma)$. We use this notation extensively.

1.3. Model identification

Clearly SEM models can have many parameters, and hence, the identification of parameters in the model is an important issue. Model identification is discussed in detail in Bollen (1989) and especially in Bekker et al. (1994). The concept of model degrees of freedom is essential to understand identification. Let p be the number of observed variables. The number of non-redundant elements in the mean vector and covariance matrix is $p + p(p + 1)/2$. Then the degrees of freedom in SEM is given by $df = p(p + 1)/2 + p - q_1$ for MCSA; $df = p(p + 1)/2 - q_2$ for

CSA, where q_1 and q_2 are the number of parameters to be estimated. When the model *df* is positive, that is, when the number of non-redundant elements in the means and covariance matrix exceed the number of parameters, the model is said to be *over-identified*; when the model *df* is negative, the model is said to be *under-identified*; and when the model *df* is exactly zero, the model is said to be *just-identified*. Here, note that over-identification does not necessarily guarantee that the model can be identified. Over-identified models, if identified, are testable; under-identified models cannot be tested; and just-identified models also cannot be tested but simply represent a mapping of the data into an equivalent model structure.

Generic necessary conditions for model identification are given in many introductory textbooks (e.g., Raykov and Marcoulides, 2006). These are as follows:

(i)   There are constraints to determine the scale of each of independent latent variables, which is typically done by either setting one of the coefficients to a fixed constant for each latent independent variable, or setting the variance of each to a fixed constant.
(ii) *df* needs to be non-negative ($df \geq 0$, that is, the model is not under-identified).
(iii) There are at least two (sometimes three) observed variables for each latent variable.

Note that the above three generic conditions are necessary but not sufficient conditions. Therefore, satisfying these conditions does not necessarily guarantee model identification. As we discuss next, identification serves as one of the regularity conditions for estimation of parameters.

2. Estimation and evaluation

2.1. Regularity conditions

The following regularity conditions are typical.

(i)   *Compactness*: The true parameter vector $\boldsymbol{\theta}_0$ belongs to a compact subset of the multi-dimensional (q-dimensional) Euclidian space, where q is the number of parameters; $\boldsymbol{\theta}_0 \in \boldsymbol{\Theta} \subset \boldsymbol{R}^q$.
(ii) *Identification*: The model structure is identified; $\boldsymbol{\beta}(\boldsymbol{\theta}) = \boldsymbol{\beta}(\boldsymbol{\theta}_0)$ implies $\boldsymbol{\theta} = \boldsymbol{\theta}_0$.
(iii) *Differentiability*: $\boldsymbol{\beta}(\boldsymbol{\theta})$ is twice continuously differentiable.
(iv) *Rank condition 1*: The matrix of partial derivatives $\dot{\boldsymbol{\beta}} = \partial \boldsymbol{\beta}(\boldsymbol{\theta})/\partial \boldsymbol{\theta}'$ is of full rank.
(v)   *Rank condition 2*: The covariance matrix of $(\boldsymbol{x}_i' \{vech((\boldsymbol{x}_i-\boldsymbol{\mu}_0)(\boldsymbol{x}_i-\boldsymbol{\mu}_0)')\}')'$ is of full rank.

Note that (1) Conditions (i) and (ii) are required for the consistency of the parameter estimates; (2) Conditions (iii) and (iv) are required for asymptotic normality; (3) Condition (v) is needed for the parameter estimates or the test statistics for the overall model to have proper asymptotic distributions; and (4) Condition (v) is typically satisfied in real data unless there are artificial dependencies among variables. These conditions imply that the information matrix is positive definite. In practice, rank deficiency in the estimated information matrix provides a clue as to lack of identification of the model (see e.g., Browne, 1984; Shapiro, 1984; Kano, 1986; Yuan and Bentler, 1997a for further discussions on regularity conditions in SEM).

2.2. Estimation methods and the corresponding fit functions

(1) *Estimation methods*: Based on a sample of size n, we may estimate the unstructured population mean vector and covariance matrix by $\bar{x}$ and S. Currently, there are four major estimation methods in SEM based on these unstructured estimates. They are: (i) LS (least squares), (ii) GLS (generalized least squares), (iii) ML (maximum likelihood), and (iv) ADF (asymptotic distribution free) (Browne, 1984). The first three are variants of methods routinely used in other areas of statistics such as multiple regression. The LS method is distribution free. The GLS and ML method are based on the assumption of multivariate normality of the variables to be analyzed. The ADF method, a minimum χ^2 method (see Ferguson, 1958, 1996), was developed to provide correct statistics regardless of the distribution of variables.

(2) *Fit functions*: For each estimation method there is a so-called fit function or discrepancy function to be minimized using some algorithm. The fit functions for MCSA are:

(i) LS : $F_{\text{LS}} = (\bar{x} - \boldsymbol{\mu}(\boldsymbol{\theta}))'(\bar{x} - \boldsymbol{\mu}(\boldsymbol{\theta})) + (1/2)tr(S - \boldsymbol{\Sigma}(\boldsymbol{\theta}))^2$, where $tr(A)$ is the trace operator of a square matrix A.

(ii) GLS : $F_{\text{GLS}} = (\bar{x} - \boldsymbol{\mu}(\boldsymbol{\theta}))'S^{-1}(\bar{x} - \boldsymbol{\mu}(\boldsymbol{\theta})) + (1/2)tr(\boldsymbol{\Sigma}(\boldsymbol{\theta})S^{-1} - I_{\text{p}})^2$;

(iii) ML : $F_{\text{ML}} = (\bar{x} - \boldsymbol{\mu}(\boldsymbol{\theta}))'\boldsymbol{\Sigma}(\boldsymbol{\theta})^{-1}(\bar{x} - \boldsymbol{\mu}(\boldsymbol{\theta})) + tr(S\boldsymbol{\Sigma}(\boldsymbol{\theta})^{-1}) - \log|S\boldsymbol{\Sigma}(\boldsymbol{\theta})^{-1}| - p$, where $|A|$ is the determinant of a matrix A.

(iv) ADF : $F_{\text{ADF}} = (t - \boldsymbol{\beta}(\boldsymbol{\theta}))'\hat{V}^{-1}(t - \boldsymbol{\beta}(\boldsymbol{\theta}))$,

where $t = (\bar{x}', s')'$, $s = vech(S)$, and V is the asymptotic covariance matrix of t which is expressed as a partitioned matrix $\begin{pmatrix} V_1 & V_{12} \\ V_{21} & V_2 \end{pmatrix}$, where $V_1 = \boldsymbol{\Sigma}$, the elements of V_{12} are $E\{(x_i-\mu_i)(x_j-\mu_j)(x_k-\mu_k)\}$, $V_{21} = V'_{12}$, and the elements of V_2 are $E\{(x_i-\mu_i)(x_j-\mu_j)(x_k-\mu_k)(x_l-\mu_l)\}-\sigma_{ij}\sigma_{kl}$ (cf., Bentler, 1995, pp. 211–212). Clearly, the ADF method assumes the existence of the finite fourth-order moments. Since these may be hard to estimate, the use of ADF requires a huge sample size (see e.g. Hu et al., 1992).

Clearly these fit functions simplify in CSA without a mean structure. For (i)–(iii), in CSA the first term can be dropped, since with a "saturated" mean structure, $\hat{\mu} = \bar{x}$. In CSA with ADF, the fit function in (iv) is reduced to $F_{\text{ADF}} = (s - \boldsymbol{\sigma}(\boldsymbol{\theta}))'\hat{V}_2^{-1}(s - \boldsymbol{\sigma}(\boldsymbol{\theta}))$.

2.3. Maximum likelihood estimation with normal data

Because a maximum likelihood estimator (MLE) is known to have some good properties, we further discuss parameter estimation and model evaluation by

ML. First, we summarize the results for ML with normal data. Under the null hypothesis of correct model structure:

(i) *Test statistic*: The test statistic

$$T_{ML} = (n-1)F_{ML} \tag{13}$$

is known to converge in distribution to a χ^2 distribution with $df = p(p+1)/2 + p - q_1$ for MCSA and with $df = p(p+1)/2 - q_2$ for CSA, where n is the sample size.

(ii) *Asymptotic normality*: When the data are from a multivariate normal distribution with true population mean vector and true population covariance matrix, the estimators are *consistent* and *asymptotic normal*, that is,

$$\sqrt{n}(\hat{\theta} - \theta_0) \rightarrow N(0, \Omega_{ML}), \tag{14}$$

where the covariance matrix is $\Omega_{ML} = (\dot{\beta}' W^* \dot{\beta})^{-1}$ with the weight matrix $W^* = \begin{pmatrix} \Sigma^{-1} & 0 \\ 0 & W \end{pmatrix}$ with $W = (1/2)D'_p(\Sigma^{-1} \otimes \Sigma^{-1})D_p$, where the duplication matrix D_p (Magnus and Neudecker, 1999) is defined such that $\text{vec}(\Sigma) = D_p\text{vech}(\Sigma)$. To compute MLEs we need to employ some algorithm for optimization, see e.g., Lee and Jennrich (1979) and Yuan and Bentler (2000b), among others.

Test statistics based on the other estimation methods are also possible. The simplest case is with GLS, where $T_{GLS} = (n-1)F_{GLS}$. Browne (1974) showed that for CSA with normal data, T_{GLS} and T_{ML} are asymptotically equivalent. This was extended to the MCSA by Yuan and Chan (2005), who showed that the asymptotic equivalence of T_{GLS} and T_{ML} does not depend on the distribution of data but on the correctness of the model structure. That is, the asymptotic equivalence holds for MCSA as long as the model is specified correctly. Similarly, the estimators $\hat{\theta}_{ML}$ and $\hat{\theta}_{GLS}$ are asymptotically equivalent.

2.4. Maximum likelihood estimation with non-normal data

(1) *Consistency and asymptotic normality*: It is natural to question whether ML is still valid if the data are not from a multivariate normal distribution. It has been shown that:

(i) *Consistency*: The parameter estimates are still consistent as long as $\beta(\theta)$ is identified and correctly specified.

(ii) *Asymptotic normality*: With non-normal data, asymptotic normality still holds with a modified covariance matrix of the estimator as follows:

$$\sqrt{n}(\hat{\theta} - \theta_0) \rightarrow N(0, \Omega_{SW}), \tag{15}$$

with the sandwich-type covariance matrix

$$\Omega_{SW} = (\dot{\beta}' W^* \dot{\beta})^{-1}(\dot{\beta}' W^* V W^* \dot{\beta})(\dot{\beta}' W^* \dot{\beta})^{-1}, \tag{16}$$

where V and W^* were defined above. The sandwich-type covariance matrix was originated in Huber (1967) and it has been used in SEM by many researchers (e.g., Bentler, 1983; Bentler and Dijkstra, 1985; Browne, 1984; Browne and Arminger, 1995; Satorra and Bentler, 1994; Shapiro, 1983; Yuan and Bentler, 1997b). Note that when the data are from a multivariate normal distribution, $W^* = V^{-1}$ in Eq. (16) and Ω_{SW} is reduced to Ω_{ML} in Eq. (14).

(2) *Satorra–Bentler rescaled statistic*: For CSA (i.e., with saturated means) with correctly specified models, T_{ML} can be approximated by a weighted sum of independent χ^2 distributions with 1 degree of freedom, that is

$$T_{ML} \to \sum_{i=1}^{df} \kappa_i \chi^2_{i(1)} \quad \text{as} \quad n \to \infty, \tag{17}$$

where κ_i's are the nonzero eigenvalues of UV_2, with

$$U = W - W\dot{\sigma}(\dot{\sigma}' W\dot{\sigma})^{-1}\dot{\sigma}' W, \tag{18}$$

(cf. e.g. the appendix of Yuan et al., 2002). When data are normal, the weights κ_i's are all 1 and T_{ML} approaches a χ^2 distribution with $df = p(p+1)/2 - q_2$. For CSA, Satorra and Bentler (1988, 1994, 2001) observed the relation $tr(UV_2) = \sum_{i=1}^{df} \kappa_i$ and proposed

$$T_{RML} = T_{ML}/\hat{\kappa} \quad \text{with} \quad \hat{\kappa} = tr(\hat{U}\hat{V}_2)/df, \tag{19}$$

which is known as the *Satorra–Bentler rescaled statistic*. Simulation studies (Curran et al., 1996; Hu et al., 1992; Yuan and Bentler, 1998a) have shown that this rescaled statistic works quite well under a variety of conditions. Technically, however, the Satorra–Bentler rescaled statistic only corrects the scaling such that the expected ML test statistic matches the degrees of freedom of the model, i.e., $E(T_{ML}) = df$. It does not correct the distributional shape to that of χ^2 (Yuan and Bentler, 1998a; Bentler and Yuan, 1999). Satorra and Bentler also proposed an adjusted statistic that corrects the variance in addition to the mean.

Similarly to CSA, for MCSA with correctly specified models, T_{ML} can be approximated by the weighted sum of independent χ^2 distributions with 1 degree of freedom, with the weights being the nonzero eigenvalues of U^*V where

$$U^* = W^* - W^*\dot{\beta}(\dot{\beta}' W^*\dot{\beta})^{-1}\dot{\beta}' W^* \tag{20}$$

(Yuan and Bentler, 2006). Thus the Satorra–Bentler rescaled statistic for MCSA can be defined as a simple extension of that for CSA, that is, $T_{ML} = T_{ML}/\hat{\kappa}^*$ with $\hat{\kappa}^* = tr(\hat{U}^*\hat{V})/df$ with $df = p(p+1)/2 + p - q_1$. Clearly this is of the same form as in CSA.

(3) *Corrected ADF and F-statistics*: With normal distribution-based MLE from non-normal data, Browne (1984) proposed a residual-based ADF statistic in the context of CSA. Unlike the Satorra–Bentler rescaled statistic, the residual-based ADF statistic asymptotically follows a χ^2 distribution regardless of the distribution form of the data. However, like the ADF statistic, the residual-based ADF statistic needs a huge sample size to have its behavior described by a χ^2 distribution. In the context of MCSA, a corrected ADF statistic and an F-statistic were developed by Yuan and Bentler (1997a) and

Yuan and Bentler (1999c), respectively. Their residual-based versions were given in Yuan and Bentler (1998a). All the four statistics are asymptotically distribution free and also perform well with finite sample sizes that are commonly encountered in practice (Bentler and Yuan, 1999).

(4) *Finite mixtures*: When the distribution is very different from normality, use of finite mixtures may be appropriate. See e.g., Yung (1997) and Hoshino (2001) on this point. Finite mixture SEMs have become very popular (e.g., Lubke and Muthén, 2005), but they are problematic to use and can falsely discover typologies when none exist (Bauer and Curran, 2003, 2004).

2.5. Robustness

Although we made a distinction between methods based on normal distribution theory and distribution-free methods, there are times where normal theory statistics can be used because they are robust to violation of distributional assumptions. Anderson and Amemiya (1988) and Amemiya and Anderson (1990) established the asymptotic robustness of SEM in the factor analysis context, namely that when (i) factors and error vector are independent and (ii) the elements of the error vector are also independent, then T_{ML} asymptotically follows a χ^2 distribution and information-based standard errors for factor loadings will be correct. The results were generalized in various direction by Browne and Shapiro (1988), Kano (1992), Mooijaart and Bentler (1991), Satorra (1992, 2002), Satorra and Bentler (1990), and Yuan and Bentler (1999a, 1999b). Unfortunately, there are two problems in applications. It is hard to know whether these independence conditions are met in any real data situation. Also, this is an asymptotic theory, and it is hard to know when it will work with moderate sample sizes.

Another approach to estimation with non-normal data is to employ a method that does not make a strong assumption such as multivariate normality. Historically, elliptical distributions provided the first generalization of non-normality used in SEM (e.g., Bentler and Berkane, 1985; Browne and Shapiro, 1988; Kano et al., 1993; Shapiro and Browne, 1987; Tyler, 1983; see Fang et al., 1990, on elliptical distributions). Elliptical distributions include heavy-tailed distributions with different degrees of multivariate kurtosis (Mardia, 1970) such as the multivariate *t*-distribution, however, they have a drawback of not allowing any skewed distributions. A more general distribution that allows heterogeneous kurtosis parameters also has been developed for CSA (Kano et al., 1990).

In classical statistics, case weighting to achieve robust statistics has a long history (see e.g. Huber, 1964, 1981; Hampel et al., 1986). This methodology has been extended to SEM (Yuan and Bentler, 1998c). A promising approach to robust procedures in SEM is based on M-estimators. Maronna (1976) obtained the properties of the M-estimators for the population mean vector and covariance matrix. The two commonly used weight functions for the M-estimators are (i) Huber-type weights and (ii) weights based on multivariate *t*-distribution. The robust transformation by Yuan et al. (2000) is a useful robust procedure based on the M-estimator approach that can be applied to SEM (see also Yuan et al., 2004, and the appendix of Yuan, 2005). Their robust transformation can be used in a variety of situations (e.g., Hayashi and Yuan, 2003). Concretely speaking the M-estimators are defined as follows: Let

$$d(x_i, \mu, \Sigma) = [(x_i - \mu)'\Sigma^{-1}(x_i - \mu)]^{1/2}, \tag{21}$$

with

$$\mu = \sum_{i=1}^{n} u_1(d_i)x_i / \sum_{i=1}^{n} u_1(d_i), \tag{22}$$

$$\Sigma = \sum_{i=1}^{n} u_2(d_i^2)(x_i - \mu)(x_i - \mu)'/n. \tag{23}$$

The weight functions are defined through a tuning parameter ρ that gives the percentage of influential cases we want to control, and r is a constant determined through $P(\chi_p^2 > r^2) = \rho$. Then the weight functions u_1 and u_2 are given by

$$u_1(d_i) = 1 \qquad \text{if} \quad d_i \le r,$$
$$ r/d_i \quad \text{if} \quad d_i > r, \tag{24}$$

$$u_2(d_i) = \{u_1(d_i)\}^2/\varphi, \tag{25}$$

where φ is a constant determined by ρ through $E\{\chi_p^2 u_2(\chi_p^2)\} = p$. Note that equations (22) and (23) can be solved by iteration, and let $\hat{\mu}$ and $\hat{\Sigma}$ be the solution of (22) and (23), respectively. Yuan et al. (2004) proposed to choose ρ based on empirical efficiency by applying the bootstrap to the transformed sample (Yuan et al., 2000)

$$x_i^{(p)} = \sqrt{u_{2i}}(x_i - \hat{\mu}), \tag{26}$$

where $u_{2i} = u_2\{d_2(x_i, \hat{\mu}, \hat{\Sigma})\}$; the optimal ρ corresponds to the most efficient parameter estimates. Yuan et al. (2000) and Yuan and Hayashi (2003) proposed alternative rationales for choosing ρ. Other approaches to robust SEM are developed in Yuan and Bentler (1998b, 2000b) and Yuan et al. (2004). For other forms of M-estimator, see e.g., Campbell (1980).

2.6. Misspecification and power

(1) *Model misspecification*: Any model is only an approximation to the truth. This implies that we inevitably encounter misspecified models in SEM. Misspecified models are known to create: (i) biases to parameter estimates; (ii) inconsistent standard errors; and (iii) an invalid asymptotic distribution of the χ^2 test statistic (White, 1982). A brief summary of research on model misspecification in SEM is as follows:

   (i) *Consistency*: Many parameter estimates in CSA and MCSA are still consistent even when the model is misspecified (Yuan et al., 2003; Yuan and Bentler, 2006).

(ii) *Convergence in distribution*: The test statistics under misspecified models can be approximated by the non-central χ^2 distribution. However, a problem in this approximation is that it requires the assumption of a sequence of local alternative hypotheses, which may not be realistic in practice. Alternatively, we can employ the asymptotic normal distribution (Vuong, 1989; Yanagihara et al., 2005; Yuan et al., 2007). Based on the approach by Vuong (1989), Yuan et al. (2007) derived the following normal approximation:

$$\sqrt{n}(T_{\mathrm{ML}}/n - \mu) \to N(0, \omega_{\mathrm{ML}}^2), \tag{27}$$

where $\mu = F_{\mathrm{ML}} + tr(U_*V)/n$ and ω_{ML}^2 is quite involved; the formulas for U_* and ω_{ML}^2 are given in Yuan et al. (in press). Here, note that the second term $tr(U_*V)/n$ substantially improves the normal approximation. For additional recent research, see Li and Bentler (2006).

(2) *Power*: Misspecification of the model means that the null hypothesis $\beta = \beta(\theta)$ on the mean and covariance structure is wrong. Thus, it is tightly connected with the concept of power. There are two main approaches to obtaining power in SEM:

(i) *Non-central χ^2 distribution*: Among the approaches to obtain power, the most common approach is based on a non-central χ^2 distribution. The references include Satorra and Saris (1985); Saris and Satorra (1993); Kim (2005); MacCallum et al. (1996); Hancock (2001). The Satorra and Saris (1985) approach requires a specification of the model under the alternative hypothesis, which can be quite complicated in a heavily parameterized model. Later they relaxed the requirement (Saris and Satorra, 1993). MacCallum et al. (1996) developed an approach where the degree of misspecification can be measured by the RMSEA fit index (see below), which does not require specification of specific alternative values for various parameters. In addition to testing the standard exact fit null hypothesis, they also discussed assessment of "close" fit. Statistical justifications for such approach are only recently being developed (Li and Bentler, 2006).

(ii) *Bootstrap approach*: A problem in using the non-central χ^2 distribution to evaluate power is that the meaning of a non-centrality parameter is not clear when the behavior of the test statistic cannot be described by a χ^2 variates (Yuan and Marshall, 2004). Because of its flexibility, the bootstrap has frequently been used in SEM (Beran and Srivastava, 1985; Bollen and Stine, 1993; Yung and Bentler, 1996; Yuan and Hayashi, 2006), and recently, it has been used to develop a promising approach to power (Yuan and Hayashi, 2003). On the bootstrap in general, see e.g., Beran (1986) or Davison and Hinkley (1997). According to Yuan and Hayashi (2003), for data sets with heavy tails, the bootstrap can be applied to a transformed sample by a downweighting procedure as in (26) (Yuan et al., 2000), which has the advantage of not requiring the assumption that the data come from a multivariate normal distribution.

Besides methods based on the non-central χ^2 distribution or the bootstrap, there are other approaches to power such as simulation (see e.g., Muthén and Muthén, 2002, and Mooijaart, 2003).

2.7. Fit indices

Besides the test statistics T, there exist numerous so-called fit indices to measure the degree of overall fit of a model to data. χ^2 tests inherently have the following two major problems in practice. The first problem is that $T = (n-1)F$ increases as n increases. As a result, any model structure null hypothesis such as (12) will tend to be rejected when the sample size n gets large enough, yet the model may be good enough for practical purposes. Another problem is that in SEM, the role of null and alternative hypothesis is reversed compared to classical hypothesis testing. As the positer of a model (such as (12)), we hope to retain the null hypothesis. Because of these shortcomings, fit indices based on test statistics have been developed. The statistical properties of some fit indices are known (e.g., Ogasawara, 2001), and simulation studies are needed to fully understand the behaviors of various fit indices (see e.g., Hu and Bentler, 1998, 1999). While many fit indices have been proposed, only a few are frequently used (McDonald and Ho, 2002) and we limit our discussion to those.

There are several ways to classify fit indices (e.g., Tanaka, 1993). Recently, Yuan (2005) classified fit indices based on their distributional assumptions. For convenience, we classify fit indices into the following four categories: (i) residual-based; (ii) independence-model-based; (iii) root mean square error of approximation; and (iv) information-criterion-based fit indices. The first two types are only appropriate to covariance structures.

(1) *Residual-based fit indices* (see e.g., Jöreskog and Sörbom, 1981): The following three are all the functions of the residuals $S - \Sigma(\hat{\theta})$.
   (i) *Standardized root mean square residual (SRMR)*: As the name shows, SRMR is the square root of the sum of squares of the residuals in a correlation metric. SRMR is given by

$$\text{SRMR} = \sqrt{\frac{2}{p(p+1)} \sum_{i \leq j} \{s_{ij} - \sigma_{ij}(\hat{\theta})\}^2 / s_{ii}s_{jj}}, \tag{28}$$

where $\sigma_{ij}(\hat{\theta})$ is the (i, j) element of $\Sigma(\hat{\theta})$. Obviously, when the value of SRMR is small and close to zero, the fit is good.
   (ii) *Goodness of fit index (GFI)*: GFI has been compared to a squared multiple correlation in multiple regression. GFI is given by

$$\text{GFI} = 1 - \frac{tr[\{\Sigma(\hat{\theta})^{-1}(S - \Sigma(\hat{\theta}))\}^2]}{tr[\{\Sigma(\hat{\theta})^{-1}S\}^2]}. \tag{29}$$

When the value of GFI is close to 1, the fit is good.
   (iii) *Adjusted goodness of fit index (AGFI)*: AGFI corresponds to the squared multiple correlation adjusted for degrees of freedom. AGFI is given by

$$\text{AGFI} = 1 - \frac{p(p+1)(1 - GFI)}{p(p+1) - 2q_2}. \tag{30}$$

When the value of AGFI is close to 1, the fit is good. AGFI is always less than or equal to GFI.

(2) *Independence-model-based fit indices*: The independence model is defined as model in which the covariance structure is diagonal: $\Sigma_I = \text{diag}(\sigma_{11}, \ldots, \sigma_{pp})$. Clearly the independence model is the smallest (i.e., most constrained) model in SEM. In contrast, the largest model is the saturated model (Bentler and Bonett, 1980). The idea of these 0–1 fit indices is to locate the current model along a line between the independence model and the saturated model, where 0 is a model no better than the independence model and 1 is a model as good as the saturated model. Let T_M and T_I be the test statistics under the current model and the independence model, respectively, and let df_M and df_I be the associated degrees of freedom.

(i) *Normed fit index* (*NFI*; Bentler and Bonett, 1980): NFI is given by the relative location of the current model between the saturated model with $T_S = 0$ and the independence model T_I:

$$\text{NFI} = 1 - \frac{T_M}{T_I}. \tag{31}$$

NFI ranges between 0 and 1, and a value of NFI close to 1 means a good fit. An advantage of this index is that it can be defined even if T is only a descriptive statistic that has no known distribution.

(ii) *Non-normed fit index* (*NNFI*; Bentler and Bonett, 1980; Tucker and Lewis, 1973): Originally, Tucker and Lewis (1973) proposed what is now called the Tucker–Lewis index (TLI) in the context of exploratory factor analysis. NNFI is an extension of TLI to SEM. When the sample size n is not large, NFI is known to have a drawback of not approaching 1 even if the current model is correct. NNFI corrects this drawback by introducing the model degrees of freedom, as follows:

$$\text{NNFI} = 1 - \frac{(T_M/d_M) - 1}{(T_I/d_I) - 1}. \tag{32}$$

When the current model is correct, the expected value of T_M should be close to its degrees of freedom df_M. Thus, T_M/df_M should be close to 1. However, NNFI can exceed 1.

(iii) *Comparative fit index* (*CFI*; Bentler, 1990): Bentler (1990) proposed to use population non-centrality parameters to define an index like (31):

$$\text{CFI} = 1 - \frac{\tau_M}{\tau_I}. \tag{33}$$

In practice, CFI is estimated using $\hat{\tau}_M = \max\{T_M - df_M, 0\}$ and $\hat{\tau}_I = \max\{T_M - df_M, T_I - df_I, 0\}$. Obviously, CFI is always between zero and 1. It avoids the underestimation of NFI and the overestimation of NNFI. In this category of fit indices, CFI is the most frequently reported one.

(3) *Root mean square error of approximation* (*RMSEA*; Steiger and Lind, 1980; Browne and Cudeck, 1993): First introduced by Steiger and Lind (1980) for

exploratory factor analysis, the RMSEA became popular due to Browne and Cudeck (1993). As a population index it is given as

$$\text{RMSEA}_{\text{pop}} = \sqrt{\tau_{\text{M}}/df}, \tag{34}$$

which can be interpreted as the square root of population misfit per degree of freedom. When the value of RMSEA is small, the fit is good, and for the same degree of misfit as measured by τ_{M}, models with higher df fit better. In practice, RMSEA is computed as

$$\text{RMSEA} = \sqrt{\max\{(T_{\text{M}} - df_{\text{M}})/(n \cdot df_{\text{M}}), 0\}}. \tag{35}$$

Yuan (2005) pointed out that an implicit assumption in RMSEA is that T_{M} under the alternative hypothesis is distributed as a non-central χ^2 with the non-centrality parameter τ_{M} equal to the sample size n times the value measured by the fit function. For this to be true, we need to assume that the concept of a sequence of local alternative hypotheses makes sense. However, this holds only when the true population covariance matrix is sufficiently close to the hypothesis $\Sigma(\theta)$. According to Yuan (2005), the distribution of the sample RMSEA is unknown in general. Any probability or confidence interval attached to RMSEA, as printed out in software, has little justification for real data or even simulated data from a normal distribution. Nonetheless, applied researchers keep using it in practice to assess the fit of their model.

(4) *Information-criterion-based fit indices*: The goodness of fit of several different models can be compared with the information criteria AIC (e.g., Akaike, 1974, 1987), CAIC (Bozdogan, 1987), and BIC (Schwarz, 1978), defined as follows:

$$\text{AIC} = T_{\text{ML}} + 2q, \tag{36}$$

$$\text{CAIC} = T_{\text{ML}} + (1 + \log n)q, \tag{37}$$

$$\text{BIC} = T_{\text{ML}} + (\log n)q, \tag{38}$$

respectively, where q is the number of parameters (either q_1 or q_2 depending on the model). Assuming that the model makes sense theoretically, the model with the smallest information criterion may be chosen.

2.8. Modification of the model

When an initial model has a poor fit, it may be desirable to modify the model to improve the fit. In principle, for nested models this can be accomplished by a model comparison procedure based on the χ^2 difference test such as $T_{\text{D}} = T_{\text{ML1}} - T_{\text{ML2}}$, where T_{ML1} is the test statistic for a more restricted model and T_{ML2} is the test for a more general model. However, this would require specifying various pairs of models and estimating both models in a pair. In SEM, two types of well-known tests, the Lagrange Multiplier (LM) or score test and the Wald test, are frequently used in addition or instead of a difference test. They only require estimation of one model, either the more restricted model in the case of the LM test, or the more general model in case of the Wald test. More importantly, both tests are available in an exploratory methodology where a search procedure can be used to find alternative parameters that may influence model fit (see e.g., Lee and Bentler, 1980; Bentler and Dijkstra, 1985; Lee, 1985; Bentler, 1986; Satorra, 1989; Chou and Bentler, 1990, 2002).

(1) *LM test or Score test*: When we would like to know which paths may be added to improve the fit of a model, i.e., which restricted parameters in a model should perhaps be freed and estimated, we can employ the score test (Rao, 1947, 1973) or its equivalent, the LM test (Aitchison and Silvey, 1958). When considering a single parameter to free, asymptotically the LM test follows a χ^2 distribution with 1 *df* (Satorra, 1989). A large χ^2 indicates that the restriction is not consistent with the data, that a better model most likely can be obtained when the parameter is freed, and that the model test statistic (e.g., T_{ML}) then would decrease by an amount approximately equal to the LM test value. Then the model can be re-estimated, and the procedure repeated. However, the tests can also be applied sequentially before re-estimating the model. In this way it is a multivariate LM test with *df* equal to the number of restrictions being tested. The multivariate test can be implemented in a forward stepwise procedure where the parameter making the biggest improvement in fit is added first, a next parameter is added that yields the largest increment in fit after controlling the influence of the first, etc. (Bentler, in press). For a comparison of these two approaches, see e.g., Green et al. (1999). In some SEM software, the LM test is called the modification index (Sörbom, 1989). Under the null hypothesis that the model differentiating parameters are zero in the population, LM tests are asymptotically χ^2 distributed, but this may not be true when applied in a search methodology. In small samples, parameters may be chosen that capitalize on chance, i.e., the method may identify restrictions to release that do not hold up well in cross-validation (e.g., MacCallum et al., 1992).

(2) *Wald test*: If we have a model that fits but seems to have unnecessary parameters, standard errors can be used to find and eliminate particular nonsignificant parameters. The Wald test (Wald, 1943) is a multivariate generalization that allows testing a set of parameters simultaneously to see if they are sufficiently unimportant that they could be eliminated. Again this methodology has been implemented in a search fashion. The procedure corresponds to backward elimination in multiple regression, that is, the least significant parameter is removed first, residuals are computed, then next least significant parameter is removed, and so on until a set is obtained that is simultaneously not significant. This implies that removal of those parameters from the model may increase the test statistic (e.g., T_{ML}), but only by a small amount. Like the LM test, under the null hypothesis that the model parameters are zero in the population, and with an *a priori* selection of parameters to test, the Wald test asymptotically follows the χ^2 distribution with either 1 *df* or as many *df*'s as there are parameters being tested (see e.g., Satorra,

1989). Again, however, this test procedure can be misleading in small samples when used empirically to search for unimportant parameters.

(3) *A word of caution*: The asymptotic distribution of the difference test T_D in SEM was studied theoretically by Steiger et al. (1985). In theory, the more general model need not be true for the distribution of T_D to be asymptotically χ^2. However, recent research has shown that when the more general model is false, tests such as T_D perform very badly in small to medium sized samples and cannot be relied upon (Yuan and Bentler, 2004a; Maydeu-Olivares and Cai, 2006). Clearly the same caution should be used with LM and Wald tests. This is not a trivial matter because in practice, even the best model may not fit statistically (see fit indices above).

3. Extensions of SEM

3.1. Extensions

So far, we have discussed SEM for the simplest case of only linear latent variable models for one standard sample from a population. However, the SEM paradigm has been extended in many different directions so that more complicated model and data structures can be handled effectively. This includes the ability to handle incomplete data, nonlinear relations among latent variables, multiple samples, hierarchical data structures, categorical variables, and so on. Here we just give a flavor of some of these developments.

3.2. Multi-group SEM

The most typical extension of SEM is to the multiple-group case, where parts of models or entire models may be held to be equal across groups in order to determine similarities or differences among samples or populations. A typical example is the two-group case, where males vs. females may be compared. Multi-group SEM was originated by Jöreskog (1971) and Sörbom (1974), and has been further developed by Bentler et al. (1987), Lee and Tsui (1982), and Muthén (1989a, 1989b). Yuan and Bentler (2001) gave a unified approach to multi-group SEM under non-normality and with missing data. Thus, we follow their notation.

(1) *Test statistic and fit function*: Suppose we have m groups with sample sizes $n_j, j = 1, \ldots, m$. Let $N = n_1 + \cdots + n_m$ be the total sample size including all the m groups. The parameters from the m groups can be arranged as $\theta = (\theta_1', \ldots, \theta_m')'$. Then the test statistics is given by

$$T_{\text{ML}}^m = N \cdot F_{\text{ML}}^m, \tag{39}$$

where

$$F_{\text{ML}}^m = \sum_{j=1}^m \frac{n_j}{N} ([\hat{\mu}_j - \mu_j(\theta_j)]' \Sigma_j^{-1}(\theta_j)[\hat{\mu}_j - \mu_j(\theta_j)])$$
$$+ tr[\hat{\Sigma}_j \Sigma_j^{-1}(\theta_j)] - \log |\hat{\Sigma}_j \Sigma_j^{-1}(\theta_j)| - p) \tag{40}$$

is a weighted sum of the fit functions from each group. Obviously, when there are no constraints on parameters, the degrees of freedom is m times the degrees of freedom for the model for each group. More typically, the fit function will be optimized under r constraints in the form of $h(\theta) = 0$, and the df will be adjusted accordingly. In addition to likelihood ratio tests of nested models, multi-group version of the Satorra–Bentler rescaled statistic (Satorra, 2000) and the sandwich-type covariance matrix exist to handle distributional violations. In addition, normal theory or generalized LM tests can be used to test the significance of the constraints.

(2) *Constraints and invariance*: As noted, multi-group SEM typically will involve constraints on the parameters because it is natural to evaluate whether path coefficients are the same among m groups. If we can assume the existence of the same latent variable(s) among the groups in the populations, we say that factorial invariance exists in the populations (see e.g., Meredith, 1993, and Millsap, 1997, on factorial invariance). However, there are different levels of factorial invariance (Horn et al., 1983). For example, when the test using the test statistic of the form (39) (without any equality constraints among the groups) is not rejected, we say that we could not reject *configural* invariance. When the structure of path coefficients is identical across groups in the populations, we say that *metric* invariance holds. We can put equality constraints also on the residual variances and/or factor correlations among the groups and can test for the factorial invariance under stronger conditions. A concrete example of these ideas is the confirmatory factor model, where each group has a structure such as (12). If the structure of factor loadings is equal across groups, we have metric invariance even if the remaining parameter matrices differ. Equality of the factorial structure implies that the same latent factors are measured in each group.

(3) *Mean structure*: When considering a factor model such as (6) for each group, it is possible to fix μ and Λ as common across all groups, but to have $E(\xi) = \mu_\xi$ differ across groups. This implies that the same latent factors are being measured in the groups, but that they differ in their level on the trait. For example, a natural question to ask might be whether there is any significant difference in factor means between males vs. females. Because factor means can have any location unit, one group's vector of factor means μ_ξ is set to zero. Without such a constraint, the model is usually non-identified.

3.3. Growth curve models

In medical and epidemiological research, many research designs are longitudinal in nature and the consistency or change of individuals across time is a key focus. We can imagine a line or curve connecting all the repeated observations of a given individual across time, and dozens or hundreds of such lines or curves to represent the entire sample. When the repeated measures are obtained a few to a dozen times, such data can be analyzed using SEM as a procedure to characterize mean trends in these curves as well as individual differences and their anteced-ents, correlates, or consequences. In this field, the methodology is known as growth curve modeling, see e.g., Bentler (2005) or Stoel (2003) for summaries, or Bollen and Curran (2006) and Duncan et al. (2006) for text-length treatments. In the simplest model setup, this methodology represents a special case of (4)–(5) or (6)–(11) and it amounts to an application of MCSA. For example, we may take $x = \mu + \Lambda\xi + \varepsilon$, but consider $\mu = 0$ so that the mean information is carried by μ_ξ. Then there are some features unique to growth curve SEM that are worth noting.

(1) The x_i will represent a quantitative variable repeatedly measured across time, and the latent factors ξ are interpreted as representing important features of the shapes of the growth curves across time. There are many ways to code shapes, but a standard one is to consider the starting point or "intercept," the linear trend (commonly referred to as "slope"), or a higher order curve feature such as a "quadratic" trend. When the repeatedly measured variable represents a substantive construct (such as "depression"), the factors represent time trends in that construct (e.g., "depression").
(2) A given latent factor, say the slope ξ_j, has scores for every individual in the sample. Each of those scores represents the given trend in scores for that individual, e.g., for slope it can be considered to be a coefficient to represent that person's linear trend across time. Some persons may be growing rapidly, and others not at all, and these individual differences show up in the variance of ξ_j. The corresponding factor mean $\mu_{\xi(j)}$ represents the average trend in the data, e.g., it would be the group average slope or linear trend. Predictors, correlates, and consequences of ξ_j can also be determined.
(3) Since factor loadings are weights attached to the factors to predict a variable, those for a given factor, such as the jth column of Λ, contains weights that represent time. Unlike standard factor analysis, the coefficients in Λ are taken to be known *a priori* in accord with the coding of time. Different factors code different aspects of time, such as the starting point, or linear or quadratic changes across time. In particular, (i) the path coefficients from the intercept factor to the observed variables are set to an equal constant, typically to 1; (ii) the factor loadings for the linear slope factor are set proportional to time elapsed. For example, if the time differences are equal among the observed variables, the path to the initial measure may take the value of 0, that to the second measure the value of 1, that to the third measure gets the value of 2, etc.; (iii) likewise, paths from the quadratic factor may be coded as $(0^2, 1^2, 2^2, \ldots) = (0, 1, 4, \ldots)$; (iv) because raw polynomial coefficients become very large as time elapses and as the degree of polynomials increase, standardized coefficients can be used. For example, for three equally spaced observed variables, the coefficients from the intercept, linear, and quadratic factors are $(0.577, 0.557, 0.555)$, $(-0.707, 0, 0.707)$, and $(0.408, -0.816, 0.408)$, respectively. This is one example of orthogonal polynomials (see e.g., Maxwell and Delaney, 2004, Chapter 6); (v) alternative approaches to the linear slope factor exist, such as spline factors by Meredith and Tisak (1990) and the piecewise linear model (Raudenbush and Bryk, 2002, p. 178). Also, since a model with fixed nonzero factor loadings may be hard to fit, researchers sometimes free these loadings. This leads to a different interpretation of time trends, and thus needs to be done with caution (see e.g., Bentler, 2005).

3.4. Multilevel SEM

Multilevel analysis, also called hierarchical linear modeling, is a statistical technique for analyzing data collected from a hierarchical sampling scheme such as
level-1 observations (e.g., students) nested within level-2 observations (e.g.,
classes). The number of levels can be extended, though a large sample size at the
highest level is required for stable estimation. Most multi-level analyses are two-
level. Some general references for multi-level analysis include Goldstein (2003),
Raudenbush and Bryk (2002), and Reise and Duan (2003). SEM can be used to
estimate parameters for multi-level data, and this approach is especially useful
when latent variables are involved, e.g., Bentler and Liang (2003), Bentler et al.
(2005), du Toit and du Toit (2002), Goldstein and McDonald (1988), McDonald
and Goldstein (1989), Lee (1990), Lee and Poon (1998), Lee et al. (1995), Lee and
Shi (2001), Lee and Song (2001), Liang and Bentler (2004), Muthén (1994, 1997),
Poon and Lee (1994), and Yuan and Bentler (2002, 2003, 2004b).

   According to Liang and Bentler (2004) and Bentler et al. (2005), two-level
SEM can be formulated as

$$\begin{pmatrix} \mathbf{z}_g \\ \mathbf{y}_{gi} \end{pmatrix} = \begin{pmatrix} \mathbf{z}_g \\ \mathbf{v}_g \end{pmatrix} + \begin{pmatrix} \mathbf{0} \\ \mathbf{v}_{gi} \end{pmatrix}, \tag{41}$$

where $\mathbf{z}_g$ ($p_2 \times 1$) is a vector of *i.i.d.* level-2 observations ($g = 1, \ldots, G$), and $\mathbf{y}_{gi}$
($p_1 \times 1$) is a vector of level-1 observations ($i = 1, \ldots, N_g$) from the same cluster or
group (level-2 unit), and $p = p_1 + p_2$. Under the model, the observed $\mathbf{y}_{gi}$ are
decomposed into a part exhibiting between-cluster variation $\mathbf{v}_g$ and a part
exhibiting within-cluster variation $\mathbf{v}_{gi}$.

   Note that for a fixed group g, $\mathbf{y}_{gi}$ are *i.i.d.*, while for all i's and g's, $\mathbf{y}_{gi}$ are not
independent. In Eq. (41), we typically assume: (i) $\mathbf{z}_g$ and $\mathbf{v}_g$ are independent of $\mathbf{v}_{gi}$;
(ii) $\mathbf{z}_g$ and $\mathbf{v}_g$ are correlated. Let us introduce further notation: $\boldsymbol{\mu}_z = E(\mathbf{z}_g)$,
$\boldsymbol{\mu}_y = E(\mathbf{y}_{gi}) = E(\mathbf{v}_g)$, $\boldsymbol{\Sigma}_{zz} = Cov(\mathbf{z}_g)$, $\boldsymbol{\Sigma}_B = Cov(\mathbf{v}_g)$, $\boldsymbol{\Sigma}_{Wi} = Cov(\mathbf{v}_{gi})$ typically
assumed to be homogeneous across clusters with $\boldsymbol{\Sigma}_{Wi} = \boldsymbol{\Sigma}_W$, and $\boldsymbol{\Sigma}_{zy} = Cov(\mathbf{z}_g,$
$\mathbf{y}_{gi}) = Cov(\mathbf{z}_g, \mathbf{v}_g)$. Under a SEM structure, we can further structure the within-
cluster covariance matrix, for example, as a confirmatory factor model (see (12))
as in:

$$\boldsymbol{\Sigma}_w = \boldsymbol{\Lambda}_W \boldsymbol{\Phi}_W \boldsymbol{\Lambda}'_W + \boldsymbol{\Psi}_W. \tag{42}$$

   More generally, the means and covariances in multi-level SEM are $\boldsymbol{\mu} = \begin{pmatrix} \boldsymbol{\mu}_z \\ \boldsymbol{\mu}_y \end{pmatrix}$,
$\tilde{\boldsymbol{\Sigma}}_B = \begin{pmatrix} \boldsymbol{\Sigma}_{zz} & \boldsymbol{\Sigma}_{zy} \\ \boldsymbol{\Sigma}_{yz} & \boldsymbol{\Sigma}_B \end{pmatrix}$, and $\boldsymbol{\Sigma}_W$, and any of these vectors and matrices can be further
structured as in (4)–(5) or (10)–(11).

   Parameter estimation methods such as ML have been developed for multilevel
SEM. For ML estimation based on Gauss–Newton or Fisher scoring algorithms,
see du Toit and du Toit (2002), Goldstein and McDonald (1988), Lee (1990), and
McDonald and Goldstein (1989). Muthén (1994, 1997) proposed an approximate
ML estimator commonly called Muthén's ML, or MUML. MUML has the

advantage of easier calculation and faster convergence than full ML estimation. When level-1 samples are equal in size, MUML is equivalent to full ML estimation. Yuan and Hayashi (2005) analytically studied the statistical properties of MUML and identified further conditions for MUML to be close to ML. The EM algorithm (Dempster et al., 1977) also has been applied by Raudenbush (1995) and Lee and Poon (1998). The approach of Lee and Poon (1998) was further extended by Bentler and Liang (2003) and Liang and Bentler (2004). Finally, just as ML test statistics in simple SEM can lead to distorted χ^2 tests and standard error estimates under non-normality, the same can occur if level-1 or level-2 observations are not multivariate normal. Corrected test statistics for this situation, and the study of robustness of multilevel SEM can be found in Yuan and Bentler (2003, 2004b, 2005a, 2005b).

3.5. Nonlinear SEM

In multiple regression, the dependent variable can be a nonlinear function of the independent variables by the use of polynomial and/or interaction terms. This is straightforward. On the contrary, in SEM it has been a difficult task to connect a dependent latent variable with independent latent variables in a nonlinear fashion. Efforts to construct and estimate a nonlinear SEM have been made for the last 20 years. Early works include Kenny and Judd (1984), Bentler (1983), Mooijaart (1985), and Mooijaart and Bentler (1986). The Kenny–Judd model, a particular simple nonlinear model that includes an interaction term, has been intensively studied. More recent works include Bollen (1996), Bollen and Paxton (1998), Jöreskog and Yang (1996), Klein and Moosbrugger (2000), Lee et al. (2004), Lee and Zhu (2000, 2002), Marsh et al. (2004), Wall and Amemiya (2000, 2001, 2003), Yang Jonsson (1998). The Bollen–Paxton and Klein–Moosbrugger approaches seem to be especially attractive. The Wall–Amemiya approach seems to be the most theoretically defensible under a wide range of conditions, since it yields consistent estimates under distributional violations. The Bayesian approaches of Lee and his colleagues are the most promising for small samples. However, to the best of the authors' knowledge, no general SEM software incorporates the Wall–Amemiya or Lee approaches.

4. Some practical issues

4.1. Treatment of missing data

Missing data are encountered frequently in data analysis, and this problem certainly also arises in the context of SEM. Rubin (1976) and Little and Rubin (2002) are general references on the missing data problem, while Allison (2002) provides a non-technical account. It is useful to discuss this topic by considering Rubin's (1976) missing data mechanisms: (1) *MCAR* (missing completely at random): Missingness of the data is independent of both the observed and the missing values; (2) *MAR* (missing at random): Missingness of the data is independent of the missing values but can depend on the observed values; (3) *NMAR* (not missing at random): Misssingness depends on the missing values themselves. While unprincipled methods such as listwise deletion require MCAR data for

appropriate inference, most methodological developments on missing data in
SEM focus on the normal theory ML procedure because it allows the weaker
MAR mechanism. When the data are from a multivariate normal distribution
and the missing data mechanism is either MCAR or MAR, the MLE is consistent
and asymptotically normal. However, note that MAR mechanism may not be
ignorable when using the wrong density to perform the ML estimation. Yuan
(2006) employed the normal density to model a non-normal distribution with
missing data and gave sufficient conditions under which consistent MLE will be
guaranteed when data are MAR.

The references on missing data related to ML include Arbuckle (1996),
Jamshidian and Bentler (1999), Lee (1986), Muthén et al. (1987), and Tang and
Bentler (1998). When missingness occurs in the context of non-normal data, the
classical ML methodology has to be extended to provide corrections to test statistics and standard errors. References include Arminger and Sobel (1990), Savalei
and Bentler (2005), Yuan and Bentler (2000a), and Yuan (2006) mentioned above.

Because of its importance in the missing data context, we describe one
approach using the EM algorithm (Dempster et al., 1977) to obtaining MLE in
this context. Let x_i be the ith case including both observed variables x_{io} and
missing variables x_{im}. That is, $x_i = (x_{io}', x_{im}')'$. Corresponding to the partition of
x_i, let $\mu = (\mu_o', \mu_m')'$ and $\Sigma = \begin{pmatrix} \Sigma_{oo} & \Sigma_{om} \\ \Sigma_{mo} & \Sigma_{mm} \end{pmatrix}$ be the partitioned population mean
vector and the covariance matrix.

(1) *E-step*: Then, under the normal distribution assumption, the conditional
     expectation of $E(x_{im}|x_{io})$ and $E(x_{im}x_{im}'|x_{io})$ are given by:

$$E(x_{im}|x_{io}) = \mu_m + \Sigma_{mo}\Sigma_{oo}^{-1}(x_{io} - \mu_o), \tag{43}$$

$$E(x_{im}x_{im}'|x_{io}) = (\Sigma_{mm} - \Sigma_{mo}\Sigma_{oo}^{-1}\Sigma_{om}) + E(x_{im}|x_{io})E(x_{im}|x_{io})'. \tag{44}$$

These Eqs (43) and (44) are incorporated in

$$E(x_i|x_{io}) = (x_{io}', E(x_{im}|x_{io})')', \tag{45}$$

$$E(x_ix_i'|x_{io}) = \begin{pmatrix} x_{io}x_{io}' & x_{io}E(x_{im}|x_{io})' \\ E(x_{im}|x_{io})x_{io}' & E(x_{im}x_{im}'|x_{io}) \end{pmatrix}, \tag{46}$$

respectively.

(2) *M-step*: Let $\bar{x} = (1/n)\sum_{i=1}^{n}E(x_i|x_{io})$ and $S = (1/n)\sum_{i=1}^{n}E(x_ix_i'|x_{io}) - \bar{x}\,\bar{x}'$.
     Then the M-step consists of minimizing the ML fit function:

$$F_{\mathrm{ML}} = (\bar{x} - \mu(\theta))'\Sigma(\theta)^{-1}(\bar{x} - \mu(\theta)) + tr(S\Sigma(\theta)^{-1}) - \log|S\Sigma(\theta)^{-1}| - p \tag{47}$$

with respect to θ. Further details can be found in Jamshidian and Bentler
(1999). More general methods based on Markov chain Monte Carlo
(MCMC) methods (e.g., Lee et al., 2003; Song and Lee, 2002) hold promise
for improved inference in small samples. Robert and Casella (2004) provide
an overview of MCMC methods.

It would be desirable to be able to evaluate whether data are MCAR, MAR, or NMAR. With regard to MCAR, it is possible to evaluate whether the various patterns of missing data are consistent with sampling from a single normal population. This can be done by testing homogeneity of means, covariances, or homogeneity of both means and covariances (Kim and Bentler, 2002). It is difficult to find general approaches to testing MAR and NMAR, although specific models for NMAR have been proposed and evaluated (Tang and Lee, 1998; Lee and Tang, 2006).

4.2. Treatment of categorical dependent variables

So far, we have assumed that the observed variables are continuous. This may not always hold true in practice. Categorical variables are frequently used in medical and epidemiological research. First of all, note that no special methods are needed if the categorical variables are independent variables. It is common that independent variables are categorical in multiple regression, and SEM can handle such variables by dummy coding as is done in multiple regression. Second, if a dependent categorical variable is ordered and has at least 4 or 5 categories as in a typical Likert scale, treating it as a continuous variable will create few serious problems (e.g., Bentler and Chou, 1987). The remaining case is when a dependent categorical variable is either binary or with three categories. Even three-category data treated continuously can perform well enough (Coenders et al., 1997), but we do not recommend it as routine practice. General accounts on how to treat such dependent categorical variables in the context of exploratory factor analysis, and hence to SEM more generally, are given by Flora and Curran (2004), Jöreskog and Moustaki (2001), and Moustaki (2001). Approaches can be categorized into two major types (see Jöreskog and Moustaki, 2001).

(1) *Underlying variable approach*: The idea that the observed correlation between categorical variables does not optimally represent the correlation between continuous latent variables that may have given rise to the observed categories is about a century old. The tetrachoric correlation was developed to describe the correlation between two underlying continuous normal variables that are categorized into binary variables. Extensions of tetrachorics to polychoric and polyserial correlations (see Poon and Lee, 1987) provided the foundation for an SEM approach (Muthén, 1978, 1984). In this approach either a sample polychoric or polyserial correlation between variables is computed from bivariate marginal likelihoods for given thresholds, which are estimated from the univariate marginal distribution. After polychoric or polyserial correlations have been computed, their asymptotic covariance matrix is computed and used in an ADF-type estimation method to estimate the covariance structure. Because ADF requires large sample sizes, inefficient estimates such as least squares estimates can be computed, and the results corrected for misspecification using Satorra–Bentler type procedures. Related approaches were given by Jöreskog (1994), Lee et al. (1990, 1992, 1995), and Lee and Song (2003). This methodology is implemented in most major SEM software.

(2) *Generalized latent variable model approach*: This approach stems from the models for educational tests called the item response theory (Baker and Kim, 2004). In this approach, conditional on the latent variables, the response model is identical to a generalized linear model (McCullagh and Nelder, 1989). The linear latent predictors are then connected with a dependent variable via a link function, which takes care of the categorical nature of the dependent variable. References on this approach include Bartholomew and Knott (1999), Maydeu-Olivares (2001, 2005), and Skrondal and Rabe-Hesketh (2004).

4.3. Further practical information

(1) *Software*: Finally, we provide some practical information. Because of the complexity of optimization algorithm(s) required in SEM, we recommend that applied researchers use existing SEM software such as Amos (http://www.spss.com/amos/), EQS (Bentler, in press; http://www.mvsoft.com/), Lisrel (Jöreskog and Sörbom, 2001; http://www.ssicentral.com/), Mplus (Muthén and Muthén, 2001; http://www.statmodel.com/), or SAS Proc Calis (http://www.sas.com/). It is possible to learn to use the software of choice from the associated program manuals or from some textbooks mentioned in the introduction. Both sources provide many examples of worked problems. Amos and EQS are especially easy to learn to use due to their graphical interface that allows model specification via path diagrams.

(2) *Computational difficulties*: We do not want to overemphasize the ease of use of SEM. A well thought-out model with many variables can be difficult to fit because such a model may be misspecified in hundreds of ways. When a model is complex, and starting values are poor, the iterative calculations may not be able to optimize the statistical function involved, i.e., non-convergence may occur. Also, a related practical problem may be that one or more residual variances may be estimated negatively or held to a zero boundary, called an improper solution (or a Heywood case; see e.g., Boomsma, 1985, Chen et al., 2001, Kano, 1998, Rindskopf, 1984, or van Driel, 1978). In these situations, simplifying the model, improving start values, or other strategies such as fitting submodels may be needed to provide meaningful as well as statistically adequate solutions. In general, SEM modeling will require subject-matter experts to cooperate with statistical experts.

Acknowledgement

This work was supported in part by grants P01 DA01070 and K05 DA00017 from the National Institute on Drug Abuse awarded to Peter Bentler and also by NSF grant DMS04-37167 awarded to Ke-Hai Yuan.

References

Aitchison, J., Silvey, S.D. (1958). Maximum likelihood estimation of parameters subject to restraints. *Annals of Mathematical Statistics* **29**, 813–828.

Akaike, H. (1974). A new look at the statistical model identification. *IEEE Transactions on Automatic Control* **19**, 716–723.

Akaike, H. (1987). Factor analysis and AIC. *Psychometrika* **52**, 317–332.

Allison, P.D. (2002). *Missing Data*. Sage, Thousand Oaks, CA.

Amemiya, Y., Anderson, T.W. (1990). Asymptotic chi-square tests for a large class of factor analysis models. *Annals of Statistics* **18**, 1453–1463.

Anderson, T.W., Amemiya, Y. (1988). The asymptotic normal distribution of estimators in factor analysis under general conditions. *Annals of Statistics* **16**, 759–771.

Arbuckle, J.L. (1996). Full information estimation in the presence of incomplete data. In: Marcoulides, G.A., Schumacker, R.E. (Eds.), *Advanced Structural Equation Modeling: Issues and Techniques*. Erlbaum, Mahwah, NJ, pp. 243–277.

Arminger, G., Sobel, M.E. (1990). Pseudo-maximum likelihood estimation of mean and covariance structures with missing data. *Journal of the American Statistical Association* **85**, 195–203.

Baker, F.B., Kim, S-H. (2004). *Item Response Theory: Parameter Estimation Techniques*, 2nd ed. Marcel Dekker, New York.

Bartholomew, D.J., Knott, M. (1999). *Latent Variable Models and Factor Analysis*, 2nd ed. Arnold, London.

Batista-Foguet, J.M., Coenders, G., Ferragud, M.A. (2001). Using structural equation models to evaluate the magnitude of measurement error in blood pressure. *Statistics in Medicine* **20**, 2351–2368.

Bauer, D.J., Curran, P.J. (2003). Distributional assumptions of growth mixture models: Implications for overextraction of latent trajectory classes. *Psychological Methods* **8**, 338–363.

Bauer, D.J., Curran, P.J. (2004). The integration of continuous and discrete latent variable models: Potential problems and promising opportunities. *Psychological Methods* **9**, 3–29.

Bekker, P.A., Merckens, A., Wansbeek, T.J. (1994). *Identification, Equivalent Models, and Computer Algebra*. Academic Press, Boston.

Bentler, P.M. (1982). Linear systems with multiple levels and types of latent variables. In: Jöreskog, K.G., Wold, H. (Eds.), *Systems Under Indirect Observation: Causality, Structure, Prediction*. North-Holland, Amsterdam, pp. 101–130.

Bentler, P.M. (1983). Some contributions to efficient statistics in structural models: Specification and estimation of moment structures. *Psychometrika* **48**, 493–517.

Bentler, P.M. (1986). *Lagrange Multiplier and Wald tests for EQS and EQS/PC*. BMDP Statistical Software, Los Angeles.

Bentler, P.M. (1990). Comparative fit indexes in structural models. *Psychological Bulletin* **107**, 238–246.

Bentler, P.M. (1995). *EQS Structural Equation Program Manual*. Multivariate Software, Inc, Encino, CA.

Bentler, P.M. (2005). Latent growth curves. In: Werner, J. (Ed.), *Zeitreihenanalysen*. Logos, Berlin, pp. 13–36.

Bentler, P.M. (in press). EQS 6 *Structural Equations Program Manual*. Multivariate Software, Encino, CA.

Bentler, P.M., Berkane, M. (1985). Developments in the elliptical theory generalization of normal multivariate analysis. *Proceedings of the Social Statistics Section, American Statistical Association*. Alexandria, VA, 291–295.

Bentler, P.M., Bonett, D.G. (1980). Significance tests and goodness of fit in the analysis of covariance structures. *Psychological Bulletin* **88**, 588–606.

Bentler, P.M., Chou, C-P. (1987). Practical issues in structural modeling. *Sociological Methods and Research* **16**, 78–117.

Bentler, P.M., Dijkstra, T. (1985). Efficient estimation via linearization in structural models. In: Krishnaiah, P.R. (Ed.), *Multivariate Analysis VI*. North-Holland, Amsterdam, pp. 9–42.

Bentler, P.M., Lee, S-Y., Weng, L-J. (1987). Multiple population covariance structure analysis under arbitrary distribution theory. *Communication in Statistics – Theory and Method* **16**, 1951–1964.

Bentler, P.M., Liang, J. (2003). Two-level mean and covariance structures: Maximum likelihood via an EM algorithm. In: Reise, S.P., Duan, N. (Eds.), *Multilevel Modeling: Methodological Advances, Issues, and Applications*. Erlbaum, Mahwah, NJ, pp. 53–70.

Bentler, P.M., Liang, J., Yuan, K-H. (2005). Some recent advances in two-level structural equation models: Estimation, testing, and robustness. In: Fan, J., Li, G. (Eds.), *Contemporary Multivariate Analysis and Experimental Designs – in Celebration of Professor Kai-Tai Fang's 65th Birthday*. World Scientific, Hackensack, NJ, pp. 99–120.

Bentler, P.M., Stein, J.A. (1992). Structural equation models in medical research. *Statistical Methods in Medical Research* **1**, 159–181.

Bentler, P.M., Weeks, D.G. (1980). Linear structural equations with latent variables. *Psychometrika* **45**, 289–308.

Bentler, P.M., Yuan, K-H. (1999). Structural equation modeling with small samples: Test statistics. *Multivariate Behavioral Research*. NewYork **34**, 181–197.

Beran, R. (1986). Simulated power functions. *Annals of Statistics* **14**, 151–173.

Beran, R., Srivastava, M.S. (1985). Bootstrap tests and confidence regions for functions of a covariance matrix. *Annals of Statistics* **13**, 95–115.

Berkane, M. (Ed.) (1997). Latent Variable Modeling and Applications to Causality. Springer, New York.

Bollen, K.A. (1989). *Structural Equations with Latent Variables*. Wiley, New York.

Bollen, K.A. (1996). An alternative two stage least squares (2SLS) estimator for latent variable equations. *Psychometrika* **61**, 109–121.

Bollen, K.A. (2002). Latent variables in psychology and the social sciences. *Annual Review of Psychology* **53**, 605–634.

Bollen, K.A., Curran, P.J. (2006). *Latent Curve Models: A Structural Equation Approach*. Wiley, New York.

Bollen, K.A., Paxton, P. (1998). Two-stage least squares estimation of interaction effects. In: Schumacker, R.E., Marcoulides, G.A. (Eds.), *Interaction and Nonlinear Effects in Structural Equation Modeling*. Erlbaum, Mahwah, NJ, pp. 125–151.

Bollen, K.A., Stine, R. (1993). Bootstrapping goodness of fit measures in structural equation models. In: Bollen, K.A., Long, J.S. (Eds.), *Testing Structural Equation Models*. Sage, Newbury Park, CA, pp. 111–135.

Boomsma, A. (1985). Nonconvergence, improper solutions, and starting values in LISREL maximum likelihood estimation. *Psychometrika* **50**, 229–242.

Bozdogan, H. (1987). Model selection and Akaike's information criteria (AIC): The general theory and its analytical extensions. *Psychometrika* **52**, 345–370.

Browne, M.W. (1974). Generalized least-squares estimators in the analysis of covariance structures. *South African Statistical Journal* **8**, 1–24.

Browne, M.W. (1984). Asymptotic distribution-free methods for the analysis of covariance structures. *British Journal of Mathematical and Statistical Psychology* **37**, 62–83.

Browne, M.W., Arminger, G. (1995). Specification and estimation of mean and covariance structure models. In: Arminger, G., Clogg, C.C., Sobel, M.E. (Eds.), *Handbook of Statistical Modeling for the Social and Behavioral Sciences*. Plenum, New York, pp. 185–249.

Browne, M.W., Cudeck, R. (1993). Alternative ways of assessing model fit. In: Bollen, K.A., Long, J.S. (Eds.), *Testing Structural Equation Models*. Sage, Newbury Park, CA, pp. 136–162.

Browne, M.W., Shapiro, A. (1988). Robustness of normal theory methods in the analysis of linear latent variate models. *British Journal of Mathematical and Statistical Psychology* **41**, 193–208.

Byrne, B.M. (2006). *Structural Equation Modeling with EQS: Basic Concepts, Applications, and Programming*, 2nd ed. Erlbaum, Mahwah, NJ.

Campbell, N.A. (1980). Robust procedures in multivariate analysis I: Robust covariance estimation. *Applied Statistics* **29**, 231–237.

Chen, F., Bollen, K.A., Paxton, P., Curran, P.J., Kirby, J.B. (2001). Improper solutions in structural equation models: Causes, consequences, and strategies. *Sociological Methods and Research* **29**, 468–508.

Chou, C-P., Bentler, P.M. (1990). Model modification in covariance structure modeling: A comparison among likelihood ratio, Lagrange multiplier, and Wald tests. *Multivariate Behavioral Research* **25**, 115–136.

Chou, C-P., Bentler, P.M. (2002). Model modification in structural equation modeling by imposing constraints. *Computational Statistics and Data Analysis* **41**, 271–287.

Coenders, G., Satorra, A., Saris, W.E. (1997). Alternative approaches to structural modeling of ordinal data: A Monte Carlo study. *Structural Equation Modeling* **4**, 261–282.

Curran, P.J., West, S.G., Finch, J.F. (1996). The robustness of test statistics to nonnormality and specification error in confirmatory factor analysis. *Psychological Methods* **1**, 16–29.

Davis, P.J., Reeves, J.L., Hastie, B.A., Graff-Radford, S.B., Naliboff, B.D. (2000). Depression determines illness conviction and pain impact: A structural equation modeling analysis. *Pain Medicine* **1**, 238–246.

Davison, A.C., Hinkley, D.V. (1997). *Bootstrap Methods and their Application.* Cambridge University Press, New York.

Dempster, A.P., Laird, N.M., Rubin, D.B. (1977). Maximum likelihood estimation from incomplete data via the EM algorithm (with discussion). *Journal of the Royal Statistical Society B* **39**, 1–38.

Dishman, R.K., Motl, R.W., Saunders, R.P., Dowda, M., Felton, G., Ward, D.S., Pate, R.R. (2002). Factorial invariance and latent mean structure of questionnaires measuring social-cognitive determinants of physical activity among black and white adolescent girls. *Preventive Medicine* **34**, 100–108.

Duncan, S.C., Duncan, T.E., Hops, H. (1998). Progressions of alcohol, cigarette, and marijuana use in adolescence. *Journal of Behavioral Medicine* **21**, 375–388.

Duncan, T.E., Duncan, S.C., Strycker, L.A. (2006). *An Introduction to Latent Variable Growth Curve Modeling*, 2nd ed. Erlbaum, Mahwah, NJ.

Dunn, G., Everitt, B., Pickles, A. (1993). *Modelling Covariances and Latent Variables Using EQS.* Chapman and Hall, London.

du Toit, S.H.C., du Toit, M. (2002). Multilevel structural equation modeling. In: de Leeuw, J., Kreft, I.G.G. (Eds.), *Handbook of Quantitative Multilevel Analysis.* Kluwer Academic, Boston.

Fang, K-T., Kotz, S., Ng., K.W. (1990). *Symmetric Multivariate and Related Distributions.* Chapman and Hall, London.

Ferguson, T. (1958). A method of generating best asymptotically normal estimates with application to estimation of bacterial densities. *Annals of Mathematical Statistics* **29**, 1046–1062.

Ferguson, T. (1996). *A Course in Large Sample Theory.* Chapman and Hall, London.

Flora, D.B., Curran, P.J. (2004). An empirical evaluation of alternative methods of estimation for confirmatory factor analysis with ordinal data. *Psychological Methods* **9**, 466–491.

Goldstein, H. (2003). *Multilevel Statistical Models*, 3rd ed. Arnold, London.

Goldstein, H., McDonald, R.P. (1988). A general model for the analysis of multilevel data. *Psychometrika* **53**, 435–467.

Green, S.B., Thompson, M.S., Poirier, J. (1999). Exploratory analyses to improve model fit: Errors due to misspecification and strategy to reduce their occurrence. *Structural Equation Modeling* **6**, 113–126.

Hampel, F.R., Ronchetti, E.M., Rousseeuw, P.J., Stahel, W.A. (1986). *Robust Statistics: The Approach Based on Influence Functions.* Wiley, New York.

Hancock, G.R. (2001). Effect size, power, and sample size determination for structured means modeling and MIMIC approaches to between-groups hypothesis testing of means on a single latent construct. *Psychometrika* **66**, 373–388.

Hayashi, K., Yuan, K-H. (2003). Robust Bayesian factor analysis. *Structural Equation Modeling* **10**, 525–533.

Hays, R.D., Revicki, D., Coyne, K. (2005). Application of structural equation modeling to health outcomes research. *Evaluation and the Health Professions* **28**, 295–309.

Horn, J.L., McArdle, J., Mason, R. (1983). When is invariance not invariant: A practical scientist's look at the ethereal concept of factor invariance. *Southern Psychologist* **1**, 179–188.

Hoshino, T. (2001). Bayesian inference for finite mixtures in confirmatory factor analysis. *Behaviormetrika* **28**, 37–63.

Hu, L.T., Bentler, P.M. (1998). Fit indices in covariance structure modeling: Sensitivity to under-parameterized model misspecification. *Psychological Methods* **3**, 424–453.

Hu, L.T., Bentler, P.M. (1999). Cutoff criteria for fit indexes in covariance structure analysis: Conventional criteria versus new alternatives. *Structural Equation Modeling* **6**, 1–55.

Hu, L.T., Bentler, P.M., Kano, Y. (1992). Can test statistics in covariance structure analysis be trusted? *Psychological Bulletin* **112**, 351–362.

Huber, P.J. (1964). Robust estimation of a location parameter. *Annals of Mathematical Statistics* **35**, 73–101.

Huber, P.J. (1967). The behavior of maximum likelihood estimates under nonstandard conditions. In: *Proceedings of the Fifth Berkeley Symposium on Mathematical Statistics and Probability.* University of California Press, Berkeley, CA, pp. 221–233.

Huber, P.J. (1981). *Robust Statistics*. Wiley, New York.

Jamshidian, M., Bentler, P.M. (1999). Using complete data routines for ML estimation of mean and covariance structures with missing data. *Journal Educational and Behavioral Statistics* **23**, 21–41.

Jöreskog, K.G. (1969). A general approach to confirmatory maximum likelihood factor analysis. *Psychometrika* **34**, 183–202.

Jöreskog, K.G. (1971). Simultaneous factor analysis in several populations. *Psychometrika* **36**, 409–426.

Jöreskog, K.G. (1994). On the estimation of polychoric correlations and their asymptotic covariance matrix. *Psychometrika* **59**, 381–389.

Jöreskog, K.G., Moustaki, I. (2001). Factor analysis of ordinal variables: A comparison of three approaches. *Multivariate Behavioral Research* **36**, 347–387.

Jöreskog, K.G., Sörbom, D. (1979). *Advances in Factor Analysis and Structural Equation Models*. Abt Books, Cambridge, MA.

Jöreskog, K.G., Sörbom, D. (1981). *LISREL 5: Analysis of linear structural relationships by maximum likelihood and least squares methods*. Research report 81–8, Department of Statistics, University of Uppsala, Uppsala, Sweden.

Jöreskog, K.G., Sörbom, D. (2001). *LISREL 8 User's Reference Guide*. Scientific Software International, Lincolnwood, IL.

Jöreskog, K.G., Yang, F. (1996). Nonlinear structural equation models: The Kenny–Judd model with interaction effects. In: Marcoulides, G.A., Schumacker, R.E. (Eds.), *Advanced Structural Equation Modeling: Issues and Techniques*. Erlbaum, Mahwah, NJ, pp. 57–88.

Kano, Y. (1986). Conditions on consistency of estimators in covariance structure model. *Journal of the Japan Statistical Society* **16**, 75–80.

Kano, Y. (1992). Robust statistics for test-of-independence and related structural models. *Statistics and Probability Letters* **15**, 21–26.

Kano, Y. (1998). Improper solutions in exploratory factor analysis: Causes and treatments. In: Rizzi, A., Vichi, M., Bock, H. (Eds.), *Advances in Data Sciences and Classification*. Springer-Verlag, Berlin, pp. 375–382.

Kano, Y., Berkane, M., Bentler, P.M. (1990). Covariance structure analysis with heterogeneous kurtosis parameters. *Biometrika* **77**, 575–585.

Kano, Y., Berkane, M., Bentler, P.M. (1993). Statistical inference based on pseudo-maximum likelihood estimators in elliptical populations. *Journal of the American Statistical Association* **88**, 135–143.

Kenny, D.A., Judd, C.M. (1984). Estimating the nonlinear and interactive effects of latent variables. *Psychological Bulletin* **96**, 201–210.

Kim, K. (2005). The relationship among fit indexes, power, and sample size in structural equation modeling. *Structural Equation Modeling* **12**, 368–390.

Kim, K.H., Bentler, P.M. (2002). Tests of homogeneity of means and covariance matrices for multivariate incomplete data. *Psychometrika* **67**, 609–624.

Klein, A., Moosbrugger, H. (2000). Maximum likelihood estimation of latent interaction effects with the LMS method. *Psychometrika* **65**, 457–474.

Kline, R.B. (2005). *Principles and Practice of Structural Equation Modeling*, 2nd ed. Guilford Press, New York.

Lawley, D.N., Maxwell, A.E. (1971). *Factor Analysis as a Statistical Method*, 2nd ed. American Elsevier, New York.

Lee, S-Y. (1985). On testing functional constraints in structural equation models. *Biometrika* **72**, 125–131.

Lee, S-Y. (1986). Estimation for structural equation models with missing data. *Psychometrika* **51**, 93–99.

Lee, S-Y. (1990). Multilevel analysis of structural equation models. *Biometrika* **77**, 763–772.

Lee, S-Y. (Ed.) (2007). Handbook of Latent Variable and Related Models. Elsevier, Amsterdam.

Lee, S-Y., Bentler, P.M. (1980). Some asymptotic properties of constrained generalized least squares estimation in covariance structure models. *South African Statistical Journal* **14**, 121–136.

Lee, S-Y., Jennrich, R.I. (1979). A study of algorithms for covariance structure analysis with specific comparisons using factor analysis. *Psychometrika* **44**, 99–113.

Lee, S-Y., Poon, W.Y. (1998). Analysis of two-level structural equation models via EM type algorithms. *Statistica Sinica* **8**, 749–766.

Lee, S-Y., Poon, W.Y., Bentler, P.M. (1990). Full maximum likelihood analysis of structural equation models with polytomous variables. *Statistics and Probability Letters* **9**, 91–97.

Lee, S-Y., Poon, W.Y., Bentler, P.M. (1992). Structural equation models with continuous and polytomous variables. *Psychometrika* **57**, 89–106.

Lee, S-Y., Poon, W.Y., Bentler, P.M. (1995). A two-stage estimation of structural equation models with continuous and polytomous variables. *British Journal of Mathematical and Statistical Psychology* **48**, 339–358.

Lee, S-Y., Shi, J.Q. (2001). Maximum likelihood estimation of two-level latent variables model with mixed continuous and polytomous data. *Biometrics* **57**, 787–794.

Lee, S-Y., Song, X.Y. (2001). Hypothesis testing and model comparison in two-level structural equation models. *Multivariate Behavioral Research* **36**, 639–655.

Lee, S-Y., Song, X.Y. (2003). Maximum likelihood estimation and model comparison of nonlinear structural equation models with continuous and polytomous variables. *Computational Statistics and Data Analysis* **44**, 125–142.

Lee, S-Y., Song, X.Y., Lee, J.C.K. (2003). Maximum likelihood estimation of nonlinear structural equation models with ignorable missing data. *Journal of Educational and Behavioral Statistics* **28**, 111–124.

Lee, S-Y., Song, X.Y., Poon, W.Y. (2004). Comparison of approaches in estimating interaction and quadratic effects of latent variables. *Multivariate Behavioral Research* **39**, 37–67.

Lee, S-Y., Tang, N-S. (2006). Bayesian analysis of nonlinear structural equation models with nonignorable missing data. *Psychometrika* **71**, 541–564.

Lee, S-Y., Tsui, K.L. (1982). Covariance structure analysis in several populations. *Psychometrika* **47**, 297–308.

Lee, S-Y., Zhu, H.T. (2000). Statistical analysis of nonlinear structural equation models with continuous and polytomous data. *British Journal of Mathematical and Statistical Psychology* **53**, 209–232.

Lee, S-Y., Zhu, H.T. (2002). Maximum likelihood estimation of nonlinear structural equation models. *Psychometrika* **67**, 189–210.

Li, L., Bentler, P.M. (2006). Robust statistical tests for evaluating the hypothesis of close fit of misspecified mean and covariance structural models. *UCLA Statistics Preprint No. 494* (http://preprints.stat.ucla.edu/).

Liang, J., Bentler, P.M. (2004). A new EM algorithm for fitting two-level structural equation models. *Psychometrika* **69**, 101–122.

Little, R.J.A., Rubin, D.B. (2002). *Statistical Analysis with Missing Data*, 2nd ed. Wiley, New York.

Loehlin, J.C. (2004). *Latent Variable Models: An Introduction to Factor, Path, and Structural Equation Analysis*, 4th ed. Erlbaum, Mahwah, NJ.

Lubke, G., Muthén, B. (2005). Investigating population heterogeneity with factor mixture models. *Psychological Methods* **10**, 21–39.

MacCallum, R.C., Austin, J.T. (2000). Applications of structural equation modeling in psychological research. *Annual Review of Psychology* **51**, 201–226.

MacCallum, R.C., Browne, M.W., Sugawara, H.M. (1996). Power analysis and determination of sample size for covariance structure modeling. *Psychological Methods* **1**, 130–149.

MacCallum, R.C., Roznowski, M., Necowitz, L.B. (1992). Model modifications in covariance structure analysis: The problem of capitalization on chance. *Psychological Bulletin* **111**, 490–504.

Magnus, J.R., Neudecker, H. (1999). *Matrix Differential Calculus with Applications in Statistics and Econometrics*, revised ed. Wiley, New York.

Marcoulides, G.A., Schumacker, R.E. (eds.) (1996). Advanced Structural Equation Modeling: Issues and Techniques. Erlbaum, Mahwah, NJ.

Marcoulides, G.A., Schumacker, R.E. (eds.) (2001). New Developments and Techniques in Structural Equation Modeling. Erlbaum, Mahwah, NJ.

Mardia, K.V. (1970). Measures of multivariate skewness and kurtosis with applications. *Biometrika* **57**, 519–530.

Maronna, R.A. (1976). Robust M-estimators of multivariate location and scatter. *Annals of Statistics* **4**, 51–67.

Marsh, H.W., Wen, Z., Hau, K.T. (2004). Structural equation models of latent interactions: Evaluation of alternative estimation strategies and indicator construction. *Psychological Methods* **9**, 275–300.

Maruyama, G.M. (1998). *Basics of Structural Equation Modeling*. Sage, Thousand Oaks, CA.

Maxwell, S.E., Delaney, H.D. (2004). *Designing Experiments and Analyzing Data: A Model Comparison Perspective*, 2nd ed. Erlbaum, Mahwah, NJ.

Maydeu-Olivares, A. (2001). Multidimensional item response theory modeling of binary data: Large sample properties of NOHARM estimates. *Journal of Educational and Behavioral Statistics* **26**, 51–71.

Maydeu-Olivares, A. (2005). Linear IRT, nonlinear IRT, and factor analysis: A unified framework. In: Maydeu-Olivares, A., McArdle, J.J. (Eds.), *Contemporary Psychometrics*. Erlbaum, Mahwah, NJ.

Maydeu-Olivares, A., Cai, L. (2006). A cautionary note on using G^2(dif) to assess relative model fit in categorical data analysis. *Multivariate Behavioral Research* **41**, 55–64.

McCullagh, P., Nelder, J.A. (1989). *Generalized Linear Models*, 2nd ed. Chapman and Hall, London.

McDonald, R.P., Goldstein, H. (1989). Balanced versus unbalanced designs for linear structural relations in two-level data. *British Journal of Mathematical and Statistical Psychology* **42**, 215–232.

McDonald, R.P., Ho, R.M. (2002). Principles and practice in reporting structural equation analyses. *Psychological Methods* **7**, 64–82.

Meredith, W. (1993). Measurement invariance, factor analysis and factorial invariance. *Psychometrika* **58**, 525–543.

Meredith, W., Tisak, J. (1990). Latent curve analysis. *Psychometrika* **55**, 107–122.

Millsap, R.E. (1997). Invariance in measurement and prediction: Their relationship in the single-factor case. *Psychological Methods* **2**, 248–260.

Mooijaart, A. (1985). Factor analysis for non-normal variables. *Psychometrika* **50**, 323–342.

Mooijaart, A. (2003). Estimating the statistical power in small samples by empirical distributions. In: Yanai, H., Okada, A., Shigemasu, K., Kano, Y., Meulman, J.J. (Eds.), *New Development in Psychometrics*. Springer-Verlag, Tokyo, pp. 149–156.

Mooijaart, A., Bentler, P.M. (1986). Random polynomial factor analysis. In: Diday, E., Escoufier, Y., Lebart, L., Pages, J., Schektman, Y., Tomassone, R. (Eds.), *Data Analysis and Informatics IV*. Elsevier Science, Amsterdam, pp. 241–250.

Mooijaart, A., Bentler, P.M. (1991). Robustness of normal theory statistics in structural equation models. *Statistica Neerlandica* **45**, 159–171.

Moustaki, I. (2001). A review of exploratory factor analysis for ordinal categorical data. In: Cudeck, R., du Toit, S., Sörbom, D. (Eds.), *Structual Equation Modeling: Present and Future*. Scientific Software International, Lincolnwood, IL.

Muthén, B. (1978). Contributions to factor analysis of dichotomous variables. *Psychometrika* **43**, 551–560.

Muthén, B. (1984). A general structural equation model with dichotomous, ordered categorical, and continuous latent variable indicators. *Psychometrika* **49**, 115–132.

Muthén, B. (1989a). Multiple group structural modelling with nonnormal continuous variables. *British Journal of Mathematical and Statistical Psychology* **42**, 55–62.

Muthén, B. (1989b). Latent variable modeling in heterogeneous populations. *Psychometrika* **54**, 557–585.

Muthén, B. (1994). Multilevel covariance structure analysis. *Sociological Methods and Research* **22**, 376–398.

Muthén, B. (1997). Latent variable modeling of longitudinal and multilevel data. In: Raftery, A. (Ed.), *Sociological Methodology 1997*. Blackwell Publishers, Boston, pp. 453–480.

Muthén, B., Kaplan, D., Hollis, M. (1987). On structural equation modeling with data that are not missing completely at random. *Psychometrika* **52**, 431–462.

Muthén, L.K., Muthén, B. (2001). *Mplus User's Guide*, 2nd ed. Muthen & Muthen, Los Angeles, CA.

Muthén, L.K., Muthén, B. (2002). How to use a Monte Carlo study to decide on sample size and determine power. *Structural Equation Modeling* **9**, 599–620.

Ogasawara, H. (2001). Approximations to the distributions of fit indices for misspecified structural equation models. *Structural Equation Modeling* **8**, 556–574.

Peek, M.K. (2000). Structural equation modeling and rehabilitation research. *American Journal of Physical Medicine and Rehabilitation* **79**, 301–309.

Penny, W.D., Stephan, K.E., Mechelli, A., Friston, K.J. (2004). Comparing dynamic causal models. *NeuroImage* **22**, 1157–1172.

Poon, W.Y., Lee, S-Y. (1987). Maximum likelihood estimation of multivariate polyserial and polychoric correlation coefficient. *Psychometrika* **52**, 409–430.

Poon, W.Y., Lee, S-Y. (1994). A distribution free approach for analysis of two-level structural equation model. *Computational Statistics and Data Analysis* **17**, 265–275.

Rao, C.R. (1947). Large sample tests of statistical hypotheses concerning several parameters with applications to problems of estimation. *Proceedings of the Cambridge Philosophical Society* **44**, 50–57.

Rao, C.R. (1973). *Linear Statistical Inference and Its Applications*, 2nd ed. Wiley, New York.

Raudenbush, S.W. (1995). Maximum likelihood estimation for unbalanced multilevel covariance structure models via the EM algorithm. *British Journal of Mathematical and Statistical Psychology* **48**, 359–370.

Raudenbush, S.W., Bryk, A.S. (2002). *Hierarchical Linear Models*, 2nd ed. Sage, Newbury Park, CA.

Raykov, T., Marcoulides, G.A. (2006). *A First Course in Structural Equation Modeling*, 2nd ed. Erlbaum, Mahwah, NJ.

Reise, S.P., Duan, N. (Eds.) (2003). *Multilevel Modeling: Methodological Advances, Issues, and Applications*. Erlbaum, Mahwah, NJ.

Rindskopf, D. (1984). Structural equation models: Empirical identification, Heywood cases, and related problems. *Sociological Methods and Research* **13**, 109–119.

Robert, C.P., Casella, G. (2004). *Monte Carlo Statistical Methods*, 2nd ed. Springer, New York.

Rubin, D.B. (1976). Inference and missing data (with discussions). *Biometrika* **63**, 581–592.

Saris, W.E., Satorra, A. (1993). Power evaluations in structural equation models. In: Bollen, K.A., Long, J.S. (Eds.), *Testing Structural Equation Models*. Sage, Newbury Park, CA, pp. 181–204.

Satorra, A. (1989). Alternative test criteria in covariance structure analysis: A unified approach. *Psychometrika* **54**, 131–151.

Satorra, A. (1992). Asymptotic robust inferences in the analysis of mean and covariance structures. *Sociological Methodology* **22**, 249–278.

Satorra, A. (2000). Scaled and adjusted restricted tests in multi-sample analysis of moment structures. In: Heijmans, D.D.H., Pollock, D.S.G., Satorra, A. (Eds.), *Innovations in Multivariate Statistical Analysis: A Festschrift for Heinz Neudecker*. Kluwer Academic, Dordrecht, pp. 233–247.

Satorra, A. (2002). Asymptotic robustness in multiple group linear-latent variable models. *Econometric Theory* **18**, 297–312.

Satorra, A., Bentler, P.M. (1988). Scaling corrections for chi-square statistics in covariance structure analysis. In: *American Statistical Association 1988 Proceedings of Business and Economics Sections*. American Statistical Association, Alexandria, VA, pp. 308–313.

Satorra, A., Bentler, P.M. (1990). Model conditions for asymptotic robustness in the analysis of linear relations. *Computational Statistics and Data Analysis* **10**, 235–249.

Satorra, A., Bentler, P.M. (1994). Corrections to test statistics and standard errors in covariance structure analysis. In: von Eye, A., Clogg, C.C. (Eds.), *Latent Variables Analysis: Applications for Developmental Research*. Sage, Thousand Oaks, CA, pp. 399–419.

Satorra, A., Bentler, P.M. (2001). A scaled difference chi-square test statistic for moment structure analysis. *Psychometrika* **66**, 507–514.

Satorra, A., Saris, W. (1985). Power of the likelihood ratio test in covariance structure analysis. *Psychometrika* **50**, 83–90.

Savalei, V., Bentler, P.M. (2005). A statistically justified pairwise ML method for incomplete non-normal data: A comparison with direct ML and pairwise ADF. *Structural Equation Modeling* **12**, 183–214.

Schumacker, R.E., Marcoulides, G.A. (Eds.) (1998). *Interaction and Nonlinear Effects in Structural Equation Modeling*. Erlbaum, Mahwah, NJ.

Schwarz, G. (1978). Estimating the dimension of a model. *Annals of Statistics* **6**, 461–464.

Shapiro, A. (1983). Asymptotic distribution theory in the analysis of covariance structures (a unified approach). *South African Statistical Journal* **17**, 33–81.

Shapiro, A. (1984). A note on the consistency of estimators in the analysis of moment structures. *British Journal of Mathematical and Statistical Psychology* **37**, 84–88.

Shapiro, A., Browne, M.W. (1987). Analysis of covariance structures under elliptical distributions. *Journal of the American Statistical Association* **82**, 1092–1097.

Shipley, B. (2000). *Cause and Correlation in Biology*. Cambridge University Press, New York.

Skrondal, A., Rabe-Hesketh, S. (2004). *Generalized Latent Variable Modeling: Multilevel, Longitudinal, and Structural Equation Models*. Chapman & Hall, London.

Song, X.Y., Lee, S-Y. (2002). Analysis of structural equation model with ignorable missing continuous and polytomous data. *Psychometrika* **67**, 261–288.

Sörbom, D. (1974). A general method for studying differences in factor means and factor structures between groups. *British Journal of Mathematical and Statistical Psychology* **27**, 229–239.

Sörbom, D. (1989). Model modification. *Psychometrika* **54**, 371–384.

Steiger, J.H., Lind, J.M. (1980). Statistically based tests for the number of common factors. Paper presented at the Annual Meeting of the Psychometric Society. Iowa City, IA.

Steiger, J.H., Shapiro, A., Browne, M.W. (1985). On the multivariate asymptotic distribution of sequential chi-square statistics. *Psychometrika* **50**, 253–264.

Stoel, R.D. (2003). *Issues in Growth Curve Modeling*. TT-Publikaties, Amsterdam.

Tanaka, J.S. (1993). Multifaceted conceptions of fit in structural equation models. In: Bollen, K.A., Long, J.S. (Eds.), *Testing Structural Equation Models*. Sage, Newbury Park, CA, pp. 10–39.

Tang, M.L., Bentler, P.M. (1998). Theory and method for constrained estimation in structural equation models with incomplete data. *Computational Statistics and Data Analysis* **27**, 257–270.

Tang, M.L., Lee, S-Y. (1998). Analysis of structural equation model with non-ignorable missing data. *Computational Statistics and Data Analysis* **27**, 33–46.

Tucker, L.R., Lewis, C. (1973). A reliability coefficient for maximum likelihood factor analysis. *Psychometrika* **38**, 1–10.

Tyler, D.E. (1983). Robustness and efficiency properties of scatter matrices. *Biometrika* **70**, 411–420.

van den Oord, E.J. (2000). Framework for identifying quantitative trait loci in association studies using structural equation modeling. *Genetic Epidemiology* **18**, 341–359.

van Driel, O.P. (1978). On various causes of improper solutions in maximum likelihood factor analysis. *Psychometrika* **43**, 225–243.

Vuong, Q.H. (1989). Likelihood ratio tests for model selection and nonnested hypotheses. *Econometrica* **57**, 307–333.

Wald, A. (1943). Tests of statistical hypotheses concerning several parameters when the number of observations is large. *Transactions of the American Mathematical Society* **54**, 426–482.

Wall, M.M., Amemiya, Y. (2000). Estimation for polynomial structural equation models. *Journal of the American Statistical Association* **95**, 920–940.

Wall, M.M., Amemiya, Y. (2001). Generalized appended product indicator procedure for nonlinear structural equation analysis. *Journal of Educational and Behavioral Statistics* **26**, 1–29.

Wall, M.M., Amemiya, Y. (2003). A method of moments technique for fitting interaction effects in structural equation models. *British Journal of Mathematical and Statistical Psychology* **56**, 47–64.

White, H. (1982). Maximum likelihood estimation of misspecified models. *Econometrica* **50**, 1–25.

Yanagihara, H., Tonda, T., Matsumoto, C. (2005). The effects of nonnormality on asymptotic distributions of some likelihood ratio criteria for testing covariance structures under normal assumption. *Journal of Multivariate Analysis* **96**, 237–264.

Yang Jonsson, F. (1998). Modeling interaction and nonlinear effects: A step-by-step Lisrel example. In: Schmacker, R.E., Marcoulides, G.A. (Eds.), *Interaction and Nonlinear Effects in Structural Equation Modeling*. Erlbaum, Mahwah, NJ, pp. 17–42.

Yuan, K-H. (2005). Fit indices versus test statistics. *Multivariate Behavior Research* **40**, 115–148.

Yuan, K-H. (2006). Normal theory ML for missing data with violation of distribution assumptions (Under review).

Yuan, K-H., Bentler, P.M. (1997a). Mean and covariance structure analysis: Theoretical and practical improvements. *Journal of the American Statistical Association* **92**, 767–774.

Yuan, K.-H., Bentler, P.M. (1997b). Improving parameter tests in covariance structure analysis. *Computational Statistics and Data Analysis* **26**, 177–198.

Yuan, K.-H., Bentler, P.M. (1998a). Normal theory based test statistics in structural equation modeling. *British Journal of Mathematical and Statistical Psychology* **51**, 289–309.

Yuan, K.-H., Bentler, P.M. (1998b). Robust mean and covariance structure analysis. *British Journal of Mathematical and Statistical Psychology* **51**, 63–88.

Yuan, K.-H., Bentler, P.M. (1998c). Structural equation modeling with robust covariances. *Sociological Methodology* **28**, 363–396.

Yuan, K.-H., Bentler, P.M. (1999a). On normal theory and associated test statistics in covariance structure analysis under two classes of nonnormal distributions. *Statistica Sinica* **9**, 831–853.

Yuan, K.-H., Bentler, P.M. (1999b). On asymptotic distributions of normal theory MLE in covariance structure analysis under some nonnormal distributions. *Statistics and Probability Letters* **42**, 107–113.

Yuan, K.-H., Bentler, P.M. (1999c). F-tests for mean and covariance structure analysis. *Journal of Educational and Behavioral Statistics* **24**, 225–243.

Yuan, K.-H., Bentler, P.M. (2000a). Three likelihood-based methods for mean and covariance structure analysis with nonnormal missing data. *Sociological Methodology* **30**, 167–202.

Yuan, K.-H., Bentler, P.M. (2000b). Robust mean and covariance structure analysis through iteratively reweighted least squares. *Psychometrika* **65**, 43–58.

Yuan, K.-H., Bentler, P.M. (2001). A unified approach to multigroup structural equation modeling with nonstandard samples. In: Marcoulides, G.A., Schumacker, R.E. (Eds.), *Advanced Structural Equation Modeling: New Developments and Techniques*. Erlbaum, Mahwah, NJ, pp. 35–56.

Yuan, K.-H., Bentler, P.M. (2002). On normal theory based inference for multilevel models with distributional violations. *Psychometrika* **67**, 539–561.

Yuan, K.-H., Bentler, P.M. (2003). Eight test statistics for multilevel structural equation models. *Computational Statistics and Data Analysis* **44**, 89–107.

Yuan, K.-H., Bentler, P.M. (2004a). On chi-square difference and z-tests in mean and covariance structure analysis when the base model is misspecified. *Educational and Psychological Measurement* **64**, 737–757.

Yuan, K.-H., Bentler, P.M. (2004b). On the asymptotic distributions of two statistics for two-level covariance structure models within the class of elliptical distributions. *Psychometrika* **69**, 437–457.

Yuan, K.-H., Bentler, P.M. (2005a). Asymptotic robustness of the normal theory likelihood ratio statistic for two-level covariance structure models. *Journal of Multivariate Analysis* **94**, 328–343.

Yuan, K.-H., Bentler, P.M. (2005b). Asymptotic robustness of standard errors in multilevel structural equation models. *Journal of Multivariate Analysis* **94**, 328–343.

Yuan, K.-H., Bentler, P.M. (2006). Mean comparison: Manifest variable versus latent variable. *Psychometrika* **71**, 139–159.

Yuan, K.-H., Bentler, P.M., Chan, W. (2004). Structural equation modeling with heavy tailed distributions. *Psychometrika* **69**, 421–436.

Yuan, K.-H., Chan, W. (2005). On nonequivalence of several procedures of structural equation modeling. *Psychometrika* **70**, 791–798.

Yuan, K.-H., Chan, W., Bentler, P.M. (2000). Robust transformation with applications to structural equation modeling. *British Journal of Mathematical and Statistical Psychology* **53**, 31–50.

Yuan, K.-H., Fung, W.K., Reise, S. (2004). Three Mahalanobis-distances and their role in assessing unidimensionality. *British Journal of Mathematical and Statistical Psychology* **57**, 151–165.

Yuan, K.-H., Hayashi, K. (2003). Bootstrap approach to inference and power analysis based on three statistics for covariance structure models. *British Journal of Mathematical and Statistical Psychology* **56**, 93–110.

Yuan, K.-H., Hayashi, K. (2006). Standard errors in covariance structure models: Asymptotics versus bootstrap. *British Journal of Mathematical and Statistical Psychology* **59**, 397–417.

Yuan, K.-H., Hayashi, K. (2005). On Muthen's maximum likelihood for two-level covariance structure models. *Psychometrika* **70**, 147–167.

Yuan, K.-H., Hayashi, K., Bentler, P.M. (2007). Normal theory likelihood ratio statistic for mean and covariance structure analysis under alternative hypotheses. *Journal of Multivariate Analysis* **98**, 1262–1282.

Yuan, K.-H., Marshall, L.L. (2004). A new measure of misfit for covariance structure models. *Behaviormetrika* **31**, 67–90.

Yuan, K.-H., Marshall, L.L., Bentler, P.M. (2002). A unified approach to exploratory factor analysis with missing data, nonnormal data, and in the presence of outliers. *Psychometrika* **67**, 95–122.

Yuan, K.-H., Marshall, L.L., Bentler, P.M. (2003). Assessing the effect of model misspecifications on parameter estimates in structural equation models. *Sociological Methodology* **33**, 241–265.

Yung, Y.-F. (1997). Finite mixtures in confirmatory factor-analysis models. *Psychometrika* **62**, 297–330.

Yung, Y.-F., Bentler, P.M. (1996). Bootstrapping techniques in analysis of mean and covariance structures. In: Marcoulides, G.A., Schumacker, R.E. (Eds.), *Advanced Structural Equation Modeling: Techniques and Issues*. Erlbaum, Hillsdale, NJ, pp. 195–226.

Handbook of Statistics, Vol. 27
ISSN: 0169-7161
© 2007 Elsevier B.V. All rights reserved
DOI: 10.1016/S0169-7161(07)27014-2

8

Statistical Modeling in Biomedical Research: Longitudinal Data Analysis

Chengjie Xiong, Kejun Zhu, Kai Yu and J. Philip Miller

Abstract

This chapter discusses some major statistical methods for longitudinal data analysis in biomedical research. We have provided a detailed review to some of the most used statistical models for the analyses of longitudinal data and relevant design issues based on these models. Our focus is on the conceptualization of longitudinal statistical models, the assumptions associated with them, and the interpretations of model parameters. It is not our intention to present the detailed theory on statistical estimations and inferences for these models in this chapter. Instead, we have presented the implementations for some of these basic longitudinal models in SAS through real-world applications.

1. Introduction

Why should longitudinal studies in biomedical research be conducted? The answer to this question depends on the study objectives in biomedical research. There is a fundamental difference between a longitudinal study and a cross-sectional study. Cross-sectional studies are those in which individuals are observed only once. Most surveys are cross-sectional, as are studies to construct reference ranges. Longitudinal studies, however, are those that investigate changes over time, possibly in relation to an intervention. Therefore, the primary characteristic of a longitudinal study is that study subjects are measured repeatedly through time. The major advantage of a longitudinal study is its capacity to separate what in the context of population studies are called *cohort* and *age* effects (Diggle et al., 2002). Outcome variables in the longitudinal studies may be continuous measurements, counts, dichotomous, or categorical indicators, and in many cases, outcomes may even be multivariate as well. Covariates in the longitudinal studies may also be continuous measurements, counts, dichotomous, or categorical indicators, and in many cases, covariate may be time varying as well. As an example, in the study of healthy ageing and Alzheimer's disease (AD), the understanding of natural history of AD requires a longitudinal design and the corresponding appropriate analysis. One of the primary objectives in these studies is to model the cognitive function as a function of baseline age, the time lapse from the baseline, the disease status, and other possible risk factors. For the purpose of demonstration, we consider a simple case and let $Y(a,t)$ be the cognitive function at time lapse t from the baseline (i.e., $t = 0$ at baseline) for a subject whose baseline age is a. Assume that the expected value of $Y(a,t)$ is a linear function of both baseline age a and the time lapse t from the baseline, i.e.,

$$EY(a, t) = \beta_0 + \beta_1 a + \beta_2 t.$$

The standard interpretation of β_1 is the expected change of cognitive function at the baseline (or at the same time t during the longitudinal course) for two subjects whose baseline age is 1 year apart. The standard interpretation of β_2 is the expected change of cognitive function per time unit for the same subject during the longitudinal course of the study. The crucial difference between β_1 and β_2 is that β_1 measures a between-subject or a cross-sectional change, whereas β_2 measures a within-subject or a longitudinal change. If only cross-sectional cognitive measures are available, i.e., the study is measured only at baseline, then $t = 0$ and $EY(a, t) = \beta_0 + \beta_1 a$. Therefore, any statistical inferences from the cross-sectional data can only be made on β_1, i.e., the cross-sectional rate of change. On the other hand, if longitudinal cognitive measures are available, then statistical inferences can be made on both β_1 and β_2. Therefore, longitudinal studies enable not only the estimation of cross-sectional rate of change based on baseline age, but also the estimation of the rate of intra-individual change based on the time lapse in the study.

Another main study objective for a longitudinal study is to relate intra-subject rate of change over time to individual characteristics (e.g., exposure, age, etc.), or to an experimental condition. In the above example, studying the healthy ageing and AD, many potential risk factors in addition to baseline age could affect not only the cognitive status of subjects at baseline but also the rate of cognitive decline after the baseline. These risk factors range from demographics such as gender and education to genetic status (i.e., Apolipoprotein E genotypes) and to relevant biomarkers and imaging markers. In addition, the stage or the severity of AD could also be an important factor affecting the rate of further cognitive decline. In general, therapeutic trials of AD are longitudinal, and the most crucial scientific question to be addressed in these trials is whether the therapeutic treatment is efficacious in slowing the cognitive and functional decline of AD patients. Therefore, the rate of cognitive decline in AD clinical trials is modeled as a function of treatment received. More specifically, let β_2^t be the expected rate of cognitive decline over time for subjects randomly assigned to receive a therapeutic treatment, and let β_2^c be the expected rate of cognitive decline over time for control subjects. The longitudinal nature of the study allows the statistical test on whether β_2^t is the same as β_2^c and the statistical estimation on the difference between these two rates of cognitive decline.

As in all biomedical studies, there are two major statistical components in longitudinal studies: statistical design and statistical analysis. This chapter will review some of the most used statistical models for the analyses of longitudinal data and relevant design issues based on these models. Throughout this chapter, we will focus on the conceptualization of basic longitudinal statistical models, the basic assumptions these models are based on, and the interpretations of model parameters. It is not our intention to present the detailed theory on statistical estimations and inferences based on these models. Instead, we will present the implementations for some of these basic longitudinal models in SAS through real-world applications. For detailed statistical theory on the parameter estimation and inferences from these models, readers are referred to some of the excellent references in longitudinal statistical methods such as Diggle et al. (2002), Fitzmaurice et al. (2004), Verbeke and Molenberghs (2000), and Singer and Willett (2003).

2. Analysis of longitudinal data

The defining characteristic of longitudinal data analysis is the fact that the response variable or variables are repeatedly measured on the same individuals over time and therefore the resulting responses on the same individuals are statistically correlated. Whereas much of the focus in the analysis of longitudinal data is on the mean response over time, the correlation among the repeated measures plays a crucial role and cannot be ignored. Generally, there are two approaches for modeling the mean response over time. The first approach is the analysis of response profile in which repeated measures analysis of variance or covariance serves as special examples. The important feature of analysis of response profile is that it allows for an unstructured pattern of mean response over time, i.e., no specific time trend is assumed. Because the analysis of response profile treats times of measurements as levels of a discrete study factor, it is especially useful when the objective of the study is to make statistical inferences at individual times or to compare mean responses among different time points. On the other hand, this approach to the analysis of longitudinal data is generally only applicable to the case when all individuals under study are measured at the same set of time points and the number of time points is usually small compared to the sample size.

Another common approach to analyze longitudinal data is based on a parametric growth curve for the mean response over time. Because this approach assumes a parametric function of time, it generally has the advantage of a much smaller number of parameters in the model as compared to the analysis of response profile and provides a very parsimonious summary of trend over time in the mean response, and therefore is especially useful when the objective of the study is to make statistical inferences on certain parameters from the parametric curve. As an example, if a linear trend is appropriate to model the mean response over time, two parameters, the intercept and the slope over time, completely characterize the entire mean response over time. Because the slope parameter measures the rate of change in mean response over time, it could be the primary interest in the statistical inference. In contrast to the analysis of response profile, the longitudinal analysis based on a parametric or semi-parametric growth curve does not require the study subjects be measured at the same set of time points, nor even the same number of repeated measures among different subjects.

2.1. Analysis of response profiles

When all individuals under study are measured at the same set of time points, the vector of longitudinal means over time is usually called the mean response profile. The analysis of response profiles is especially useful when there is a one-way treatment structure and when there is no pilot information on the mean response profiles over time among different treatment groups. This method assumes no specific structure on the mean response profile and nor on the covariance structure of the repeated measures.

Assume a longitudinal study in which the treatment factor has a total of u levels and the response variable Y is measured at each of the v time points. For the ith treatment group, $i = 1, 2, \ldots, u$ and kth time point, $i = 1, 2, \ldots, v$, let μ_{ik} be the mean of the response variable. Let $\mu^i = (\mu_{i1}, \mu_{i2}, \ldots, \mu_{iv})^t$ (superscript t stands for the matrix transpose) be the response profile for the ith treatment group. In general, the most important question in this type of longitudinal study is whether the response profiles are parallel among different treatment groups, which are the same as whether there exists an interaction between the treatment factor and the time factor. Mathematically, let $d^i = \mu^i - \mu^1 = (d_{i1}, d_{i2}, \ldots, d_{iv})^t$ be the vector of mean difference profile between the ith treatment group and the first treatment group (i.e., the reference group). If there is no interaction between the treatment factor and the time factor, then the hypothesis $H_0 : d_{i1} = d_{i2} = \cdots = d_{iv}$ holds for $i = 2, 3, \ldots, u$. The test of this hypothesis has a degree of freedom equal to $(u-1)(v-1)$. Notice that the null hypothesis of no interaction between the treatment factor and the time factor is equivalent to

$$H_0 : \Delta = (\delta_{22}, \delta_{23}, \ldots, \delta_{2v}, \delta_{32}, \delta_{33}, \ldots, \delta_{3v}, \ldots, \delta_{u2}, .\delta_{u3}, \ldots, \delta_{uv})^t = 0,$$

where $\delta_{ik} = d_{ik} - d_{i1}$, $i = 2, 3, \ldots, u$, and $k = 2, 3, \ldots, v$.

When analyzing response profiles, it is generally assumed that the response vector $Y_j = (y_1, y_2, \ldots, y_v)^t$ follows a multivariate normal distribution (Graybill, 1976) and that the covariance matrix of response vector $Y_j = (y_i, y_2, \ldots, y_v)^t$ is unstructured, although it is required to be symmetric and positive-definite. When longitudinal data are observed, the maximum likelihood (ML) estimates or the restricted maximum likelihood (REML) estimates $\hat{\Delta} = (\hat{\delta}_{22}, \hat{\delta}_{23}, \ldots, \hat{\delta}_{2v}, \hat{\delta}_{32}, \hat{\delta}_{33}, \ldots, \hat{\delta}_{3v}, \ldots, \hat{\delta}_{u2}, .\hat{\delta}_{u3}, \ldots, \hat{\delta}_{uv})^t$ can then be obtained (Diggle et al., 2002). Further, assume that the covariance matrix of $\hat{\Delta}$ can be estimated by $\hat{\Sigma}_{\hat{\Delta}}$. Then the test of interaction effect between the treatment factor and the time factor can be carried out through the standard Wald test by computing

$$\chi^2 = \hat{\Delta}^t \left(\hat{\Sigma}_{\hat{\Delta}} \right)^{-1} \hat{\Delta}.$$

At a significance level of $\alpha(0 < \alpha < 1)$, this test rejects the null hypothesis when $\chi^2 > \chi^2_\alpha((u-1)(v-1))$, where $\chi^2_\alpha((u-1)(v-1))$ is the upper $100\alpha\%$ percentile of the χ^2 distribution with $(u-1)(v-1)$ degrees of freedom.

Likelihood-ratio test can also be used to test the interaction effect between the treatment factor and the time factor. This requires fitting two models with and without the constraint of the null hypothesis. Without the constraint (also called the full model), this amounts to the standard sampling theory of multivariate normal distributions, and the likelihood function L_{full} can be readily computed through the standard ML estimates of mean response vector and covariance matrices. Under the null hypothesis (also called the reduced model), another maximization procedure is needed to find the ML estimates of mean response vector and covariance matrices, and the likelihood function $L_{reduced}$ under the null hypothesis can be obtained. Finally, the likelihood-ratio test of interaction effect between the treatment factor and the time factor can be carried out by computing

$$LRT = 2\log(L_{full}) - 2\log(L_{reduced}),$$

and further by comparing it to the upper $100\alpha\%$ percentile of the χ^2 distribution with $(u-1)(v-1)$ degrees of freedom. Depending on the results from the statistical test on the interaction effect between the treatment factor and the time factor, one can proceed to test the main effects for both the treatment factor and the time factor, as well as the pairwise comparisons between different levels of the treatment factor at given time points and between different levels of the time factor at given treatment levels.

An analysis of response profiles can be implemented in SAS through the following codes, where TREATMENT is the classification variable of the treatment factor, TIME is the classification variable for the time factor, and ID is the identification for subjects under the study:

```
PROC MIXED DATA = ; CLASSES ID TREATMENT TIME;
MODEL Y = TREATMENT TIME TREATMENT*TIME;
REPEATED TIME/TYPE = UN SUBJECT = ID R RCORR;
LSMEANS TREATMENT TIME TREATMENT*TIME/PDIFF;
RUN;
```

When the number of time points is relatively large, the omnibus test with $(u-1)(v-1)$ degrees of freedom on the interaction effect might become rather insensitive to the specific departures from parallelism and therefore have a rather low statistical power to detect the treatment differences. There are several different ways that more powerful tests on the interaction effect could be derived. In a two-arm randomized clinical trial consisting of a novel therapeutic treatment and a placebo, by the nature of randomization, the treated group and the placebo group should have the same mean response at the baseline. Therefore, it might make sense to examine the treatment difference by comparing the difference between the mean response over all time points beyond the baseline and the mean response at the baseline. More specifically, if there are 6 time points used in the study (coded as 1,2,3,4,5,6 with 1 = baseline), one would assess the effect of the novel treatment (coded as 2) as compared to the placebo (coded as 1) by testing $H_0 : ((\mu_{22} + \mu_{23} + \mu_{24} + \mu_{25} + \mu_{26})/5) - \mu_{21} = ((\mu_{12} + \mu_{13} + \mu_{14} + \mu_{15} + \mu_{16})/5) - \mu_{11}.$

This test has 1 degree of freedom and can be implemented by the following SAS codes with a CONTRAST statement. (The CONTRAST statement could differ depending on how these factors are coded in SAS, but option E should clearly indicate whether a correct CONTRAST statement was written (SAS Institute, Inc., 1999).)

```
PROC MIXED DATA = ; CLASSES ID TREATMENT TIME;
MODEL Y = TREATMENT*TIME/NOINT;
REPEATED TIME/TYPE = UN SUBJECT = ID R RCORR;
CONTRAST '1 DF INTERACTION TEST'
TREATMENT*TIME 1 -0.2 -0.2 -0.2 -0.2 -0.2 -1 0.2 0.2 0.2 0.2 0.2/E;
RUN;
```

In addition to the insensitivity of the general test with $(u-1)(v-1)$ degrees of freedom on the interaction effect to specific departures from the parallelism, the analysis of response profiles has other limitations in the analyses of longitudinal data despite the fact it is relatively simple to understand and easy to implement. The primary limitation of this approach is the requirement that all individuals under study be measured at the same set of time points, which prevents the use of the method in unbalanced and incomplete longitudinal studies. Another limitation is the fact that the analysis does not take into account of the time ordering of the repeated measurements from the same subjects, resulting in a possible loss of power in the analysis. Further, when the number of time points is relatively large, the analysis requires the estimation of a large covariance matrix, which also partly explains the fact the omnibus test with $(u-1)(v-1)$ degrees of freedom on the interaction effect has a rather low statistical power to detect the treatment differences.

2.2. Repeated measures analysis of variance

When a longitudinal study has a simple and classical design in which all subjects are measured at the same set of time points, and the only covariates which vary over time do so by design, the repeated measure analysis of variance can be used. The rationale for the repeated measures analysis of variance is to regard time as a within-subject factor in a hierarchical design which is generally referred to as a split-plot design in agricultural research. Unlike the analysis of response profiles in which the covariance matrix from the repeated measures from the same subjects are generally assumed unstructured, the repeated measures analysis of variance allows much simpler covariance matrix structure for the repeated measures over time. However, the usual randomization requirement in a standard split-plot design is not available in the longitudinal design because allocation of times to the multiple observations from the same subjects cannot be randomized. Therefore, it is necessary to assume an underlying model for the longitudinal data, which is essentially a special case of the general linear mixed models to be discussed in the next section.

Assume again that the covariate (i.e., the study conditions or treatments) takes a total of u possibilities and the response variable Y is measured at a total of

v time points. The repeated measures analysis of variance models the response y_{ijk} for the jth subject at the ith study condition and the kth time point as

$$y_{ijk} = \mu_{ik} + p_{ij} + e_{ijk},$$

where μ_{ik} is the mean response for the ith study condition or treatment at the kth time point, p_{ij} represents the subject error, and e_{ijk} the time interval error. The standard assumptions made to this type of models are that p_{ij} are independent and identically distributed as $N(0, \sigma_p^2)$, e_{ijk} are independent and identically distributed as $N(0, \sigma_e^2)$, and that e_{ijk}'s and p_{ij}'s are statistically independent. Let $Y_{ij} = (y_{ij1}, y_{ij2}, \ldots, y_{ijv})$ be the vector of the repeated measures for the jth subject under the ith study condition. Under the above assumptions, it is straightforward to derive the covariance matrix of Y_{ij} as

$$\mathrm{Cov}(Y_{ij}) = \begin{pmatrix} \sigma_p^2 + \sigma_e^2 & \sigma_p^2 & \cdots & \sigma_p^2 \\ \sigma_p^2 & \sigma_p^2 + \sigma_e^2 & \cdots & \sigma_p^2 \\ \cdots & \cdots & \cdots & \cdots \\ \sigma_p^2 & \sigma_p^2 & \cdots & \sigma_p^2 + \sigma_e^2 \end{pmatrix}.$$

This covariance structure is called the structure of compound symmetry, which further implies that the correlation between any two repeated measures from the same subject j is $\mathrm{Corr}(Y_{ijk}, Y_{ijk'}) = \sigma_p^2/(\sigma_p^2 + \sigma_e^2)$.

The above assumptions on the variance components p_{ij} and e_{ijk} will guarantee that the usual F-tests from a standard two-way analysis of variance of a split-plot design are still valid to test the main effect of study conditions and the main effect of the time intervals, as well as the interaction effect between the study conditions and the time intervals. The more general assumptions required for the usual F-tests from a standard two-way analysis of variance to be valid requires certain forms of the covariance matrix of the measurement errors of the time intervals and of the covariance matrix of the error terms of the subjects assigned to a given study conditions. This form is called the Huynh–Feldt (H–F) condition (Huynh and Feldt, 1970). A covariance matrix Σ of dimension v by v satisfies the H–F condition if $\Sigma = \lambda I_v + \gamma J_v^t + J_v \gamma^t$, where I_v is the v by v identity matrix, J_v a v-dimensional column vector of 1's, λ an unknown constant, and γ a v-dimensional unknown column vector of parameters. The following SAS code can be used to fit the above model (where GROUP is the classification variable of study conditions):

```
PROC MIXED DATA = ; CLASS GROUP ID TIME;
MODEL Y = GROUP TIME GROUP*TIME;
RANDOM ID(GROUP);
RUN;
```

The covariance structure of compound symmetry may be inappropriate in longitudinal studies because of the constant correlation between any two repeated measures from the same subjects regardless of their time distance between the repeated measures. Many other covariance structures on the repeated measures have been proposed, most of which are motivated by the standard time series analyses and therefore might be more appropriate in longitudinal data. For example, in the following autoregressive error structure, the covariance matrix is proportional to

$$\Sigma = \begin{pmatrix} 1 & \rho & \cdots & \rho^{v-1} \\ \rho & 1 & \cdots & \rho^{v-2} \\ \cdots & \cdots & \cdots & \cdots \\ \rho^{v-1} & \rho^{v-2} & \cdots & 1 \end{pmatrix}$$

for some $-1 < \rho < +1$. This covariance matrix represents the fact that the more two repeated measures are apart in time, the less correlation are between them. Unfortunately, when such covariance matrix is assumed for the within-subject error terms on the repeated measures, the H–F condition generally no longer holds. When the H–F condition is not satisfied, the statistical comparison on the study conditions (i.e., the whole plot analysis in the standard two-way analysis of variance from a split-plot design) from the usual analysis of variance is still accurate and valid. The inferences from the within-subject comparisons, however, can only be approximated through various appropriate F-tests or t-tests. These are especially true for the tests of the main effect on time and the interactive effect between the study condition and the time factor. Multiple approximations to these tests can be used, for example, Box's correction method (Box, 1954), and those based on the Satterthwaite's approximation (Satterthwaite, 1946) to the denominator degrees of freedoms in F- and t-tests. Other types of covariance matrix on the errors of the time intervals can also be fitted to this model in SAS. SAS also provides several different options for approximating the degrees of freedoms when approximate F-tests are needed.

The following SAS code fits the repeated measures analysis of variance model with autoregressive within-subject error structure and the approximate F- and t-tests based on Satterthwaite's method:

```
PROC MIXED DATA = ; CLASS GROUP ID TIME;
MODEL Y = GROUP TIME GROUP*TIME/DDFM = SATTERTH;
RANDOM ID(GROUP);
REPEATED TIME/SUBJECT = ID TYPE = AR;
RUN;
```

2.3. General linear models and general linear mixed models

2.3.1. General linear models for longitudinal data
General linear models and general linear mixed models are statistical methodologies frequently used to analyze longitudinal data. These models recognize the likely correlation structure from the repeated measurements on same subjects over time. The general linear models are built on either explicit parametric models of the covariance structure of repeated measures over time whose validity can be checked against the available data or, where possible, to use methods of inference which are robust to misspecification of the covariance structure. Unlike

the analysis of response profiles and repeated measures analysis of variance, the general linear models and general linear mixed models do not require that the longitudinal design be balanced or completed. In many cases, especially when the sample size is relatively small or moderate with many covariate variables, a parametric structure also need to be imposed on the covariance matrix of repeated measurements over time. Many different types of covariance structures have been used in the general linear models. In general, there are essentially two most popular ways to build a structure into a covariance matrix: using serial correlation models, and using random effects. The uniform correlation model assumes a positive correlation between any two measurements on the same subject. In contrast, the exponential correlation model (also called the first-order autoregressive model, Diggle, 1990) assumes an exponential decay toward 0 for the correlation between two measurements on the same subject as the time separation between the two measurements increases. The covariance structure of repeated measures based on random effects depends on the design matrix associated with the random effects.

Let $Y_j = (y_{j1}, y_{j2}, \ldots, y_{jk_j})^t$ be the vector of longitudinal observations for the variable of interest on the jth subject over k_j different time points $T_j = (t_{j1}, t_{j2}, \ldots, t_{jk_j})^t$. Notice that here we allow not only different numbers of time points but also different design vector over time among different subjects. Let $X_{jk} = (x_{jk1}, x_{jk2}, \ldots, x_{jkp})^t$ be the p by 1 vector of covariates associated with the kth measurement on the jth subject. Notice here that the vector of covariates could be time dependent. Let $X_j = (X_{j1}, X_{j2}, \ldots, X_{jk_j})^t$ be the design matrix of the jth subject. In longitudinal data analyses, it is generally assumed that X_j contains T_j itself and possibly some other covariates. The most general assumptions of a general linear model is

(1) $(Y_1, X_1), (Y_2, X_2), \ldots, (Y_n, X_n)$ are stochastically independent, which, in the case of fixed design matrix by design, is equivalent to $(Y_1, Y_2, \ldots, Y_n)$ that are independent, where n is the sample size of subjects under study;
(2) Given X_j, $EY_j = X_j\beta$, where β is a p by 1 column vector of regression coefficients, and $\text{cov}(Y_j) = \Sigma_j$.

2.3.2. Random effects models and general linear mixed models

A general way of introducing a covariance structure on repeated measurements is through the two-stage random effects models. When study subjects are sampled from a population, various aspects of their behavior may show stochastic variation between subjects. The simplest example of this is when the general level of the response profile varies between subjects, that is, some subjects are intrinsically high responders, others low responders. The two-stage random effect model (Diggle, 1988; Laird and Ware, 1982; Vonesh and Carter, 1992) allows the individual-specific response profile or 'growth curve' for each study subject at the first stage. The second stage of the two-stage random effects models introduces the between-subjects variation of the subject-specific effects and the population parameters of the subject-specific effects. The entire process leads to the development of the general linear mixed models. The ML estimates, the REML estimates, and the method-of-moment estimators are used to estimate the

regression parameters in general linear mixed models. In addition, the general
linear mixed models not only provide the best linear unbiased estimator (BLUE)
(Graybill, 1976) for any estimable contrast of the regression parameters, but also
estimate the subject-specific effects through the best linear unbiased predictor
(BLUP) (Harville, 1977).

The major advantages of using random effects model is both to provide a way
of modeling correlation among repeated measures from the same subjects and
to derive good estimates to the subject-specific random effects. First, random
effects are useful when strict measurements protocols in biomedical studies
are not followed or when the design matrix on time was irregularly spaced and
not consistent among subjects. Although many times biomedical studies are not
designed this way, it can happen because of protocol deviation, bad timing, or
missing data. Therefore the covariance matrix in the vector of longitudinal
measurements might then depend on the individual subjects. Random effects
model can handle this type of dependence in a very natural way. More specifically, the two-stage random effects models first assume that given the subject-
specific design matrix Z_j of dimension $k_j \times q$ and the subject-specific regression
coefficients β_j of dimension $q \times 1$,

$$Y_j = Z_j \beta_j + e_j,$$

where e_j follows a multivariate normal distribution with a mean vector of 0's and
a covariance matrix equal to $\sigma^2 I_{k_j \times k_j}$ ($I_{k_j \times k_j}$ is the identity matrix of dimension k_j).
At the second stage, given subject-level covariates A_j of dimension $q \times p$ and
another set of regression coefficients β of dimension $p \times 1$, the variation among
subject-specific regression coefficients β_j is modeled by another linear function of
subject-level covariates as

$$\beta_j = A_j \beta + b_j,$$

where b_j follows another multivariate normal distribution with a mean vector of
0's and a covariance matrix D of dimension q. Other standard assumptions about
the two-stage random effects model are that the vectors (Y_j, Z_j, A_j) are independent among a sample of size n, $j = 1, 2, \ldots, n$, and that e_j and b_j are statistically independent, $j = 1, 2, \ldots, n$. Notice that the design matrix A_j at the second
stage is between-subjects and typically time independent, whereas the design
matrix Z_j at the first stage is within-subjects and could be time dependent. In fact,
Z_j usually specifies some type of growth curve model over time, such as linear or
quadratic or spline functions.

An intuitive way to think of the two-stage random effects models in a longitudinal design is that each subject has his or her own 'growth curve' which is
specified by the subject-specific regression coefficients β_j in the model from the
first stage, and the population means of subject-specific regression coefficients β_j
are given by the model at the second stage, which depends on the between-
subjects covariates A_j. Combining the model from Stage 1 and that from Stage 2
in the two-stage random effects models, it follows that

$$Y_j = X_j(A_j \beta + b_j) + e_j,$$

i.e.,

$$Y_j = (X_j A_j)\beta + Z_j b_j + e_j.$$

This final model is a special case of the general linear mixed model formulation which has the following general form:

$$Y_j = W_j \beta + Z_j b_j + e_j,$$

where b_j follows a multivariate normal distribution with a mean vector of 0's and a covariance matrix D of dimension q, e_j follows another multivariate normal distribution with a mean vector of 0's and a covariance matrix R_j, W_j and Z_j are the design matrices associated with the fixed and random effects, respectively. Although R_j could assume different structures, it is generally assumed the diagonal matrix $\sigma^2 I_{k_j}$, where I_{k_j} is the identity matrix of dimension k_j. Under this assumption, e_{ji}'s could be interpreted as measurement errors. Other standard assumptions about the general linear mixed model are that, given W_j, e_j, and Y_j are statistically independent, $j = 1, 2, \ldots, n$. In the general linear mixed models, coefficients β are called the vector of fixed effects, which are assumed the same for all individuals and can be interpreted as the population parameters. In contrast to β, b_j are called random effects and are comprised of subject-specific regression coefficients, which, along with the fixed effects, describe the mean response for the jth subject as

$$E(Y_j | b_j) = W_j \beta + Z_j b_j.$$

It is also straightforward to derive that

$$E(Y_j) = W_j \beta,$$

and

$$\Sigma_j = \mathrm{Cov}(Y_j) = Z_j D Z_j' + R_j.$$

Weighted least squares estimation and the ML or REML methods through the EM algorithm (Patterson and Thompson, 1971; Cullis and McGilchrist, 1990; Verbyla and Cullis, 1990; Tunnicliffe-Wilson, 1989; Dempster et al., 1977; Laird and Ware, 1982; Vonesh and Carter, 1992) are used to estimate the mean response and the covariance parameters. Software is readily available for ML and REML.

2.3.3. Predictions of random effects
In many longitudinal biomedical studies, subject-specific growth curve on repeated measures could be crucial information not only for investigators to understand the biological mechanism of the diseases under study, but also for clinicians to better predict the disease progression and eventually offer better care to the patients. Under the framework of the general linear mixed model, it is possible to obtain estimates to the subject-specific effects, b_j. The estimate to b_j, along with the estimates to the fixed effects, β, subsequently provides an estimate to the subject-specific longitudinal trajectories, $W_j \beta + Z_j b_j$.

The prediction of random effects can be best understood in the framework of Bayesian analysis when each random effect is treated as a random parameter whose prior is a multivariate normal distribution with a mean vector of 0's and a covariance matrix D. Given the vector of responses $Y_j = (y_{j1}, y_{j2}, \ldots, y_{jk_j})^t$, it is well known (Graybill, 1976) that the best predictor of b_j is the conditional expectation of the posterior distribution:

$$\hat{b}_j = E(b_j | Y_j).$$

The well-known Bayesian Theorem then implies that the conditional distribution of b_j, given $Y_j = (y_{j1}, y_{j2}, \ldots, y_{jk_j})^t$, is another normal distribution with mean

$$\hat{\mu}_{b_j} = DZ_j'\Sigma_j^{-1}(Y_j - W_j\beta)$$

and covariance matrix

$$\Sigma_{b_j} = Cov(b_j | Y_j) = D - DZ_j'\Sigma_j^{-1}Z_j D.$$

Because $\hat{\mu}_{b_j}$ is a linear function of the response vector $Y_j = (y_{j1}, y_{j2}, \ldots, y_{jk_j})^t$, and it can be shown that $\hat{\mu}_{b_j}$ is also an unbiased predictor to b_j and has the minimum variance in the class of unbiased linear predictors of b_j, $\hat{\mu}_{b_j}$ is therefore a BLUP of b_j. Because $\hat{\mu}_{b_j}$ is also a function of unknown parameters β, D, and Σ_j, the ML or REML estimates to these parameters can be used to obtain the empirical BLUP of b_j as

$$\hat{b}_j = \hat{D}Z_j'\hat{\Sigma}_j^{-1}(Y_j - W_j\hat{\beta}).$$

Obtaining a valid estimate to the covariance matrix of the empirical BLUP $\hat{b}_j$ turns out to be more challenging. A simple replacement of unknown parameters by their estimates in Σ_{b_j} would underestimate the variability because of the ignorance to the uncertainty in the estimate of β. Notice that

$$Cov(\hat{b}_j - b_j) = D - DZ_j'\Sigma_j^{-1}Z_j D + DZ_j'\Sigma_j^{-1}W_j$$
$$\times \left(\sum_{j=1}^{n} W_j'\Sigma_j^{-1}W_j \right)^{-1} W_j'\Sigma_j^{-1}Z_j D.$$

The standard error of the empirical BLUP $\hat{b}_j$ can be obtained by substituting the ML or REML estimates for the unknown parameters in $Cov(\hat{b}_j - b_j)$. Finally, the predicted growth curve for the jth subject is

$$\hat{Y}_j = W_j\hat{\beta} + Z_j\hat{b}_j,$$

which can be rewritten as

$$\hat{Y}_j = \left(\hat{R}_j\hat{\Sigma}_j^{-1} \right) W_j\hat{\beta} + \left(I_{k_j} - \hat{R}_j\hat{\Sigma}_j^{-1} \right) Y_j.$$

Therefore, the predictor of individual growth curve Y_j can be conceptualized as a weighted sum between the population mean growth curve $W_j\hat{\beta}$ and the observed growth curve $Y_j = (y_{j1}, y_{j2}, \ldots, y_{jk_j})^t$, which indicates some type of 'shrinkage' (James and Stein, 1961) for the predictor of individual growth curve Y_j toward the population mean growth curve $W_j\hat{\beta}$. The degree of 'shrinkage' that is reflected by the weights depends on R_j and Σ_j. In general, when the within-subject variability, R_j, is large relative to the between-subject variability, more weight is given to the population mean growth curve $W_j\beta$ than to the individual growth curve $Y_j = (y_{j1}, y_{j2}, \ldots, y_{jk_j})^t$. On the other hand, when the between-subject variability is large relative to the within-subject variability, more weight is assigned to the individually observed growth curve than to the population mean growth curve $W_j\hat{\beta}$.

We now present some applications of general linear mixed models in biomedical applications, especially in the study of AD. AD is a neurodegenerative disease which is characterized by the loss of cognitive and functional ability. It is the most common of the degenerative dementias affecting up to 47% of the population over the age of 85 (Evans et al., 1989; Herbert et al., 1995; Crystal et al., 1988; Katzman et al., 1988; Morris et al., 1991). Many neuropsychological measures and staging instruments have been used to describe the longitudinal disease progression. For example, the severity of dementia can be staged by the clinical dementia rating (CDR) according to published rules (Morris, 1993). A global CDR is derived from individual ratings in multiple domains by an experienced clinician such that CDR 0 indicates no dementia and CDR 0.5, 1, 2, and 3 represent very mild, mild, moderate, and severe dementia, respectively. A major interest in longitudinal AD research is to estimate and compare the rate of cognitive decline as a function of disease severity and other possible risk factors such as age, education, and the number of Apolipoprotein E4 alleles.

Example 1. Random intercept and random slope model at different stages of AD.

Let $Y_j = (y_{j1}, y_{j2}, \ldots, y_{jk_j})^t$ be the vector of longitudinal observations for the cognitive function on the jth subject over k_j time points $T_j = (t_{j1}, t_{j2}, \ldots, t_{jk_j})^t$ (i.e., TIME). Suppose that the growth curve over time is approximately linear for each stage of the disease as measured by CDR and that subjects stayed at the same CDR stage during the longitudinal follow-up. At the first stage of the two-stage random effects model, a linear growth curve is assumed for each subject, i.e., given the subject-specific intercept and slope over time,

$$y_{jk} = \beta_{0j} + \beta_{1j}t_{jk} + e_{jk},$$

for $k = 1, 2, \ldots, k_j$, or $Y_j = A_j\beta_j + e_j$ in the matrix form, where $A_j = (J\ T_j)$, J is the column vector of 1's, $\beta_j = (\beta_{0j}\ \beta_{1j})$, and $e_j = (e_{j1}, e_{j2}, \ldots, e_{jk_j})^t$. At the second stage, the subject-specific intercept and slope are modeled as functions of possible subject-level covariates. Because it has been well established in the literature that the rate of cognitive decline in AD is associated with the disease severity at the baseline (Storandt et al., 2002), one such subject-level covariate could be the baseline disease severity as measured by CDR. Therefore, one can model the subject-specific intercept and slope separately as a function of CDR in a standard analysis of variance (ANOVA) model (Milliken and Johnson, 1992), i.e.,

$$\beta_{0j} = \beta_{\text{CDR}}^0 + b_{0j},$$

$$\beta_{1j} = \beta_{\text{CDR}}^1 + b_{1j}.$$

One difference between here and the standard ANOVA model is that two variables (the intercept and the slope) are conceptualized from the same subjects. Therefore a correlation structure is usually required to account for the possible correlation between the intercept and the slope from the same subjects. These are generally done by assuming that the error vector $b_j = (b_{0j} \ b_{1j})^t$ follows a normal distribution with mean vector of 0's and a covariance matrix D which could be assumed completely unstructured (i.e., specified by the option TYPE = UN) or with certain structured form. The above model can be easily implemented in SAS with the following codes:

```
PROC MIXED DATA = ; CLASSES ID CDR;
MODEL Y = CDR TIME CDR*TIME /DDFM = SATTERTH;
RANDOM INT TIME/SUBJECT = ID TYPE = UN;
RUN;
```

It is important to understand the hypothesis that each term in the model is testing. The term CDR*TIME is testing the hypothesis that the mean slopes are the same across all baseline CDR groups, whereas the term CDR is testing whether the mean intercepts at TIME = 0 (i.e., the baseline) are the same across the CDR groups. The term TIME is testing the main effect of the slope over time across the CDR groups, which can in general only be interpreted if the test on CDR*TIME is not statistically significant.

If the estimates to the mean intercepts and mean slopes for each CDR and subject-specific predictions to the random effects are needed, the following SAS code can be used:

```
PROC MIXED DATA = ; CLASSES ID CDR;
MODEL Y = CDR CDR*TIME/NOINT S DDFM = SATTERTH;
RANDOM INT TIME/SUBJECT = ID TYPE = UN SOLUTION;
RUN;
```

One needs to be careful about the interpretation of the output from this new set of codes. The term CDR*TIME is no longer testing the hypothesis that the mean slopes are the same across all CDR groups, but the hypothesis that all mean slopes across CDR groups are simultaneously equal to 0. Likewise, the term CDR is no longer testing whether the mean intercepts at TIME = 0 are the same across the CDR groups, but whether all the mean intercepts are simultaneously equal to 0. Some of these hypotheses tested by this new set of codes might not be scientifically interesting, but the set of codes does offer the valid estimates to the fixed effects and random effects.

Example 2. Random intercept and random slope model at different stages of AD adjusting for the baseline age.

In Example 1, a random intercept and random slope model was used to describe the growth curve of cognitive decline across different stages of AD. It is also well known that baseline age is an important risk factor for the cognitive decline. An extended two-stage random effects model can be used to describe the rate of cognitive decline as a function of both baseline CDR and baseline age (i.e., AGE). The first stage of this model will be the same as the first stage of the model introduced in Example 1. At the second stage, where the subject-specific intercept and slope are modeled as functions of possible subject-level covariates, one can conceptualize both the subject-specific intercept and subject-specific rate of cognitive decline for each CDR stage as a linear function of baseline age in a standard analysis of covariance (ANOCOVA) model (Milliken and Johnson, 2001), i.e.,

$$\beta_{0j} = \beta_{CDR}^0 + \gamma_{CDR}^0 * AGE + b_{0j},$$

$$\beta_{1j} = \beta_{CDR}^1 + \gamma_{CDR}^1 * AGE + b_{1j}.$$

Notice here β_{CDR}^0, γ_{CDR}^0 are the intercept and slope of the subject-specific intercept as a linear function of AGE, and β_{CDR}^1, γ_{CDR}^1 are the intercept and slope of the subject-specific longitudinal rate of cognitive decline as a linear function of AGE. Again, a correlation structure is usually required to account for the possible correlation between the intercept and the slope from the first-stage model by assuming that the error vector $b_j = (b_{0j} \ b_{1j})'$ at the second stage of the model follows a normal distribution with mean vector of 0's and a covariance matrix D which could be assumed completely unstructured. The above model can be easily implemented in SAS by the following code:

```
PROC MIXED DATA = ; CLASSES ID CDR;
MODEL Y = CDR AGE CDR*AGE TIME AGETIME CDR*TIME
CDR*AGETIME /DDFM = SATTERTH;
RANDOM INT TIME/SUBJECT = ID TYPE = UN;
RUN;
```

In these codes, AGETIME is the variable created in the data set by multiplying TIME and AGE. All the terms CDR AGE CDR*AGE in the MODEL statement are modeling the intercept part of the cognitive function, whereas all the other terms in the MODEL statement are modeling the longitudinal rate of the cognitive function. More specifically, the term CDR*AGETIME here tests whether all γ_{CDR}^1 are the same across different CDR levels, the term CDR*AGE tests whether all γ_{CDR}^0 are the same across different CDR levels, and the term CDR*TIME tests whether all β_{CDR}^1 are the same across different CDR levels.

Different variations and extensions to the above models can also be used. These include the cases when either the subject-specific intercepts or subject-specific slopes but not both are assumed random and the other cases when additional risk factors for AD such as education and the number of Apolipoprotein E4 alleles are also entered into the model. There are also cases that additional random effects need to be introduced into the model. For example, with a multicenter study, centers are usually treated as a random effect to account for the possible variation among centers and the possible correlation of the measures for subjects from the same centers.

Example 3. Piecewise random coefficients model in AD.

Piecewise linear growth curves are common in many biomedical applications. In AD research, it has been well recognized that the rate of cognitive decline depends on the disease severity at the baseline (Storandt et al., 2002). This further implies that a simple linear growth curve over time is inappropriate when subjects make conversions from lower CDR level to higher CDR levels. Again let $Y_j = (y_{j1}, y_{j2}, \ldots, y_{jk_j})'$ be the vector of longitudinal observations for the cognitive function on the jth subject over k_j time points $T_j = (t_{j1}, t_{j2}, \ldots, t_{jk_j})'$. Assume that the subject begins with CDR 0 and then converts into CDR 0.5 at time $t_{jk_j^{0.5}}$, $1 < k_j^{0.5} < k_j$, the subject goes on at CDR 0.5 and makes another conversion into CDR 1 at time $t_{jk_j^1}$, $1 \leq k_j^{0.5} < k_j^1 \leq k_j$. Suppose that the growth curve over time is approximately linear at each CDR level. Then at the first stage of a two-stage random effects model, a piecewise linear growth curve connected at the CDR conversion times is assumed for each subject, i.e., given the subject-specific intercept and slopes over time,

$$y_{jk} = \beta_{0j} + \beta_j^0 t_{jk} + \beta_j^{0.5} t_{jk}^{0.5} + \beta_j^1 t_{jk}^1 + e_{jk},$$

where $t_{jk}^{0.5} = t_{jk}$ when $k \geq k_j^{0.5}$, and $t_{jk}^{0.5} = 0$ when $k < k_j^{0.5}$; and $t_{jk}^1 = t_{jk}$ when $k \geq k_j^1$, and $t_{jk}^1 = 0$ when $k < k_j^1$. Notice that the parameters in this model indicate three different rates of cognitive decline at three different CDR levels during the longitudinal follow-up. β_j^0 represents the slope of cognitive decline at CDR 0, $\beta_j^0 + \beta_j^{0.5}$ represents the slope of cognitive decline at CDR 0.5, and $\beta_j^0 + \beta_j^{0.5} + \beta_j^1$ represents the slope of cognitive decline at CDR 1. Therefore, $\beta_j^{0.5}$ represents the difference on the slope of cognitive decline between CDR 0.5 and CDR 0, and β_j^1 represents the difference on the slope of cognitive decline between CDR 1 and CDR 0.5. At the second stage, the subject-specific intercept and slopes are again modeled as a function of possible subject-level covariates. Assume that the subject-specific slopes are to be compared between subjects with at least one Apolipoprotein E4 allele (i.e., E4 positive) and those without Apolipoprotein E4 alleles (i.e., E4 negative). One can then write four analysis of variance models as

$$\beta_{0j} = \beta_{0E4} + b_{0j},$$

$$\beta_j^0 = \beta_{E4}^0 + b_j^0,$$

$$\beta_j^{0.5} = \beta_{E4}^{0.5} + b_j^{0.5},$$

and

$$\beta_j^1 = \beta_{E4}^1 + b_j^1.$$

The variation among subject-specific parameters and the correlation for within-subject parameters are modeled by assuming $b_j = \left(b_{0j} \; b_j^0 \; b_j^{0.5} \; b_j^1 \right)'$ follows a normal distribution with mean vector of 0's and a covariance matrix D which could be assumed completely unstructured. The above model could be implemented in SAS by the following codes:

```
PROC MIXED DATA = ; CLASSES ID E4;
MODEL Y = E4 T T^0.5 T^1 E4*T E4*T^0.5 E4*T^1;
RANDOM INT T T^0.5 T^1 /SUBJECT = ID TYPE = UN;
RUN;
```

In these codes, T, $T^{0.5}$, and T^1 represent t_{jk}, $t_{jk}^{0.5}$, and t_{jk}^1, respectively. All terms in above model test specific hypotheses. For example, $E4*T^{0.5}$ tests whether the difference on the rate of cognitive decline between CDR 0.5 and CDR 0 is the same between E4-positive and E4-negative subjects. The following SAS codes give estimates to the mean intercepts and mean slopes for each CDR level and subject-specific predictions to the random effects. (The ESTIMATE statement could differ depending on how these factors are coded in SAS, but option E should clearly indicate whether a correct ESTIMATE statement was written (SAS Institute, Inc., 1999.)

```
PROC MIXED DATA = ; CLASSES ID E4;
MODEL Y = E4 E4*T E4*T^0.5 E4*T^1/NOINT DDFM = SATTERTH
SOLUTION;
RANDOM INT T T^0.5 T^1 /SUBJECT = ID TYPE = UN SOLUTION;
ESTIMATE 'rate at CDR 0.5 for E4 +' E4*T 1 0 E4*T^0.5 1 0/E;
ESTIMATE 'rate difference by E4 at CDR 0.5' E4*T 1 -1 E4*T^0.5 1 -1/E;
RUN;
```

The first ESTIMATE statement gives the estimated mean rate of cognitive decline at CDR 0.5 for subjects with positive E4 (it could be for subjects with negative APOE4 depending on the code of APOE4, but the option E should indicate clearly which one is estimated). The second ESTIMATE statement estimates the mean difference on the mean rate of cognitive decline at CDR 0.5 between subjects with positive E4 and those with negative E4 and tests whether the difference is 0. Similar additional ESTIMATE statements can be written to estimate the rate of cognitive decline at CDR 1 and test whether a difference exists between E4-positive and E4-negative subjects.

2.4. Generalized linear models for longitudinal data

The generalized linear models for longitudinal data extend the techniques of general linear models. They are suited specifically for non-linear models with binary or discrete responses, such as logistic regression, in which the mean response is linked to the explanatory variables or covariates through a non-linear link function (McCullagh and Nelder, 1989; Liang and Zeger, 1986; Zeger and

Liang, 1986). Several approaches have been proposed to model longitudinal data in the framework of generalized linear models. The marginal models for longitudinal data permit separate modeling of the regression of the response on explanatory variables, and the association among repeated observations of the response for each subject. They are appropriate when inferences about the population averages are the focus of the longitudinal studies. For example, in an AD treatment clinical trial, the average difference between control and treatment is the most important, not the difference for any single subject. Marginal models are also useful in AD epidemiological studies. It could help to address what the age-specific prevalence of AD is, whether the prevalence is greater in a specific sub-population, and how the association between a specific sub-population and the AD prevalence rate changes with time. The techniques of generalized estimating equations (GEEs) can be used to estimate the regression parameters in the marginal models (Liang and Zeger, 1986; Gourieroux et al., 1984; Prentice, 1988; Zhao and Prentice, 1990; Thall and Vail, 1990; Liang et al., 1992; Fitzmaurice et al., 1993). The approach of random effects models in the setup of generalized linear model allows the heterogeneity among subjects in a subset of the entire set of the regression parameters. Two general approaches of the estimation are used in the random effects models. One is to find the marginal means and variance of the response vector and then apply the technique of GEE (Zeger and Qaqish, 1988; Gilmore et al., 1985; Goldstein, 1991; Breslow and Clayton, 1993; Lipsitz et al., 1991). The other is the likelihood approach (Anderson and Aitkin, 1985; Hinde, 1982) or the penalized quasi-likelihood (PQL) approach (Green, 1987; Laird, 1978; Stiratelli et al., 1984; McGilchrist and Aisbett, 1991; Breslow and Clayton, 1993). Another generalized linear model is the transition model for which the conditional distribution of the response at a time given the history of longitudinal observations is assumed to depend only on the prior observations with a specified order through a Markov chain. Full ML estimation can be used to fit the Gaussian autoregressive models (Tsay, 1984), and the conditional ML estimation can be used to fit logistic and log-linear models (Korn and Whittemore, 1979; Stern and Coe, 1984; Zeger et al., 1985; Wong, 1986; Zeger and Qaqish, 1988). A comprehensive description of various models for discrete longitudinal data can be found in Molenberghs and Verbeke (2005).

2.4.1. Marginal models and generalized estimating equations

In many biomedical applications the longitudinal responses are not necessarily continuous, which imply that the general linear models and general linear mixed models might not apply. For example, the presence or absence of depression and the count of panic attacks during certain time interval are all likely response variables of scientific interest. When the longitudinal responses are discrete, generalized linear models are required to relate changes in the mean responses to covariates. In addition, another component is needed to introduce the within-subject associations among the vector of repeated responses. Marginal models are one of these choices.

We again let $Y_j = (y_{j1}, y_{j2}, \ldots, y_{jk_j})^t$ be the vector of longitudinal observations for the response variable on the jth subject over k_j time points $T_j = (t_{j1}, t_{j2}, \ldots, t_{jk_j})^t$. Let $X_{jk} = (x_{jk1}, x_{jk2}, \ldots, x_{jkp})^t$ be the p by 1 vector of covariates associated with the kth measurement on the jth subject. Notice here that the vector of covariates could be time dependent. Let $X_j = (X_{j1}, X_{j2}, \ldots, X_{jk_j})'$ be the design matrix of the jth subject. A marginal model for longitudinal data specifies the following three components:

(1) The conditional expectation of Y_{jk}, given X_{jk}, is assumed to depend on the covariates through a given link function g, i.e.,

$$E(Y_{jk}|X_{jk}) = \mu_{jk}$$

and

$$g(\mu_{jk}) = X_{jk}^t \beta,$$

where β is a p by 1 vector of unknown regression parameters.
(2) The conditional variance of Y_{jk}, given X_{jk}, is assumed to depend on the mean according to some given 'variance function' V, i.e.,

$$\text{Var}(Y_{jk}|X_{jk}) = \phi V(\mu_{jk}),$$

where ϕ is an additional parameter.
(3) The conditional within-subject association among repeated responses, given the covariates, is assumed to depend on an additional set of parameters α, although it could also depend on the mean parameters.

The first two conditions in a marginal model are standard requirements from a generalized linear model (McCullagh and Nelder, 1989) relating the marginal means to a set of covariates at each individual time point. The third condition is in addition to the standard assumptions in generalized linear model, which makes the application of generalized linear model to longitudinal data possible. Notice that even if all three components are completely specified in a marginal model, the model still does not completely specify the joint distribution of the vector of repeated measures on the response variable. In fact, it will be clear later that such a complete specification of joint distribution is not needed to obtain valid asymptotic statistical inferences to the regression parameters β. The following are several examples of marginal models for longitudinal data.

Example 1: In the case of continuous response variables, the standard repeated measure analysis of variance models and the two-stage random effects models are special cases of marginal models. Here the link function is the simple identity function, i.e., $g(\mu_{jk}) = \mu_{jk}$, and the variance function is constant 1, i.e., $V = 1$. The conditional within-subject association is described by correlations among repeated measures of the response, which are independent of the mean parameters.

Example 2: In a longitudinal study to examine the longitudinal trend on the probability of depression and to relate this probability to other covariates such as gender and education, the occurrence of depression is longitudinally observed. Because Y_{jk} is binary and coded as 1 when depression occurs and 0 otherwise, the distribution of each Y_{jk} is Bernoulli which is traditionally modeled through a logit- or probit-link function, i.e., the conditional expectation of Y_{jk}, given X_{jk}, is

$E(Y_{jk}|X_{jk}) = Pr(Y_{jk} = 1|X_{jk}) = \mu_{jk}$, and the logit-link function links μ_{jk} with covariates by

$$\ln\left(\frac{\mu_{jk}}{1 - \mu_{jk}}\right) = X_{jk}^t\beta.$$

The conditional variance of Y_{jk}, given X_{jk}, is given by the 'variance function',

$$\mathrm{Var}(Y_{jk}|X_{jk}) = \mu_{jk}(1 - \mu_{jk}),$$

i.e., $\phi = 1$. The conditional within-subject association among repeated responses, given the covariates, is usually specified by an unstructured pairwise odds ratio between two repeated responses,

$$\alpha_{k_1 k_2} = \frac{Pr(Y_{jk_1} = 1, Y_{jk_2} = 1)Pr(Y_{jk_1} = 0, Y_{jk_2} = 0)}{Pr(Y_{jk_1} = 1, Y_{jk_2} = 0)Pr(Y_{jk_1} = 0, Y_{jk_2} = 1)}.$$

Example 3: In many studies of AD, psychometric tests are generally used to assess subjects' cognition longitudinally. One of these tests records the number of animals that the subject can name within a given period of time. This type of count data could be modeled by a Poisson distribution, using a log-link function. More specifically, the conditional expectation of Y_{jk}, given X_{jk}, is $E(Y_{jk}|X_{jk}) = \mu_{jk}$, and is assumed to depend on the covariates through the log-link function,

$$\ln(\mu_{jk}) = X_{jk}^t\beta.$$

The conditional variance of Y_{jk}, given X_{jk}, is given by the Poisson 'variance function',

$$\mathrm{Var}(Y_{jk}|X_{jk}) = \mu_{jk},$$

i.e., $\phi = 1$. The conditional within-subject association among repeated responses, given the covariates, is usually specified by unstructured pairwise correlations between two repeated responses,

$$\alpha_{k_1 k_2} = \mathrm{CORR}(Y_{jk_1}, Y_{jk_2}).$$

This marginal model is sometimes referred to a log-linear model.

When a marginal model is specified, the estimation of the model parameters is generally done through the GEE instead of the standard inferences based on the ML estimates. Part of the reason that a standard ML approach is not used here is that the marginal model fails to specify the joint distribution on the vector of repeated responses and therefore a likelihood function is not available. The basic idea of GEE is to find β that minimizes the following generalized sum of square (also called the objective function):

$$\sum_j [Y_j - \mu_j]^t V_j^{-1}[Y_j - \mu_j],$$

where μ_j is the vector of expectations of repeated responses for the jth subject which is a function of the regression parameters β. V_j is called the 'working' covariance matrix of Y_j and is given by

$$V_j = A_j^{1/2}\text{CORR}(Y_j)A_j^{1/2},$$

where $A_j^{1/2}$ is the diagonal matrix such that $(A_j^{1/2})^2 = A_j$, and A_j the diagonal matrix consisting of the variance of Y_{jk}, and $\text{CORR}(Y_j)$ the correlation matrix of Y_j depending on the set of parameters α's (also possibly β's). The reason that V_j is called the 'working' covariance matrix of Y_j is that it is not necessarily the same as the true covariance matrix of Y_j. The mathematical minimization of the above objective function is equivalent to finding β that solves the following GEEs:

$$\sum_j D_j^t V_j^{-1}[Y_j - \mu_j] = 0,$$

where

$$D_j = \begin{pmatrix} \partial\mu_{j1}/\partial\beta_1 & \partial\mu_{j1}/\partial\beta_2 & \cdots & \partial\mu_{j1}/\partial\beta_p \\ \partial\mu_{j2}/\partial\beta_1 & \partial\mu_{j2}/\partial\beta_2 & \cdots & \partial\mu_{j2}/\partial\beta_p \\ \cdots & \cdots & \cdots & \cdots \\ \partial\mu_{jk_j}/\partial\beta_1 & \partial\mu_{jk_j}/\partial\beta_2 & \cdots & \partial\mu_{jk_j}/\partial\beta_p \end{pmatrix}$$

is called the derivative matrix of μ_j with respect to the regression parameters β. Notice that $\mu_{jk} = g^{-1}(X_{jk}^t\beta)$, where g^{-1} is the inverse of the link function g. Although the derivative matrix is only a function of the regression parameters, the GEEs involve not only the regression parameters β but also the parameters α and ϕ. The latter are usually called nuisance parameters because they generally are not the major interest in biomedical research, but they play important roles in the inferential process. In general, the GEEs have no closed form solutions with a non-linear link function, and therefore require an iterative algorithm to approximate the solutions. The standard two-stage iterative algorithms are available for these computations and can be found in the literature (Fitzmaurice et al., 2004). These iterative algorithms begin with some seed estimates to parameters α and ϕ, and then estimate regression parameters β by solving the system of GEEs at the first stage. At the second stage of the iterative algorithms, the current estimates of β's are used to update the estimates of α and ϕ. These two-stage processes are iterated until computational convergence is achieved. These algorithms are also implemented in many standard statistical software packages.

Assume that $\hat{\beta}$ is the final solution of β to the GEEs after the two-stage iterative algorithm converges. The most appealing part of a marginal model is the fact that $\hat{\beta}$ is a consistent estimator, i.e., when the sample size is sufficiently large, $\hat{\beta}$ approaches the true regression parameters β. This is true even when the within-subject associations have been incorrectly specified in the marginal model. In other words, as long as the mean component of the marginal model is correctly specified, $\hat{\beta}$ will provide valid statistical inferences. Another important appealing property of GEE estimate $\hat{\beta}$ is the fact that it is almost as efficient as the MLE estimate, especially in the generalized linear mixed models for continuous outcome variable under the assumption of multivariate normality over repeated measures. Similar to the standard asymptotic properties of ML estimates, when the sample size is sufficiently large, $\hat{\beta}$ follows an asymptotically multivariate normal distribution with mean β and a covariance matrix which can be estimated by the so-called 'sandwich' estimator

$$\hat{\Sigma} = \hat{B}^{-1} \hat{M} \hat{B}^{-1},$$

where $\hat{B} = \Sigma_j \hat{D}_j^t \hat{V}_j^{-1} \hat{D}_j$ and $\hat{M} = \Sigma_j \hat{D}_j^t \hat{V}_j^{-1} [Y_j - \hat{\mu}_j][Y_j - \hat{\mu}_j]' \hat{V}_j^{-1} \hat{D}_j$, and the estimates $\hat{D}_j$, $\hat{V}_j$, and $\hat{\mu}_j$ are obtained by replacing β, α, and ϕ by their GEE estimates from D_j, V_j, and μ_j, respectively.

For the statistical inferences about the regression parameters β, valid standard errors can be obtained based on the above sandwich estimator $\hat{\Sigma} = \hat{B}^{-1} \hat{M} \hat{B}^{-1}$. In fact, both GEE estimate of β and the sandwich estimator to $\mathrm{Cov}(\hat{\beta})$ are robust in the sense that it is still valid even if the within-subject associations have been incorrectly specified in the marginal model. This does not imply that it is not necessary to try to specify correctly the within-subject associations in the marginal model. In fact, the correct modeling or approximation to the within-subject associations is important as far as the efficiency or the precision on the estimation of regression parameters β is concerned. It can be mathematically proved that the optimum efficiency in the estimation of regression parameters β can be obtained when the working matrix V_j is the same as the true within-subject association among repeated responses. On the other hand, the sandwich estimate is most appropriate when the study design is almost balanced and the number of subjects is relatively large and the number of repeated measures from the same subject is relatively small, especially when there are many replications on the response vectors associated with each distinct set of covariate values. When the longitudinal study designs severely deviate from these 'ideal' cases, the use of sandwich estimator for the statistical inferences might be problematic, in which case, the specification of the entire model over the repeated measures might be desired and therefore the effort to specify the correct covariance matrix become necessary.

The following is a SAS code to obtain GEE for Example 2 above in which the longitudinal trend on the probability of depression is modeled as a function of gender and time through the logit-link function. The occurrence of depression is treated as binary and longitudinally observed. The option LOGOR specifies the possible working covariance structure based on log odds ratio for the within-subject responses:

```
PROC GENMOD DESCENDING DATA = ;
CLASSES ID GENDER;
MODEL DEPRESSION = GENDER TIME GENDER*TIME/
DIST = BINOMIAL LINK = LOGIT;
REPEATED SUBJECT = ID/WITHINSUBJECT = TIME LOGOR = ;
RUN;
```

2.4.2. Generalized linear mixed effect models

The basic conceptualization of the generalized linear mixed effects models is quite similar to that of the general linear mixed effects models, although there are crucial differences in the parameter interpretations of these models. More specifically, a generalized linear mixed effects model for longitudinal data assumes the heterogeneity across subjects in the study in the entire set or a subset of the regression coefficients. In other words, the entire set or a subset of the subject-specific regression coefficients are assumed to be random variables across study subjects which follow a univariate or a multivariate normal distribution.

The generalized linear mixed effects models can also be thought of following a standard two-stage paradigm in which the first stage specifies a conditional distribution for each response Y_{jk}. More specifically, at the first stage, it is assumed that conditional on the subject-specific random effect b_j and covariates X_{jk}, the distribution of Y_{jk} belongs to a very wide family of distributions called the exponential family. The exponential family covers essentially all the important distributions used in biomedical applications. These distributions include, but are not limited to, the normal distribution, the binomial distribution, and the Poisson distribution. Let

$$\mu_{jk} = E(Y_{jk}|b_j, X_{jk}).$$

The conditional variance of Y_{jk} is given through some known variance function V

$$\text{Var}(Y_{jk}|b_j, X_{jk}) = \phi V(\mu_{jk}).$$

Further, conditional on the random effect b_j and covariates X_{jk}, Y_{jk}'s are assumed independent. The conditional mean of Y_{jk} is linked to a linear predictor through a given link function g

$$g(\mu_{jk}) = X_{jk}^t \beta + Z_{jk}^t b_j.$$

The final assumption on generalized linear mixed models is about the distribution for the random effects. It is common to assume that b_j follows a multivariate normal distribution with a mean vector of 0's and a covariance matrix D and is independent of covariates X_{jk}.

The primary difference between a generalized linear mixed model and a marginal model is that the former completely specifies the distribution of Y_j while the latter does not. It is also clear that the general linear mixed model is a special case of the generalized linear mixed models. However, the interpretations of regression parameters are also different between the marginal models and the generalized linear mixed models. Because the mean response and the within-subject association are modeled separately, the regression parameters in a marginal model are not affected by the assumptions on the within-subject associations, and therefore can be interpreted as population averages, i.e., they describe the mean response in the population and its relations with covariates. As an example, a marginal model can be used in a longitudinal study to examine the longitudinal trend on the probability of depression and to relate this probability to other covariates such as gender. Because Y_{jk} is binary and coded as 1 when depression occurs and 0 otherwise, the distribution of each Y_{jk} can be modeled through a logit-link function, i.e., the conditional expectation of Y_{jk}, given time (i.e., t_{jk}) and gender (coded numerically as GENDER), is $E(Y_{jk}|X_{jk}) = Pr(Y_{jk} = 1|X_{jk}) = \mu_{jk}$, and

$$\ln\left(\frac{\mu_{jk}}{1 - \mu_{jk}}\right) = \beta_0 + t_{jk}\beta_1 + \text{GENDER}^*\beta_2.$$

The parameter β's here have the standard population averaged interpretations. β_2 is the log odds ratio of depression between the two genders at a given time point, and β_1 is the log odds ratio of depression for each unit increase of time for a given gender. On the other hand, in a generalized linear mixed model with time (i.e., t_{jk}) and gender through the same logit link, assuming a random coefficient for the intercept and the regression coefficient (i.e., the slope) before time,

$$\ln\left(\frac{P(Y_{jk} = 1|b_j, \text{GENDER})}{1 - P(Y_{jk} = 1|b_j, \text{GENDER})}\right) = \beta_0 + t_{jk}\beta_1 + \text{GENDER}^*\beta_2 + b_{0j} + t_{jk}b_{1j},$$

where $(b_{0j}, b_{1j})'$ follows a bivariate normal distribution. The regression parameters β's now describe the subject-specific mean response and its association with covariates. β_1 is the subject-specific log odds ratio of depression for each unit increase of time because $(b_{0j}, b_{1j})'$, the random effects from the individual, and gender are fixed for the subject. The interpretation of β_2 has to be extrapolated because gender is a between-subject covariate and it is impossible to change it within a subject. Therefore, β_2 can only be interpreted as the log odds ratio of depression between two subjects of different genders who happen to have exactly the same random effects $(b_{0j}, b_{1j})'$. A SAS code to implement the above generalized linear mixed effects model is given below:

```
PROC GLIMMIX DATA = ; CLASSES ID GENDER;
MODEL DEPRESSION = GENDER TIME/DIST = BINOMIAL
LINK = LOGIT;
RANDOM INT TIME/SUBJECT = ID TYPE = UN;
RUN;
```

Much of the difference in the interpretation of the regression parameters between a marginal model and a generalized linear mixed effects model is due to the fact that the former directly specifies $E(Y_{jk}|X_{jk})$, whereas the latter specifies $E(Y_{jk}|X_{jk}, b_j)$ instead. When there is an identical link, both approaches become equivalent based on the fact $E(Y_{jk}|X_{jk}) = E_{b_j}[E(Y_{jk}|X_{jk}, b_j)]$, and the interpretation of regression parameters in the generalized linear mixed model can also be made in terms of population averages. When the link function is non-linear, however, the interpretations for the regression parameters in generalized linear mixed models are distinct from those in the marginal models. These distinctions allow different scientific questions to be addressed in longitudinal biomedical studies. Because of the subject-specific feature on the regression coefficients at least to within-subject covariates or time-varying covariates, the generalized linear mixed effects models are most useful when the primary scientific objective is to make inferences about individuals rather than the population averages in the longitudinal studies.

2.5. Missing data issues

Missing data arise in the analysis of longitudinal data whenever one or more of the sequences of measurements from subjects within the study are incomplete, in the sense that the intended measurements are not taken, are lost, or are otherwise unavailable. Missing data occur in almost all longitudinal studies, and they cause not only technical difficulties in the analysis of such data, but also deeper conceptual issues as one has to ask why the measurements are missing, and more specifically whether their being missing has any bearing on the practical and scientific objectives to be addressed by the data. A general treatment of statistical analysis with missing data along with a hierarchy of missing data mechanisms (MDM) has been proposed (Little and Rubin, 2002). MDM is classified as missing completely at random (MCAR), missing at random (MAR), or non-ignorable (NI). These are generally described in a designed study which calls for k planned observations on each subject but lesser than k are actually observed.

Let $Y_j = (y_{j1}, y_{j2}, \ldots, y_{jk})^t$ be the vector of planned longitudinal measurements for the variable of interest on the jth subject over k time points. Let $I_j = (I_{j1}, I_{j2}, \ldots, I_{jk})^t$ be the vector of indicators of observations with $I_{ji} = 1$ if the ith measurement is actually observed and $I_{ji} = 0$ otherwise. Let X_j be the vector of covariates on the jth subject, and let $f(Y_j|X_j, \beta)$ be the conditional density of Y_j given X_j and a set of parameters β, and let $f(I_j|Y_j, X_j, \psi)$ be the conditional density of I_j given (Y_j, X_j, ψ), where ψ is the parameters associated with missing data. The missing responses are said to be MCAR if

$$f(I_j|Y_j, X_j, \psi) = f(I_j|X_j, \psi),$$

i.e., given the covariates X_j, the probability of missingness does not depend on $Y_j = (y_{j1}, y_{j2}, \ldots, y_{jk})^t$, observed or not. This simply implies that the missingness is the results of a chance mechanism that does not depend on either observed or unobserved components of $Y_j = (y_{j1}, y_{j2}, \ldots, y_{jk})^t$. With missing data MCAR, it can be mathematically proved that the joint distribution of these observed y_{ji}'s is the same as the ordinary marginal distribution of these observed from Y_j. This then implies that the observed y_{ji}'s are just random samples of y_{ji}'s, and thus essentially any method of analysis will yield valid statistical inferences as long as the distribution satisfies the assumptions under which the method is justified. In a longitudinal study, if dropout from the study is not related to any factors under study, the missingness is considered MCAR.

The missing responses are said to be MAR if

$$f(I_j|Y_j, X_j, \psi) = f(I_j|Y_j^o, X_j, \psi),$$

where Y_j^o is the observed vector of $Y_j = (y_{j1}, y_{j2}, \ldots, y_{jk})^t$. The MAR implies that given the covariates, the probability of missingness depends only on the observed y_{ji}'s, but not on the missing values. With missing data MAR, it is no longer true that the joint distribution of these observed y_{ji}'s is the same as the marginal distribution of these observed from Y_j. However, it can be concluded that the contribution of the jth subject to the full likelihood as a function of β is proportional to the ordinary marginal distribution of these observed from Y_j as long as β and ψ do not share any parameters, or in another word, are functionally distinct. The implication of this result is that, as far as the statistical inferences of β are concerned, any likelihood-based methods are still valid as long as the distribution satisfies the assumptions under which the method is justified. Examples of MAR include the cases when a study protocol requires that subjects be removed from the study once the value of an outcome variable falls outside of a normal range, which implies that the missingness is related to the observed components only. In summary, whether missing data are MCAR or MAR, standard likelihood procedures can be applied to the observed data without worrying about the effect of missing to the validity of the statistical inferences. It is in this sense that both MCAR and MAR are called ignorable.

The missing responses are said to be NI or not missing at random (NMAR) if $f(I_j | Y_j, X_j, \psi)$ depends on the missing data, although it may or may not depend on Y_j^o. In a longitudinal study of cognitive function for Alzheimer's patients, the missing responses are NI if patients are not able to complete the cognitive and psychometric tests because their cognition is severely impaired. Several other examples of NI can also be found in Diggle and Kenward (1994). With missing data NI, special attention should be paid to the case when non-likelihood-based statistical inferential procedures are used. Likelihood-based inferential procedures can still be used, but generally this can only be done with the specification of the MDM. The validity of such likelihood-based inference methods depends on the validity of these specifications of MDM, $f(I_j | Y_j, X_j, \psi)$, which are generally not verifiable based on the collected data. NI missingness is also sometimes called informative, indicating the crucial role of the MDM in the analyses of this type of missing data. Other approaches have also been available in the literature that tried to relax the requirement on the precise specification of MDM when missingness is NI. Little (1993) discussed pattern-mixture models, a broad class of models that do not require precise specification of the MDM. Little and Wang (1996) extended the simple pattern-mixture model developed in Little (1994) to repeated-measures data with covariates. Little (1995) developed a model-based framework for repeated-measures data with dropouts, and placed existing literature within this framework.

The details on the analyses of missing data can be found in Little and Rubin (2002). Little and Raghunathan (1999) compared ML and summary measures approaches to longitudinal data with dropouts in a simulation study. There is also an important distinction between intermittent missing and dropout in the analysis, where the latter refers only to missing all measurements after a certain time point. If the intermittent missing values arise from a known censoring mechanism, for example, if all values below a known threshold are missing, the EM algorithm (Dempster et al., 1977) provides a possible theoretical framework for the analysis, but practical implementation for a realistic range of longitudinal data seems to be rather difficult (Laird, 1988). When the intermittent missing values do not arise from censoring, it may be reasonable to assume that they arise from mechanisms unrelated to the measurement process, and therefore are MCAR or MAR. In such cases, all likelihood-based inferences would be valid. Dropouts do not arise as a result of censoring mechanism applied to individual measurements. Often a subject's withdrawal is for reasons directly or indirectly related to the measurement process. Methods are also proposed for the statistical test of MDM (Diggle, 1989; Ridout, 1991; Cochran, 1977; Barnard, 1963). The modeling of the dropout process (Diggle and Kenward, 1994; Wu and Carroll, 1988; Wu and Bailey, 1989) highlights the practical implications of the distinctions between MCAR, MAR, and informative dropouts and provides a possible framework for routine analysis of longitudinal data with dropouts. Although complete generality in dealing with missing values in longitudinal data is not available as yet, one should be very aware of the fact that in general likelihood-based inferences will no longer be valid when the MDM is NI. The sensitivity analysis has also been recommended as a necessary step to help the analysis of missing data.

3. Design issues of a longitudinal study

In this section we focus on the response variables which are of continuous type, although the case when the longitudinally measured response variable is binary or ordinal can be worked out in a similar fashion.

As stated earlier, the major objective of a longitudinal study is to study the rate of change over time on response variables. There are different designs that can be used when planning a longitudinal study. The determination of sample sizes and the corresponding statistical powers are some of the most important issues when designing a longitudinal study. The answers to these questions depend on several factors: the primary hypotheses/objectives of the study, the statistical models used for analyzing the longitudinal data, the significance level of the primary statistical test or the confidence level of the confidence interval estimate to the rate of change over time, the statistical power desired for a statistical test, or the degree of accuracy in the confidence interval estimate to the rate of change. Most of times, analysis of response profiles, repeated measures analysis of variance, and the general linear mixed models are the major statistical models used for determining the sample sizes of longitudinal studies when the primary outcome variable is of continuous type.

When no parametric forms are assumed for the mean response profiles which are estimated and compared based on the analysis of response profiles or the repeated measures analysis of variance, the methods of sample size determination can be based on the standard analysis of response profiles and repeated measures analysis of variance. In a longitudinal study to compare multiple treatment groups over time, if repeated measures analysis of variance is used under the assumption that the covariance matrices of the measurement errors of the time intervals and the error terms of the subjects assigned to a given study conditions satisfy the H–F condition (Huynh and Feldt, 1970), the sample size determination can be further based on the F-tests or t-tests from a standard two-way analysis of variance (Chow and Liu, 2003) based on appropriate statistical tests on the primary hypothesis of the study. We consider here several types of longitudinal studies which are analyzed by the general linear mixed effects models in which a linear growth curve over time is assumed, one is to estimate the rate of change over time, and the other is to compare two subject groups on the rate of change over time.

Case 1. Estimating a single rate of change over time.

The simplest longitudinal study design is an observational study for which study subjects are followed for a certain period of time. This type of longitudinal study can be used to estimate the rate of change for the outcome variable over a certain time period. In many of these observational studies, the most important objective is to achieve an accurate estimate to the rate of change over time on some important measures for a population of subjects. Suppose that a sample of size n will be used in the study for which each subject is planned to take k repeated measures of the response variable at time points $t_1, t_2, \ldots, t_k$. Let $Y_j = (y_{j1}, y_{j2}, \ldots, y_{jk})^t$ be the vector of longitudinal measurements of the jth subject. For simplicity, we assume that changes in the mean response can be modeled by a linear trend over time and therefore the slope over time can be used to describe the rate of change. The major objective here is to obtain an accurate confidence interval estimate to the mean slope over time for the population of subjects under study. Recall that the two-stage random effects model assumes an individual growth curve for each subject at Stage 1

$$Y_{ji} = \beta_{0j} + \beta_{1j} t_i + e_{ji},$$

where e_{ji}'s are assumed to be independent and identically distributed as a normal distribution with mean 0 and variance σ_e^2. At Stage 2, the subject-specific rates of change β_{1j}'s are assumed to follow another normal distribution with mean β_1 and variance σ_b^2 and are independent of e_{ji}'s (the distribution of β_{0j} need not be used here). The major interest is in the estimation of mean change of rate β_1 in the population. The simple least square estimate to the subject-specific rate of change for the jth subject is

$$\hat{\beta}_{1j} = \frac{\sum\limits_{i=1}^{k} (t_i - \bar{t}) Y_{ji}}{\sum\limits_{i=1}^{k} (t_i - \bar{t})^2},$$

where $\bar{t} = \sum_{i=1}^{k} t_i / k$. Notice that $\hat{\beta}_{1j}$ follows a normal distribution with mean β_1 and variance σ^2, where

$$\sigma^2 = \sigma_e^2 \left\{ \sum\limits_{i=1}^{k} (t_i - \bar{t})^2 \right\}^{-1} + \sigma_b^2.$$

Therefore a $100(1-\alpha)\%$ $(0 < \alpha < 1)$ confidence interval for β_1 based on a sample of size n is $\bar{\beta}_1 \pm z_{\alpha/2}(\sigma/\sqrt{n})$, where

$$\bar{\beta}_1 = \frac{\sum_{j=1}^{n} \hat{\beta}_{1j}}{n}.$$

This gives the sample size required for achieving a confidence interval estimate of β_1 with a margin of error $\pm \delta$ as

$$n = \frac{(z_{\alpha/2}\sigma)^2}{\delta^2}.$$

If the longitudinal study is unbalanced or incomplete in which different study subjects may have different design vectors of times or even different number of time points, similar sample size formula could be derived under certain convergence assumptions on the design vectors of times.

Case 2. Estimating the difference of two rates of change over time.

A comparative longitudinal study compares the longitudinal courses of one or more response variables over two or more techniques, treatments, or levels of a covariate. In many clinical trials that evaluate the efficacy of one or more therapeutic treatments for a disease such as AD, a comparative longitudinal design is likely used to compare the treatments with placebo on the rate of change over time for a primary endpoint. Here we consider estimating the difference on the rates of change for the primary endpoint between the treated group and the placebo. The random coefficients model in this case assumes that the subject-specific slope β_{1j} follows a normal distribution with mean β_t and variance σ_{bt}^2 when the subject belongs to the treated group and another normal distribution with mean β_c and variance σ_{bc}^2 when the subject belongs to the control group. Similar to Case 1, when the subject belongs to the treated group, $\hat{\beta}_{1j}$ follows a normal distribution with mean β_t and variance σ_t^2, where

$$\sigma_t^2 = \sigma_e^2 \left\{ \sum_{i=1}^{k} (t_i - \bar{t})^2 \right\}^{-1} + \sigma_{bt}^2.$$

When the subject belongs to the control group, $\hat{\beta}_{1j}$ follows another normal distribution with mean β_c and variance σ_c^2, where

$$\sigma_c^2 = \sigma_e^2 \left\{ \sum_{i=1}^{k} (t_i - \bar{t})^2 \right\}^{-1} + \sigma_{bc}^2.$$

Therefore a $100(1-\alpha)\%$ $(0<\alpha<1)$ confidence interval for the difference $\beta_t - \beta_c$ on the mean rates of change over time between the treated group and the control group is $\bar{\beta}_t - \bar{\beta}_c \pm z_{\alpha/2} \sqrt{(\sigma_t^2/n_t) + (\sigma_c^2/n_c)}$, where

$$\bar{\beta}_i = \frac{\sum_{j=1}^{n_i} \hat{\beta}_{1j}}{n_i}$$

for $i = $ t, c, and n_t, n_c are the sample size for the treated group and the control group, respectively. Let $\lambda = n_t/n_c$ be the sample size ratio between two subject groups. This confidence interval also yields the sample sizes for the two study groups required for achieving a confidence interval estimate of $\beta_t - \beta_c$ with a margin of error $\pm\delta$ as

$$n_c = \left(\frac{\sigma_t^2}{\lambda} + \sigma_c^2\right)\left(\frac{z_{\alpha/2}}{\delta}\right)^2,$$

and $n_t = \lambda n_c$.

Case 3. Testing a hypothesis on the difference of two rates of change over time.

Along the similar arguments made in Case 2, the test statistic for testing $H_0 : \beta_t = \beta_c$ against $H_a : \beta_t - \beta_c = \Delta \neq 0$ is

$$z = \frac{\bar{\beta}_t - \bar{\beta}_c}{\sqrt{(\sigma_t^2/n_t) + (\sigma_c^2/n_c)}}.$$

The test statistic follows a standard normal distribution when the null hypothesis is true. The test therefore rejects the null hypothesis when $|z| > z_{\alpha/2}$ at a significance level of α $(0 < \alpha < 1)$. The power of the test, as a function of Δ is given by

$$P(\Delta) = 1 - \Phi\left(z_{\alpha/2} - \frac{\Delta}{\sqrt{(\sigma_t^2/n_t) + (\sigma_c^2/n_c)}}\right)$$

$$+ \Phi\left(-z_{\alpha/2} - \frac{\Delta}{\sqrt{(\sigma_t^2/n_t) + (\sigma_c^2/n_c)}}\right).$$

Therefore, the sample sizes required to achieve a statistical power of $(1-\gamma)(0 < \gamma < 1)$ is the solution to n_t and n_c such that

$$P(\Delta) = 1 - \gamma.$$

Notice that in all these sample size formulas, the length of the study, the number of repeated measures on the response variable, and the time spacing of the repeated measures all impact the statistical power through the quantity

$$f(t_1, t_2, \ldots, t_k) = \sum_{i=1}^{k}(t_i - \bar{t})^2.$$

Because this quantity is inversely related to the variance of the estimated subject-specific rate of change over time, the larger the quantity is, the smaller the variance for the estimated subject-specific slope is, the more accurate the confidence interval estimates to the mean slopes are, and the more powerful the statistical test is for comparing the two mean rates of changes over time between the treated group and the control group. Therefore, an optimal design should in theory maximize the quantity $f(t_1, t_2, \ldots, t_k)$ over the choice of $k, t_1, t_2, \ldots, t_k$. Notice that $t_k - t_1$ is the entire duration of the study. Although theoretically it should be chosen to maximize $f(t_1, t_2, \ldots, t_k)$, many economic and logistic and subject matters factors constrain the choice of $t_k - t_1$. In addition, the validity of the assumed statistical model also constrains the choice of $t_k - t_1$ in the sense that a linear growth over time might not be a reasonable assumption with a very long study duration, which is especially the case in the study of cognitive decline in Alzheimer's patients. Similarly, the number of repeated measures in a longitudinal study might also be constrained by many practical factors and cannot be freely chosen by the designers of the study. As a result, many longitudinal studies are restricted to relatively short duration with a predetermined number of repeated measures which is not chosen statistically based on an optimal design. Given that $t_k - t_1$ and k are typically chosen by some non-statistical reasons, the optimal design now relies on the choice of time spacing to maximize $f(t_1, t_2, \ldots, t_k)$. It can be mathematically proved that with an even k, $f(t_1, t_2, \ldots, t_k)$ is maximized when $k/2$ observations are taken at baseline t_1 and the other $k/2$ taken at the final time point t_k for each study subject. This mathematically optimal design, however, is not only impractical in many longitudinal studies but also completely erases the ability of verifying the validity of the linear growth curve based on the collected data. Therefore optimal longitudinal designs are sometimes based on further assumptions on the spacing of design vector of times. For example, if the researchers would want to design an equally spaced longitudinal study, then

$$f(t_1, t_2, \ldots, t_k) = \frac{(t_k - t_1)^2 k(k+1)}{12(k-1)}.$$

This function indicates the relevant influence of $t_k - t_1$ and k on the sample size computations. In general, if the linear growth curve is a valid statistical model and that the logistic and practical factors allow, an increase of either the study duration or the frequency of repeated measures will decrease the within-subject variability and improve the precision of parameter estimates or the statistical power in the test on the rate of change over time.

Missing data almost always happen in longitudinal studies. In general, the impact of missing data on sample size determination is difficult to quantify precisely because of the complexity in the patterns of missingness. The simplest conservative approach to account for the missing data in sample size determination is to first compute the sample sizes required assuming all subjects have the complete data, and then adjust the sample sizes based on an estimated rate of attrition accordingly.

Acknowledgements

The work was supported by National Institute on Aging grants AG 03991 and AG 05681 (for C.X. and J.P.M.) and AG 025189 (for C.X.). The work of K.Z. was supported by the National Natural Science Foundation, Grant # 70275101, of People's Republic of China.

266   C. Xiong et al.

References

Anderson, D.A., Aitkin, M. (1985). Variance component models with binary response: Interviewer variability. *Journal of the Royal Statistical Society, Series B* **47**, 203–210.

Barnard, G.A. (1963). Contribution to the discussion of professor Bartlett's paper. *Journal of the Royal Statistical Society, Series B* **25**, 294.

Box, G.E.P. (1954). Some theorems on quadratic forms applied in the study of analysis of variance problems. *Annals of Mathematical Statistics* **25**, 290–302.

Breslow, N.E., Clayton, D.G. (1993). Approximate inference in generalized linear mixed models. *Journal of the American Statistical Association* **88**, 9–25.

Chow, S.-C., Liu, J.-P. (2003). *Design and Analysis of Clinical Trials: Concepts and Methodologies*. Wiley, New York.

Cochran, W.G. (1977). *Sampling Techniques*. Wiley, New York.

Crystal, H., Dickson, D., Fuld, P., Masur, D., Scott, R., Mehler, M., Masdeu, J., Kawas, C., Aronson, M., Wolfson, L. (1988). Clinico-pathologic studies in dementia: Nondemented subjects with pathologically confirmed Alzheimer's disease. *Neurology* **38**, 1682–1687.

Cullis, B.R., McGilchrist, C.A. (1990). A model for the analysis of growth data from designed experiments. *Biometrics* **46**, 131–142.

Dempster, A.P., Laird, N.M., Rubin, D.B. (1977). Maximum likelihood from incomplete data via the EM algorithm (with discussion). *Journal of the Royal Statistical Society, Series B* **39**, 1–38.

Diggle, P.J. (1988). An approach to the analyses of repeated measures. *Biometrics* **44**, 959–971.

Diggle, P.J. (1989). Testing for random dropouts in repeated measurement data. *Biometrics* **45**, 1255–1258.

Diggle, P.J. (1990). *Time Series: A Biostatistical Introduction*. Oxford University Press, Oxford.

Diggle, P.J., Heagerty, P., Liang, K.-Y., Zeger, S.L. (2002). *Analysis of Longitudinal Data*, 2nd ed. Oxford University Press, New York.

Diggle, P.J., Kenward, M.G. (1994). Informative dropout in longitudinal data analysis (with discussion). *Applied Statistics* **43**, 49–93.

Evans, D.A., Funkenstein, H.H., Albert, M.S., Scheer, P.A., Cook, N.C., Chown, M.J., Hebert, L.E., Hennekens, C.H., Taylor, J.O. (1989). Prevalence of Alzheimer's disease in a community population of older persons: Higher than previously reported. *Journal of the American Medical Association* **262**, 2551–2556.

Fitzmaurice, G.M., Laird, N.M., Rotnitsky, A.G. (1993). Regression models for discrete longitudinal response (with discussion). *Statistical Science* **8**, 284–309.

Fitzmaurice, G.M., Laird, N.M., Ware, J.H. (2004). *Applied Longitudinal Analysis*. Wiley, Hoboken, NJ.

Gilmore, A.R., Anderson, R.D., Rae, A.L. (1985). The analysis of binomial data by a generalized linear mixed model. *Biometrika* **72**, 593–599.

Goldstein, H. (1991). Nonlinear likelihood approaches to variance component estimation and to related problems. *Journal of the American Statistical Association* **72**, 320–340.

Gourieroux, C., Monfort, A., Trognon, A. (1984). Pseudo-maximum likelihood methods: Theory. *Econometrica* **52**, 681–700.

Graybill, F.A. (1976). *Theory and Application of the Linear Model*. Wadsworth & Brooks, California.

Green, P.J. (1987). Penalized likelihood for general semi-parametric regression models. *International Statistical Review* **55**, 245–259.

Harville, D.A. (1977). Maximum likelihood approaches to variance component estimation and to related problems. *Journal of the American Statistical Association* **72**, 320–340.

Herbert, L.E., Scheer, P.A., Beckett, L.A., Albert, M.S., Pilgrim, D.M., Chown, M.J., Funkenstein, H.H., Evans, D.A. (1995). Age-specific incidence of Alzheimer's disease in a community population. *Journal of the American Medical Association* **273**, 1354–1359.

Hinde J. (1982). Compound Poisson regression models. In: Gilchrist R. (Ed.), *GLIM 82: Proceedings of the International Conference on Generalized Linear Models*. Springer, Berlin.

Huynh, H., Feldt, L.S. (1970). Conditions under which mean square ratios in repeated measures designs have exact F-distributions. *Journal of the American Statistical Association* **65**, 1582–1589.

James, W., Stein, C. (1961). Estimation with quadratic loss. *Proceedings of the Fourth Berkeley Symposium on Mathematical Statistics and Probability* **1**, 311–319.

Katzman, R., Terry, R., DeTeresa, R., Brown, T., Davies, P., Fuld, P., Renbing, X., Peck, A. (1988). Clinical, pathological and neurochemical changes in dementia: A subgroup with preserved mental status and numerous neocortical plaques. *Annals of Neurology* **23**, 138–144.

Korn, E.L., Whittemore, A.S. (1979). Methods for analyzing panel studies of acute health effects of air pollution. *Biometrics* **35**, 795–802.

Laird, N.M. (1978). Empirical Bayes methods for two-way tables. *Biometrika* **65**, 581–590.

Laird, N.M. (1988). Missing data in longitudinal studies. *Statistics in Medicine* **7**, 305–315.

Laird, N.M., Ware, J.H. (1982). Random-effects models for longitudinal data. *Biometrics* **38**, 963–974.

Liang, K.-Y., Zeger, S.L. (1986). Longitudinal data analysis using generalized linear models. *Biometrika* **73**, 13–22.

Liang, K.-Y., Zeger, S.L., Qaqish, B. (1992). Multivariate regression analyses for categorical data (with discussion). *Journal of the Royal Statistical Society, Series B* **54**, 3–40.

Lipsitz, S., Laird, N., Harrington, D. (1991). Generalized estimating equations for correlated binary data: Using odds ratios as a measure of association. *Biometrika* **78**, 153–160.

Little, R.J.A. (1993). Pattern-mixture models for multivariate incomplete data. *Journal of the American Statistical Association* **88**, 125–134.

Little, R.J.A. (1994). A class of pattern-mixture models for normal missing data. *Biometrika* **81**(3), 471–483.

Little, R.J.A. (1995). Modeling the drop-out mechanism in longitudinal studies. *Journal of the American Statistical Association* **90**, 1112–1121.

Little, R.J.A., Raghunathan, T.E. (1999). On summary-measures analysis of the linear mixed-effects model for repeated measures when data are not missing completely at random. *Statistics in Medicine* **18**, 2465–2478.

Little, R.J.A., Rubin, D.B. (2002). *Statistical Analysis with Missing Data*, 2nd ed. Wiley, New York.

Little, R.J.A., Wang, Y.-X. (1996). Pattern-mixture models for multivariate incomplete data with covariates. *Biometrics* **52**, 98–111.

McCullagh, P., Nelder, J.A. (1989). *Generalized Linear Models*, 2nd ed. Chapman & Hall, London.

McGilchrist, C.A., Aisbett, C.W. (1991). Restricted BLUP for mixed linear models. *Biometrical Journal* **33**, 131–141.

Milliken, G.A., Johnson, D.E. (1992). *Analysis of Messy Data, Volume 1: Designed Experiments*. Chapman & Hall/CRC, New York.

Milliken, G.A., Johnson, D.E. (2001). *Analysis of Messy Data, Volume 3: Analysis of Covariance*. Chapman & Hall/CRC, New York.

Molenberghs, G., Verbeke, G. (2005). *Models for Discrete Longitudinal Data*. Springer, New York.

Morris, J.C. (1993). The clinical dementia rating (CDR): Current version and scoring rules. *Neurology* **43**, 2412–2414.

Morris, J.C., MeKeel, D.W., Storandt, M., Rubin, E.H., Price, L., Grant, E.A., Ball, M.J., Berg, L. (1991). Very mild Alzheimer's disease: Informant-based clinical, psychometric and pathologic distinction from normal aging. *Neurology* **41**, 469–478.

Patterson, H.D., Thompson, R. (1971). Recovery of inter-block information when block sizes are unequal. *Biometrika* **58**, 545–554.

Prentice, R.L. (1988). Correlated binary regression with covariates specific to each binary observation. *Biometrics* **44**, 1033–1048.

Ridout, M. (1991). Testing for random dropouts in repeated measurement data. *Biometrics* **47**, 1617–1621.

SAS Institute, Inc. (1999). *SAS/STAT User's Guide, Version 8*, vols. 1–5. SAS Publishing, Cary, NC.

Satterthwaite, F.E. (1946). An approximate distribution of estimates of variance components. *Biometrics Bulletin* **2**, 110–114.

Singer, J.D., Willett, J.B. (2003). *Applied Longitudinal Data Analysis: Modeling Change and Event Occurrence*. Oxford University Press, New York.

Stern, R.D., Coe, R. (1984). A model fitting analysis of daily rainfall data (with discussion). *Journal of the Royal Statistical Society, Series A* **147**, 1–34.

Stiratelli, R., Laird, N.M., Ware, J.H. (1984). Random effects models for serial observations with dichotomous response. *Biometrics* **40**, 961–972.

Storandt, M., Grant, E.A., Miller, J.P., Morris, J.C. (2002). Rates of progression in mild cognitive impairment and early Alzheimer disease. *Neurology* **59**, 1034–1041.

Thall, P.F., Vail, S.C. (1990). Some covariance models for longitudinal count data with overdispersion. *Biometrics* **46**, 657–671.

Tsay, R. (1984). Regression models with time series errors. *Journal of the American Statistical Association* **79**, 118–124.

Tunnicliffe-Wilson, G. (1989). On the use of marginal likelihood in time series model estimation. *Journal of the Royal Statistical Society, Series B* **51**, 15–27.

Verbeke, G., Molenberghs, G. (2000). *Linear Mixed Models for Longitudinal Data*. Springer, New York.

Verbyla, A.O., Cullis, B.R. (1990). Modeling in repeated measures experiments. *Applied Statistics* **39**, 341–356.

Vonesh, E.F., Carter, R.L. (1992). Mixed effect nonlinear regression for unbalanced repeated measures. *Biometrics* **48**, 1–18.

Wong, W.H. (1986). Theory of partial likelihood. *Annals of Statistics* **14**, 88–123.

Wu, M.C., Bailey, K.R. (1989). Estimation and comparison of changes in the presence of informative right censoring: Conditional linear model. *Biometrics* **45**, 939–955.

Wu, M.C., Carroll, R.J. (1988). Estimation and comparison of changes in the presence of right censoring by modeling the censoring process. *Biometrics* **44**, 175–188.

Zeger, S.L., Liang, K.Y. (1986). Longitudinal data analysis for discrete and continuous outcomes. *Biometrics* **42**, 121–130.

Zeger, S.L., Liang, K.Y., Self, S.G. (1985). The analysis of binary longitudinal data with time-dependent covariates. *Biometrika* **72**, 31–38.

Zeger, S.L., Qaqish, B. (1988). Markov regression models for time series: A quasi-likelihood approach. *Biometrics* **44**, 1019–1031.

Zhao, L.P., Prentice, R.L. (1990). Correlated binary regression using a generalized quadratic model. *Biometrika* **77**, 642–648.

Handbook of Statistics, Vol. 27
ISSN: 0169-7161
DOI: 10.1016/S0169-7161(07)27016-6

9

Sequential and Group Sequential Designs in Clinical Trials: Guidelines for Practitioners

Madhu Mazumdar and Heejung Bang

Abstract

In a classical fixed sample design, the sample size is set in advance of collecting any data. The main design focus is choosing the sample size that allows the clinical trial to discriminate between the null hypothesis of no difference and the alternative hypothesis of a specified difference of scientific interest. A disadvantage of fixed sample design is that the same number of subjects will always be used regardless of whether the true treatment effect is extremely beneficial, marginal, or truly harmful relative to the control arm. Often, it is difficult to justify because of ethical concerns and/or economic reasons. Thus, specific early termination procedures have been developed to allow repeated statistical analyses to be performed on accumulating data and to stop the trial as soon as the information is sufficient to conclude. However, repeated analyses inflate the false positive error to an unacceptable level. To avoid this problem, many approaches of group sequential methods have been developed. Although there is an increase in the planned sample size under these designs, due to the sequential nature, substantial sample size reductions compared with the single-stage design is also possible not only in the case of clear efficacy but also in the case of complete lack of efficacy of the new treatment. This feature provides an advantage in utilization of patient resource. These approaches are methodologically complex but advancement in software packages had made the planning, monitoring, and analysis of comparative clinical trials according to these approaches quite simple. Despite this simplicity, the carrying on of a trial under group sequential design requires efficient logistics with dedicated team of data manager, study coordinator, biostatistician, and clinician. Good collaboration, rigorous monitoring, and guidance offered by an independent data safety monitoring committee are all indispensable pieces for its successful implementation.

In this chapter, we provide a review of sequential designs and discuss the underlying premise of all current methods. We present a recent example and an historical example to illustrate the methods discussed and to provide a flavor of the variety and complexity in decision making. A comprehensive list of softwares is provided for easy implementation along with practical guidelines. Few areas with potential for future research are also identified.

1. Introduction

Randomized clinical trial (RCT) is regarded as the gold standard for assessing the relative effectiveness/efficacy of an experimental intervention, as it minimizes selection bias and threats to validity by estimating average causal effects. There are two general approaches for designing RCT: (1) fixed sample design (FSD) and (2) group sequential design (GSD). In FSD, a predetermined number of patients (ensuring a particular power for proving a given hypothesis) are accrued, and the study outcome is assessed at the end of the trial. In contrast, a design where analyses are performed at regular intervals after a group of patients are accrued is called GSD. In comparative therapeutic trials with sequential patient entry, FSDs are often unjustified on ethical and economic grounds, and GSDs are preferred for their flexibility (Geller et al., 1987; Fleming and Watelet, 1989). Currently used methods can be classified into three categories: group sequential methods for repeated significance testing; stochastic curtailment or conditional power (Lan et al., 1982; Pepe and Anderson, 1992; Betensky, 1997) and Bayesian sequential methods (Spiegelhalter and Freedman, 1994; Fayers et al., 1997). While no single approach addresses all the issues, they do provide useful guidance in assessing the emerging trends for safety and benefit.

Trials using GSDs are common in published literature and the advantage of this kind of design is self evident by their impact (Gausche et al., 2000; Kelly et al., 2001; Sacco et al., 2001). One example of its successful use is a trial reported by Frustaci et al., where 190 sarcoma patients (a rare form of cancer) were to be accrued in order to detect a 20% difference in 2-year disease-free survival (60% on the adjuvant chemotherapy treatment arm versus 40% in the control arm undergoing observation alone) (Frustaci et al., 2001). An interim analysis was planned after half of the patients were accrued with stopping rule in terms of adjusted p-value. The trial was stopped as this criterion was met thereby saving 50% of the planned patient accrual. The observed difference was found to be 27% (72% on the treatment arm versus 45% on the control arm), 7% higher than what was hypothesized initially at the design stage. Therefore, the risk of treating additional patients with suboptimal therapy was greatly reduced.

Independent data safety monitoring committee (DSMC) with responsibilities of (1) safeguarding the interests of study patients, (2) preserving the integrity and credibility of the trial in order to ensure that future patients be treated optimally, and (3) ensuring that definitive and reliable results be available in a timely manner to the medical community has been mandated for all comparative therapeutic clinical trials sponsored by national institutes (URL: http://cancertrials.nci.nih. gov; Ellenberg, 2001). GSD provides an excellent aid to the DSMC for decision making. Other names utilized for this kind of committees playing virtually the same role are data or patient safety monitoring board (DSMB or PSMB), data monitoring and ethics committees (DMEC), and policy and data monitoring board (PDMB).

In this chapter, we start with a historical account of sequential methods and provide introduction to the underlying concept and approaches to the commonly utilized methods of inflation factor (IF) for sample size calculation and alpha spending function for monitoring the trials for early stopping. A listing of softwares is provided that has the capabilities of accommodating all of the methods discussed. A table of IF for sample size calculation of GSD is provided for quick assessment of feasibility of a trial (in regard to sample size) even before acquiring any special software for GSD. One current example is presented with standard template of a biostatistical consideration for writing study protocol, details of a stopping boundary utilized, items to be included in an interim analysis reports presented to the DSMC, and the substance included in the statistical section write-up for final dissemination in published literature. Another historical example (the BHAT trial) is discussed to highlight that the DSMC's decision to stop early was based not only on statistical group sequential boundary point, but also on a variety of other subjective considerations.

Several review papers and books from various perspectives are recommended to those who wish to learn about further details (Fleming and DeMets, 1993; Jennison and Turnbull, 2000; Sebille and Bellissant, 2003; Proschan et al., 2006).

2. Historical background of sequential procedures

The first strictly sequential method, the sequential probability ratio test, was developed during the Second World War (Wald, 1947). As its main application was the quality control of manufactured materials, its publication was only authorized after the end of the war, in 1947. Another class of sequential test is based on triangular continuation regions (Anderson, 1960). The basic idea on which these methods rely is to constantly use the available information to determine whether the data are compatible with null hypothesis, with alternative hypothesis, or insufficient to choose between these two hypotheses. In the first two cases, the trial is stopped and the conclusion is obtained whereas in the third case the trial continues. The trial is further processed until the data allows a legitimate (or per-protocol) decision between the two hypotheses. An example of a completely sequential trial can be found in Jones et al. (1982).

Armitage (1954) and Bross (1952) pioneered the concept of group sequential methods in medical field (Bross, 1952; Armitage, 1954). At first, these plans were fully sequential and did not gain widespread acceptance perhaps due to the inconvenience in their application. The problems discussed included the fact that response needs to be available soon after the treatment is started and that there would be organizational problems, such as coordination in multicenter trials and a much greater amount of work for the statistician. The shift to group sequential methods for clinical trials did not occur until the 1970s. Elfring and Schultz (1973) specifically used the term 'group sequential design' to describe their procedure for comparing two treatments with binary response (Elfring et al., 1973). McPherson (1974) suggested that the repeated significance tests of

Armitage et al. (1969) might be used to analyze clinical trial data at a small number of interim analyses (Armitage et al., 1969; McPherson, 1974). Canner (1977) used Monte Carlo simulation to find critical values of a test statistic for a study with periodic analyses of survival endpoint (Canner, 1977). However, Pocock (1977) was the first to provide clear guidelines for the implementation of the GSD attaining particular operating characteristics of type I error and power (Pocock, 1977). He made the case that most investigators do not want to evaluate results every time a couple of new patients are accrued but do want to understand the comparative merit every few months to assess if the trial is worth the time and effort and that continual monitoring does not have a remarkable benefit. More specifically, only a minor improvement is expected with more than five interim looks. A more comprehensive account of this history can be read from the excellent book by Jennison and Turnbull (2000).

3. Group sequential procedures for randomized trials

A primary difficulty in performing repeated analyses over time is the confusion about the proper interpretation of strength of evidence obtained from such evaluations. Suppose that only a single data analysis is performed after data collection has been fully completed for a trial. Then a two-sided (or one-sided if justified, e.g., non-inferiority design) significance value of $p \leq 0.05$, obtained from a test of hypothesis of no difference between an experimental therapy and a control, is usually interpreted as providing strong enough evidence that the new therapy provides an advantage. The interpretation is justified by the willingness of investigators to accept up to five false-positive conclusions in every 100 trials of regimens that, in truth, have equivalent efficacy. Unfortunately, even when a new treatment truly provides no advantage over a standard therapy, performing repeated analyses can greatly increase the chance of obtaining positive conclusions when this $p \leq 0.05$ guideline is repeatedly used.

As such, interim data safety reports pose well-recognized statistical problems related to the multiplicity of statistical tests to be conducted on the accumulating set of data. The basic problem is well known and is referred to as "sampling to a foregone conclusion" (Cornfield, 1966) and has been illustrated mathematically, pictorially or through simulations by many researchers (Fleming and Green, 1984). Specifically, in a simulation of 100 typical clinical trials of two interventions with truly equivalent efficacy that called for up to four periodic evaluations, 17 (rather than five) trials yielded false-positive conclusions (i.e. $p \leq 0.05$) in at least one analysis. The rate of false-positives continues to rise as the frequency of interim analyses rises. This serious increase in the likelihood of reaching false-positive conclusions due to misinterpretation of the strength of evidence when repeated analyses are conducted over time partly explains why many published claims of therapeutic advances have been false leads and provides the motivation for development of GSD.

A GSD first provides a schedule that relates patient accrual to when the interim analyses will occur. This schedule is conveniently expressed in terms of the proportion of the maximal possible number of patients that the trial could accrue. Second, such designs give a sequence of statistics used to test the null hypothesis, and third, they give a stopping rule defined in terms of a monotone increasing sequence of nominal significance levels at which each test will be conducted. This sequence of significance levels is carefully chosen to maintain the overall type I error at some desired level (e.g., 0.05 or 0.10) using one- or two-sided hypothesis. Either the number or the time of analyses is prespecified or the rate at which the overall significance level is "used up" is fixed in advance. Thus, undertaking group sequential trials assumes that hypothesis testing at nominal significance levels less than a prestated overall significance level will be performed, and that if results are ever extreme enough to exceed prespecified thresholds, the trial should be stopped. While such group sequential procedures differ in detail, they have certain common features.

The two commonly discussed pioneering mechanisms in GSD are given by Pocock (Pocock, 1977) and O'Brien and Fleming (OBF) (O'Brien and Fleming, 1979). Pocock adapted the idea of a repeated significance test at a constant nominal significance level to analyze accumulating data at a relatively small number of times over the course of the study. Patient entry was divided into equally sized groups and the data are analyzed after each group of observations has been collected. As an alternative, OBF proposed a test in which the nominal significance levels needed to reject the null hypothesis at sequential analyses increase as the study progresses, thus, making it more difficult to reject the null hypothesis at the earliest analysis but easier later on. Other variations to these schemes have also been developed but OBF is the most commonly utilized GSD as it fits well with the wishes of clinical trialists who do not want to stop a trial prematurely with insufficient evidence based on less reliable or unrepresentative data. There are other reasons for this preference. Historically, most clinical trials fail to show a significant treatment difference, hence from a global perspective, it is more cost-effective to use conservative designs. Indeed, even a conservative design such as OBF often shows a dramatic reduction in the average sample number (ASN or expected sample size) under the alternative hypothesis, H_A, compared to a FSD (see Table 1 for brief overview). Moreover, psychologically, it is preferable to have a nominal p-value at the end of the study for rejecting the null hypothesis, H_0, which is close to 0.05 in order to avoid the embarrassing situation where, say, a p-value of 0.03 at the final analysis would be declared non-significant.

Later, Wang et al. (1987) proposed a class of generalized formulation that encompasses Pocock and OBF methods as two extreme members.

Table 1
General properties of monitoring designs

Design	General	ASN (under H_0)	ASN (under H_A)
Fixed	Most conservative	Low	Large
OBF	Conservative, hard to stop early	Mid	Mid
Pocock	Most liberal, early stopping properties	Large	Low

Although the formulation of GSD started with binary outcomes, a generalized formulation has helped establish the wide applicability of the large sample theory for multivariate normal random variables with independent increments (i.e., standardized partial sums) to group sequential testing (Jennison and Turnbull, 1997; Scharfstein et al., 1997). This structure applies to the limiting distribution of test statistics which are fully efficient in parametric and semiparametric models, including generalized linear models and proportional hazards models (Tsiatis et al., 1995). It applies to all normal linear models, including mixed-effects models (Lee and Demets, 1991; Reboussin et al., 1992). Gange and Demets showed its applicability to the generalized estimating equation setting and Mazumdar and Liu showed the derivation for the comparative diagnostic test setting where area under the receiver operating characteristic curve is the endpoint (Mazumdar and Liu, 2003; Mazumdar, 2004). In short, almost any statistic likely to be used to summarize treatment differences in a clinical trial will justify group sequential testing with this basic structure and common mathematical formulation (Jennison and Turnbull, 2000).

3.1. Power and sample size calculation using inflation factor

Sample size computation in GSD setting involves the size of the treatment effect under some non-null hypothesis, the standard error of the estimated treatment effect at the end of the trial, and the drift of the underlying Brownian motion used to model the sequentially computed test statistics. The appropriate drift is determined by multiple factors such as the group sequential boundaries, type I error, and desired power. The theoretical background for design of group sequential trials has been discussed elsewhere (Kim and DeMets, 1992; Lan and Zucker, 1993) but the drift of commonly used GSDs can be easily translated into the corresponding IFs, provided in Table 2. The sample size approximation for a GSD in any setting is simply obtained by multiplying the sample size under the corresponding FSD by the IF provided in this table for the features of the specific GSD chosen. It is easy to note that the sample size inflation under OBF is minimal.

Table 2
Inflation Factors for Pocock and O'Brien–Fleming alpha spending functions for different total numbers of looks (K) under equal-sized increments

	$\alpha = 0.05$ (Two-sided)				$\alpha = 0.01$ (Two-sided)			
K	Spending function	Power ($1-\beta$)		K	Spending function	Power ($1-\beta$)		
		0.80	0.90	0.95			0.80	0.90	0.95
2	Pocock	1.11	1.10	1.09	2	Pocock	1.09	1.08	1.08
2	OBF	1.01	1.01	1.01	2	OBF	1.00	1.00	1.00
3	Pocock	1.17	1.15	1.14	3	Pocock	1.14	1.12	1.12
3	OBF	1.02	1.02	1.02	3	OBF	1.01	1.01	1.01
4	Pocock	1.20	1.18	1.17	4	Pocock	1.17	1.15	1.14
4	OBF	1.02	1.02	1.02	4	OBF	1.01	1.01	1.01
5	Pocock	1.23	1.21	1.19	5	Pocock	1.19	1.17	1.16
5	OBF	1.03	1.03	1.02	5	OBF	1.02	1.01	1.01

3.2. Monitoring boundaries using alpha spending functions

The earlier publications for group sequential boundaries required that the number and timing of interim analyses be fixed in advance. However, while monitoring data for real clinical trials, it was felt that more flexibility in being able to look at the data at time points dictated by the emerging beneficial or harmful trend is desired. To accommodate this capability, Lan and Demets proposed a more flexible implementation of the group sequential boundaries through an innovative 'alpha spending function' (Lan and Demets, 1983; Lan and DeMets, 1989). The spending function controls how much of the false-positive error (or false-negative error when testing to rule out benefit) can be used at each interim analysis as a function of the proportion (t^*, range 0 (study start)-1 (study end)) of total information observed. In many applications, t^* may be estimated as the fraction of patients recruited (for dichotomous outcomes) or the fraction of events observed (for time to event outcomes) out of the respective total expected. The alpha spending functions underlying OBF GSD correspond to

$$\alpha_1(t^*) = 2 - 2\Phi\left[\frac{Z_{1-(\alpha/2)}}{(t^*)^{1/2}}\right],$$

whereas the one for Pocock is described by

$$\alpha_2(t^*) = \alpha \ln[1 + (e - 1)t^*].$$

The advantage of the alpha spending function is that neither the number nor the exact timing of the interim analyses needs to be specified in advance. Only the particular spending function needs to be specified. It is useful to note that the nominal significance levels utilized in any GSD will always add up to more than the overall significance level, because with multiple significance testing the probability of rejecting the null hypothesis does not accumulate additively due to positive correlations among test statistics.

Following is a sample 'Biostatistical Consideration' write-up for a clinical trial in Germ Cell Tumor (GCT) utilizing GSD with OBF boundaries. IF approach with three total looks ($K = 3$) was chosen at design stage and a series of boundaries and sequence of significance level were computed accordingly. The option of utilizing spending function approach was also kept open, which is often the case in practice.

3.3. Design of a phase 3 study with OBF GSD: A sample template

3.3.1. Biostatistical considerations

1. *Objective and background*: The objective of this study is to compare in a prospective randomized manner the efficacy of an experimental combination regimen versus the standard regimen in previously untreated 'poor' risk GCT patients. The poor risk criterion helps identify patients who are expected to have high probability of worse outcome. It is described in the protocol and roughly depends on the primary site, histology, and specific blood markers

being high. For this kind of cancer, a patient's prognosis is considered to be favorable if their tumor completely disappears and does not come back at least for a year. The response of these patients is called durable complete responder (DCR) at one year. In the institutional database at Memorial Sloan–Kettering Cancer Center (MSKCC) of size 796 patients treated by standard therapy, the proportion of patients remaining DCR at one year for the poor risk group ($n = 141$) is 30% with a 95% confidence interval (CI) of 22.2–37.3%.

2. *Primary endpoint, power and significance level*: The major endpoint for this trial is DCR at one year where the time is computed from the day a patient is defined responder. This study is planned to detect a 20% absolute difference from the currently observed rate of 30% (30% versus 50%). We are expecting an accrual of 50 patients per year. The sample size calculation based on log-rank test for an FSD with 80% power and 5% level of significance, 195 patients will be needed. To incorporate two interim looks and a final look (so total $K = 3$) at the end of full accrual, an IF of 1.02 was multiplied to 195 requiring 199 patients ($= 1.02 \times 195$) using OBF method (O'Brien and Fleming 1979). Rounding it off to 200 patients (100 per arm), we decide to place the two interim looks at the end of second and third year and the final look at the end of fourth year as the accrual rate of 50 patients makes the length of study to be four years.

3. *Randomization*: After eligibility is established, patients will be randomized via a telephone call to the coordinating center at MSKCC clinical trial office (Phone number: XXX-XX-XXXX; 9:00 am to 5:00pm Monday through Friday). Randomization will be accomplished by the method of stratified random permuted block, where patient institution (MSKCC versus ECOG versus SWOG versus remaining participating institutions) was adopted for stratification, where ECOG denotes Eastern Cooperative Oncology Group and SWOG denotes Southwest Oncology Group.

4. *Data safety monitoring committee and interim analyses*: The data will be reviewed at designated intervals by an independent DSMC. This committee was formed with two independent oncologists and one independent biostatistician. The committee will be presented with the data summary on accrual rates, demographics and bio-chemical markers etc. and comparative analysis (using Fisher's exact test) on toxicity and DCR proportion by the principal investigator (PI) and the biostatistician on study. Survival and progression-free survival curves will be estimated only if there is an enough number of events that governs statistical power. Semi-annual reports on toxicity will be disseminated to all the participating groups.

Normalized z-statistics according to the OBF boundary to be used for stopping early if the experimental regimen looks promising are ± 3.471, ± 2.454, ± 2.004, where the corresponding sequence of nominal significance levels are 0.001, 0.014, and 0.036, respectively (East, Cytel Statistical Software). If situation emerges where these time points are not the most convenient or desirable, Lan–Demets spending function utilizing OBF boundaries will be used to compute the corresponding z-statistics and significance level. The committee is expected to use the statistical stopping rules as a guideline in addition to both medical judgment and the relevant emerging data in the literature, especially ones obtained from similar trials.

5. *Final analysis*: All toxicities will be evaluated based on the NCI common toxicity criteria and tabulated by their frequencies and proportions. Fisher's exact test will be used to compare the toxicities and adverse events by the two arms. The primary analysis, DCR-free survival curves will be estimated using Kaplan–Meier method and with appropriate follow-up, comparisons will be made using log-rank test (Kaplan and Meier, 1958; Mantel, 1966). Once the trial stops (either at interim look or at final look), standard statistical estimation and inference will be undertaken for the observed treatment difference.

3.4. Analyses following group sequential test

Analysis following a group sequential test consists of two scenarios: The first is upon conclusion of the trial after the test statistic has crossed a stopping boundary and the second is when an interval estimate of the treatment difference is desired whether the design calls for a termination or not. Tsiatis et al. (1984) have shown that in both situation, it is inappropriate to compute a 'naïve' CI, treating the data as if they had been obtained in a fixed sample size experiment. They estimated naïve CI following a five-stage Pocock's test with 5% level of significance and found their coverage to vary between 84.6% and 92.9%, depending on the true parameter value.

For the first scenario, Tsiatis et al. suggested a numerical method for calculating an exact CIs following group sequential tests with Pocock (1977) or O'Brien and Fleming (1979) boundaries based on ordering the sample space in a specific manner. They derived the CIs based on normal distribution theory, which pull the naive CIs toward zero and are no longer symmetric about the sample mean. They also commented that their method is applicable to any (asymptotically) normal test statistic which has uncorrelated increments and for which the variance can be estimated consistently. Whitehead (1986) suggested an approach for adjusting the maximum likelihood estimate as the point estimate by subtracting an estimate of the bias. Wang and Leung (1997) proposed a parametric bootstrap method for finding a bias-adjusted estimate, whereas Emerson and Fleming (1990) provide a formulation of uniformly minimum variance unbiased estimator calculated by Rao–Blackwell technique.

For the second scenario, the multiple-looks problem affects the construction of CIs just as it affects significance levels of hypothesis tests. Repeated CIs for a parameter θ are defined as a sequence of intervals I_k, $k = 1, \dots, K$, for which a simultaneous coverage probability is maintained at some level, say, $1 - \alpha$. The defining property of a $(1 - \alpha)$-level sequence of repeated CIs for θ is $P[\theta \in I_k$ for all $k = 1, \dots, K] = 1 - \alpha$ for all θ (Jennison and Turnbull, 1983, 1984, 1985). The interval I_k, $k = 1, \dots, K$, provides a statistical summary of the information about the parameter θ at the kth analysis, automatically adjusted to compensate for repeated looks at the accumulating data. As a result, repeated

CIs instead of group sequential testing can be used for monitoring clinical trials (Jennison and Turnbull, 1989).

Most conventional trials are designed to have a high probability of detecting a predefined treatment effect if such an effect truly exists. That probability is called the power of the trial. Most trials use power in the range of 0.8–0.95 for a plausible range of alternatives of interest and the sample size of the study is calculated to achieve that power. The concept of 'conditional power' comes into play when supporting evidence is sought to decide the power midstream.

3.5. Stochastic curtailment

Once the trial starts and data become available, the probability that a treatment effect will ultimately be detected can be recalculated (Halperin et al., 1982; Lan et al., 1982; Lan and Wittes, 1988). An emerging trend in favor of the treatment increases the probability that the trial will detect a beneficial effect, while an unfavorable trend decreases the probability of establishing benefit. The term 'conditional power' is often used to describe this evolving probability. The term 'power' is used because it is the probability of claiming a treatment difference at the end of the trial, but it is 'conditional' because it takes into consideration the data already observed that will be part of the final analysis. Conditional power can be calculated for a variety of scenarios including a positive beneficial trend, a negative harmful trend, or no trend at all. However, these calculations are frequently made when interim data are viewed to be unfavorable. For this scenario, it represents the probability that the current unfavorable trend would improve sufficiently to yield statistically significant evidence of benefit by the scheduled end of the trial. This probability is usually computed under the assumption that the remainder of the data will be generated from a setting in which the true treatment effect was as large as the originally hypothesized in the study protocol.

When an unfavorable trend is observed at the interim analysis, the conditional probability of achieving a statistically significant beneficial effect is much less than the initial power of the trial. If the conditional power is low for a wide range of reasonable assumed treatment effect, including those originally assumed in the protocol, this might suggest to the DSMC that there is little reason to continue the trial since the treatment is highly unlikely to show benefit. Of course, this conditional power calculation does increase the chance of missing a real benefit (false-negative or type II error) since termination eliminates any chance of recovery by the intervention. However, if the conditional power under these scenarios is less than 0.2 compared to the hypothesis for which the trial originally provided power of 0.85–0.9, the increase in the rate of false-negative error is negligible. There is no concern with false-positive error in this situation since there is no consideration of claiming a positive result. An example of its use will follow in the Beta-Blocker Heart Attack Trial (BHAT) trial description later in this chapter.

3.6. Bayesian monitoring

The Bayesian approach for monitoring accumulating data considers unknown parameters to be random and to follow probability distributions (Spiegelhalter et al., 1986; Freedman et al., 1994; Parmar et al., 1994; Fayers et al., 1997). The investigators specify a prior distribution(s) describing the uncertainty in the treatment effect and other relevant parameters. These prior distributions are developed based on previous data and beliefs. It is quantified through a distribution of possible values and is referred to as the prior distribution. The observed accumulating data are used to modify the prior distribution and produce a posterior distribution, a distribution that reflects the most current information on the treatment effect, taking into account the specified prior as well as the accumulated data. This posterior distribution can then be used to compute a variety of summaries including the predictive probability that the treatment is effective. In 1966, Cornfield introduced the idea of Bayesian approach to monitoring clinical trial (Cornfield, 1966). Although, interest has recently increased in its use (Kpozehouen et al., 2005) and availability of computational tools have made it more feasible to use, these methods are still not widely utilized.

3.7. Available softwares

Softwares for implementing GSDs have been developed and commercialized since the early 1990s. Extended descriptions of these softwares are available through their user's guide and some review papers (Emerson, 1996; Wassmer and Vandemeulebroecke, 2006). Most of the computational tools employ the recursive numerical integration technique that takes advantage of a quadrature rule of replacing integral by a weighted sum for probabilistic computations (Armitage et al., 1969; Jennison and Turnbull, 2000).

Here, we provide a comprehensive listing of appropriate links for free self-executable softwares as well as codes written in FORTRAN, SAS, Splus, and R languages. FORTRAN source code used in the textbook by Jennison and Turnbull (2000) can be downloaded from Dr. Jennison's homepage on http://people.bath.ac.uk/mascj/book/programs/general. The code provides continuation regions and exit probabilities for classical GSDs including those proposed by Pocock (1977), O'Brien and Fleming (1979), Wang and Tsiatis (1987) and Pampallona and Tsiatis (1994). In addition, the spending function approach according to Lan and Demets (1983) is implemented. Another implementation in FORTRAN of the spending function approach is available for use under UNIX and MS-DOS. It can be downloaded from http://www.biostat.wisc.edu/landemets/ as a stand-alone program with a graphical user interface, while details of methodologies and algorithms are found in Reboussin et al. (2000). These codes provide computation of boundaries and exit probabilities for any trial based on normally or asymptotic normally distributed test statistics with independent increments, including those in which patients give a single continuous or binary response, survival studies, and certain longitudinal designs. Interim analyses need not be equally spaced, and their number need not be specified in advance via flexible alpha spending mechanism. In addition to boundaries, power computations, probabilities associated with a given set of boundaries, and CIs can also be computed.

The IML (Interactive Matrix Language) module of SAS® features the calls SEQ, SEQSCALE, and SEQSHIFT that perform computations for group sequential tests. SEQ calculates the exit probabilities for a set of successive continuation intervals. SEQSCALE scales these continuation regions to achieve a specified overall significance level and also returns the corresponding exit probabilities. SEQSHIFT computes the non-centrality parameter for a given power.

S-PLUS that is commercially available provides a package for designing, monitoring, and analyzing group sequential trials through its $S + SeqTrial^{TM}$ module. It makes use of the unifying formulation by Kittelson et al. (Kittelson and Emerson, 1999), including all classical GSDs, triangular tests (Whitehead, 1997), and the spending function approach. It offers the calculation of continuation regions, exit probabilities, power, sample size distributions, overall p-values and adjusted point estimates and CIs, for a variety of distributional assumptions. It comes with a graphical user interface and very good documentation, which can be downloaded from http://www.insightful.com/products/seqtrial/default.asp.

In R (http://www.r-project.org/), cumulative exit probabilities of GSDs can be computed by the function seqmon. It implements an algorithm proposed by Schoenfeld (2001) and the documentation and packages are freely downloadable at http://www.maths.lth.se/help/R/.R/library/seqmon/html/seqmon.html.

PEST, version 4 offers a wide range of scenarios, including binary, normal, and survival endpoints, and different types of design. The main focus of PEST is the implementation of triangular designs. Sequential designs from outside PEST can also be entered and analyzed. Besides the planning tools, the software offers a number of analysis tools including interim monitoring and adjusted p-values, CIs, and point estimates for the final analysis. An important and unique feature of PEST is that interim and final data can be optionally read from SAS data sets. More information about the software can be found at http://www.rdg.ac.uk/mps/mps_home/software/software.htm#PEST%204.

East of Cytel Statistical Software and Services (http://www.cytel.com/Products/East/) is the most comprehensive package for planning and analyzing group sequential trials. The software provides a variety of capabilities of advanced clinical trial design, simulation and monitoring, and comes with extensive documentation including many real data examples. Tutorial sessions for East are frequently offered during various statistical meetings and conferences and educational settings.

"PASS 2005 Power Analysis and Sample Size" is distributed by NCSS Inc. This software supplies the critical regions and the necessary sample sizes but it is not yet possible to apply a sequential test to real data in the sense of performing an adjusted analysis (point estimates, CIs, and p-values). Documentation and a free download are available on http://www.ncss.com./passsequence.html.

"ADDPLAN Adaptive Designs-Plans and Analyses" (http://www.addplan.com/) is designed for the purpose of planning and conducting a clinical trial based on an adaptive group sequential test design. New adaptive (flexible) study designs allow for correct data-driven re-estimation of the sample size while controlling the type I error rate. Redesigning the sample size in an interim analysis based on the results observed so far considerably improves the power of the trial since the best available information at hand is used for the sample size adjustment. The simulation capabilities for specific adaptation rules are also provided.

The choice of software is based on the users' need and the complexity of design. The freely available softwares are often enough to implement basic functions to be used in standard or popular designs and to perform associated data analyses outlined in this chapter unless special features are required.

3.8. Data safety monitoring committee

Early in the development of modern clinical trial methodology, some investigators recognized that, despite the compelling ethical needs to monitor the accumulating results, repeated review of interim data raised some problems. It was recognized that knowledge of the pattern of the accumulating data on the part of investigators, sponsors, or trial participants, could affect the course of the trial and the validity of the results. For example, if investigators were aware that the interim trial results were favoring one of the treatment groups, they might be reluctant to continue to encourage adherence to all regimens in the trial, or to continue to enter patients in the trial, or they may alter the types of patients they would consider accrual. Furthermore, influenced by financial or scientific conflicts of interest, investigators, or the sponsor might take actions that could diminish the integrity and credibility of the trial. A natural and practical approach to dealing with this problem is to assign sole responsibility for interim monitoring of data on safety and efficacy to a committee whose members have no involvement in the trial, no vested interest in the trial results, and sufficient understanding of the trial design, conduct, and data-analytical issues to interpret interim analyses with appropriate caution. These DSMCs consisting of members from variety of background (clinical, statistical, ethical, etc.) have become critical components of virtually all clinical trials.

For the above example, an independent DSMC consisting of three members with background in oncology (one from community hospital and one from specialized center) and biostatistics met every year to discuss the progress of the trial. The outcome comparison was only presented when an interim analysis with OBF was allowed. Below we present a list of items that were included in the interim report for this trial. This is a typical template for a clinical trial and could be useful in other scenarios.

Items included in the interim report:

1. Brief outline of the study design
2. Major protocol amendments with dates (or summary) if applicable
3. Enrollment by arm and year and center (preferably, updated within a month of the DSMC meeting date)
4. Information on eligibility criterion violation or crossover patients
5. Summary statistics (e.g., mean/median) on follow-up times of patients
6. Frequency tables of baseline characteristics (demographics, toxicity, and adverse event summary, laboratory test summary, precious treatment) of the full cohort
7. Comparative analysis of primary and secondary endpoints (when data mature)
8. Subgroup analyses and analyses adjusted for baseline characteristics (and some secondary outcomes data, if any)

9. Comparative analysis of adverse event and toxicity data
10. Comparative analysis of longitudinal lab values.

The GCT study referred above struggled with accrual of patients and remained open for 10 years instead of the four years planned initially. To improve accrual rate, new centers were added and the patient eligibility was expanded. DSMC met annually and approved these actions. The first DSMC meeting where outcome data were compared was at 6th year after study start instead of the 2nd year. Lan–Demets with OBF boundary was utilized to compute the appropriate boundary but the boundary was not crossed. DSMC deliberations continued with concern for the accrual rate but since the experimental regimen utilizing autologus bone marrow transplant was quite a novel and unique approach and it was added to the standard therapy, the DSMC did not feel any harm to patients and decided to keep the trial open. More assertive accrual plans were adopted but when many of these plans failed to improve accrual, the study was at last closed at 219 patients (in contrast, $N = 270$ in the original plan).

3.8.1. Details included in the final paper (on design and primary analysis)
The final write-up or summary report needs to include as much details as possible about the original design (including sample size/power calculation), modifications, rationale for modification, decisions by DSMC, and conclusions. Here's part of the 'Statistical Methods' section from the final paper related to the GCT study (Motzer et al., 2007):

> The trial was designed with the proportion of patients with durable complete response (DCR) at one year from entry onto the trial as the primary endpoint. The original study population to be enrolled on this study was poor-risk GCT patients only. We had planned to accrue 200 patients (100 per arm) to detect a 20% difference in DCR rate at one year (an improvement from 30% to 50%) with a 5% level of significance and 80% power. However, as the trial progressed, the accrual rate was far lower than our expectation of 50 poor-risk patients per year. Also during this time, an international effort brought along a newly developed but broadly accepted risk group classification and it was felt that the intermediate-risk group patients with poor markers (lactate dehydrogenase greater than 3 times upper limit of normal) would benefit from the treatment under investigation. Therefore it was decided to extend the study to this modified intermediate risk group from the poor risk classification utilized before. Based on a historical one-year DCR rate of 45% in the poor and intermediate risk groups combined, we then modified our target accrual to 218 patients to detect an improvement of 20% with the same level and power.
>
> A final modification to the study was implemented in 2002 after a new center CALGB was added to the study and accrual at that center began. At that point, it was our hope to be able to address the original question of interest in the poor-risk group of patients. We planned to accrue 270 patients, consisting of 216 poor-risk patients (200 per original calculation + 16 to account for withdrawals) and 54 intermediate-risk patients. However, as accrual did not meet our expectations even with the additional cooperative group participating, the study was closed in August of 2003. The data were reviewed annually

by an independent DSMC. Initially, the design included an O'Brien and Fleming stopping rule with the sequence of nominal significance levels of 0.001, 0.014, and 0.036 for the two interim analyses and the final analysis, respectively. A formal comparative interim analysis on DCR proportion and overall survival was presented in May 2000 based on a recalculated boundary utilizing Lan–Demets spending function. The decision was to continue the trial as the boundary was not crossed and no ethical conflict was found since the experimental regimen was an autologus bone marrow transplant regimen on top of the standard therapy. The study was at last stopped in 2003 due to not being able to improve accrual rate.

3.9. Historical example of GSD use

It is always educational to look back on the trials that were planned with GSD and benefited from it. Two excellent books by DeMets et al., 2006 and Ellenberg et al., 2006 provide essential and in-depth reading materials for clinical trialists starting in this field. An example considered by these books and many other publications is described below to show the multifaceted decision process that goes into the deliberation of DSMB.

The BHAT compared the beta-blocker propranolol against placebo in patients who had a myocardial infarction recently. The statistical design called for enrollment of 4,020 patients, aged 30–69 years, who had a myocardial infarction 5–21 days prior to randomization. The primary objective of the study was to determine if long-term administration of propranolol would result in a difference in all-cause mortality. The design utilized O'Brien–Fleming boundary with alpha level set at two-tailed 0.05, 90% power, and three-year average follow-up. The attempt was to detect a 21.25% relative change in mortality, from a three-year rate of 17.46% in the control (placebo) group to 13.75% in the intervention group, which were obtained from earlier studies (Furberg and Friedwald, 1978; Anderson et al., 1979) after taking non-adherence into account (Byington, 1984).

Enrollment began in 1978 and a total of 3,837 participants were accrued instead of the planned 4,020. This reduced the power slightly from the planned 90% to 89%. The PDMB first reviewed the data in May 1979. Subsequent data reviews were to occur approximately every six months, until the scheduled end of the trial in June 1982. At the *October, 1979* meeting of the PDMB, the log-rank z-value exceeded the conventional 1.96 critical value for a nominal p of 0.05 but was far from significance due to the conservative nature of the O'Brien–Fleming boundaries early in the study. PDMB recommended continuation of the trial.

At the meeting in *April 1981*, the PDMB reviewed not only the accumulating BHAT data but the results of the timolol trial that had just been published. This trial of 1,884 survivors of an acute myocardial infarction showed a statistically significant reduction in all-cause mortality, from 16.2% to 10.4%, during a mean follow-up of 17 months. At this point, BHAT was no longer enrolling patients, but follow-up was continuing. The PDMB recommended that BHAT continues, primarily because, despite the timolol findings, the BHAT data did not show convincing evidence of benefit. Not only had the monitoring boundary not been crossed, but the long-term effect on mortality and possible adverse events was unknown. Importantly, all patients in BHAT had been in the trial for at least six months post-infarction, and there was no evidence that beta-blockers started after that time produced benefit. Thus, there was not an ethical concern about leaving the participants on placebo. The PDMB advised that the study investigators be informed of the timolol results. However, it also advised that because there had been conflicting results from other beta-blocker trials, the positive results of the timolol trial should not preclude the continuation of BHAT. Furthermore, timolol was not available for sale in the United States then. At its *October 1981* data review, the PDMB noted that the upper OBF boundary had been crossed. The normalized log-rank statistic was then 2.82, which exceeded the boundary value of 2.23. In addition to the monitoring boundaries, the PDMB considered a number of factors in its recommendation to stop early:

> 1) Conditional power calculations indicated that there was little likelihood that the conclusions of the study would be changed if follow-up were to continue; 2) The gain in precision of the estimated results for the first two years would be tiny, and only modest for the third year; 3) The results were consistent with those of another beta-blocker trial; 4) There would be potential medical benefits to both study participants on placebo and to heart attack patients outside the study; 5) Other characteristics, such as subgroup examinations and baseline comparability, confirmed the validity of the findings; 6) The consent form clearly called for the study to end when benefit was known. Following points in favor of continuing until the scheduled end were considered but were not found to weigh enough in favor of not stopping: 1) Even though slight, there remained a chance that the conclusions could change; 2) Because therapy would be continued indefinitely, it would be important to obtain more long-term (4 year) data; 3) It would be important to obtain more data on subgroups and secondary outcomes; 4) The results of a study that stopped early would not be as persuasive to the medical community as would results from a fully powered study that went to completion, particularly given the mixed results from previous trials.

> Lessons learnt from these experiences are that 1) O'Brien-Fleming approach to sequential boundaries could prove very helpful in fostering a cautious attitude with regard to claiming significance prematurely. Even though conventional significance was seen early in the study, the use of sequential boundaries gave the study added credibility and probably helped make it persuasive to the practicing medical community; 2) The use of conditional power added to the persuasiveness of the results, by showing the extremely low likelihood that the conclusions would change if the trial were to continue to its scheduled end; 3) The decision-making process involves many factors, only some of which are statistical (Friedman et al., 2003).

4. Steps for GSD design and analysis

4.1. Classical design

> *Step 1*: Decide the number of maximum looks (or groups) K and the choice of boundary (that can be indexed by shape parameter, Δ (Wang and Tsiatis, 1987).

Remark:
  a) The gain in ASN is most dramatic when going from $K = 1$ (i.e., the fixed sample size design) to $K = 2$. Beyond $K = 5$, there is relatively little change in ASN.
  b) The choice of K may be dictated by some practicality such as the frequency of the DSMC meetings that is feasible.
  c) $\Delta = 0$ for OBF and $\Delta = 0.5$ for Pocock.
Step 2: Compute the sample size for fixed design as you would ordinarily do (using significance level, power, and effect size). Multiply by the appropriate IF.
Step 3: After computing the maximum sample size, divide it into K equal group sizes and conduct interim analyses after each group. Reject H_0 at the first interim analysis where the test statistic using all the accumulated data exceeds the boundary values computed. Alternatively, we can translate the boundaries to the corresponding nominal p-values at each look and conduct the test using p-values.

4.2. Information-based design

Step 1: Specify level of significance, power, K and alternative of interest (γ).
Remark:
You specify K at the design stage but you may deviate from this at the time of analysis.
Step 2: Choose a spending function and stopping boundary (Lan and DeMets spending function with OBF or Pocock or other boundaries).
Step 3: Compute maximum information (MI) required to have a specific power as $MI = (z_{1-\alpha/2} + z_{1-\beta/\gamma})^2 \times IF$.
Step 4: The first time the data are monitored, say, at time t_1, compute the proportion of information compared to MI. Then find the first boundary value. If the test statistic exceeds the boundary computed, stop and reject H_0. If not, continue to next monitoring time.
Step 5: At time t_2, compute the ratio of observed information and MI. Then perform the testing.
Step 6: Continue in this fashion, if necessary, until the final analysis, at which point you use up the remaining significance level.
Remark:
With this strategy, you are guaranteed a level alpha test regardless of how often or when you look at the data prior to obtaining MI.

5. Discussion

In RCTs designed to assess the efficacy and safety of medical interventions, evolving data are typically reviewed on a periodic basis during the conduct of the study. These interim reviews are especially important in trials conducted in the setting of diseases that are life-threatening or result in irreversible major morbidity. Such reviews have many purposes. They may identify unacceptably slow rates of accrual or high rates of ineligibility determined after randomization, protocol violations that suggest that clarification of or changes to the study protocol are needed or unexpectedly high dropout rates that threaten the trial's ability to produce unbiased results. The most important purpose, however, is to ensure that the trial remains appropriate and safe for the individuals who have been or are still to be enrolled. Efficacy results must also be monitored to enable benefit-to-risk assessments to be made. Repeated statistical testing of the primary efficacy endpoint was seen to increase the chance of false-positive rate. The methods of adjusting the significance levels at each interim analysis so that the overall false-positive rate stays at an acceptable level gave rise to GSDs. The field has been developing for past 30 years and is now quite mature with various methods with well-studied operating characteristics and availability of an array of user-friendly software.

One new field of applications has been cluster-randomized trials (CRTs). CRTs have been used increasingly over the past two decades to measure the effects of health interventions applied at the community level. Excellent reviews and books are written by Donner et al. and Murray (Donner and Brown, 1990; Murray, 1998; Donner and Klar, 2000). Recently, Zou et al. (2005) developed group sequential methods that can be applied to CRT. Although the design aspect is well characterized and related computer program is available upon request, effect estimation following this group sequential test remains a topic of future research. This method is not yet used prospectively on a clinical trial. Development of methodology for novel design such as the split-cluster design could also be a useful addition to this field (Donner and Klar, 2004).

Adaptive designs in the context of group sequential testing allow modifications of particular aspects of the trials (such as inappropriate assumptions, excessive cost, or saving in time) after its initiation without undermining the validity and integrity of the trial. Some developments have been made to combine the advantages of adaptive and of classical group sequential approaches. Although research has been ongoing in this field, it still remains a field of research priority (Tsiatis and Mehta, 2003; Jennison and Turnbull, 2005; Kuehn, 2006; Wassmer, 2006).

There are some settings where GSDs may not be appropriate. For example, when the endpoint assessment time is lengthy relative to the recruitment period, there might be enough interim results to perform an analysis only after all or most subjects have been recruited and treated, thereby potentially rendering the GSD irrelevant. Most other large studies will benefit from having planned look at the data as trial progresses. Quite surprisingly, we found that many large trials follow FSD (Cooper et al., 2006; Cotton et al., 2006; Nicholls et al., 2006). A systematic literature search to assess the percentage of studies that would benefit from GSD but is not currently planning to use it would be interesting. This effort could also identify additional areas for further research or need for expanded exposure of these designs among practitioners.

Acknowledgement

We thank Ms. Anita Mesi for her excellent help with the published literature management using endnote software and past collaborators, Dr. Robert Motzer, and Ms. Jennifer Bacik, for many discussions on this topic. Partial support for this work came from the following grants: CERTs (AHRQ RFA-HS-05-14), CIPRA (NIAID U01 AI058257), R25 CA105012, and Cornell Institute of Clinical Research (supported by Tolly Vinik Trust).

References

Anderson, M., Bechgaard, P., Frederiksen, J. (1979). Effect of Alprenolol on mortality among patients with definite or suspected acute myocardial infarction: Preliminary results. *Lancet* **2**, 865–868.
Anderson, T. (1960). A modification of the sequential probability ratio test to reduce the sample size. *Ann Math Stat* **31**, 165–197.
Armitage, P. (1954). Sequential tests in prophylactic and therapeutic trials. *Quarterly Journal of Medicine* **23**, 255–274.
Armitage, P., McPherson, C.K., Rowe, B.C. (1969). Repeated significance tests on accumulating data. *Journal of Royal Statistical Society. Series A* **132**, 235–244.
Betensky, R.A. (1997). Early stopping to accept H(o) based on conditional power: Approximations and comparisons. *Biometrics* **53**(3), 794–806.
Bross, I. (1952). Sequential medical plans. *Biometrics* **8**, 188–205.
Byington, R. (1984). Beta-Blocker Heart Attack Trial: Design, methods, and baseline results. *Controlled Clinical Trials* **5**, 382–437.
Canner, P.L. (1977). Monitoring treatment differences in long-term clinical trials. *Biometrics* **33**(4), 603–615.
Cooper, C.J., Murphy, T.P. et al. (2006). Stent revascularization for the prevention of cardiovascular and renal events among patients with renal artery stenosis and systolic hypertension: Rationale and design of the CORAL trial. *American Heart Journal* **152**(1), 59–66.
Cornfield, J. (1966). A Bayesian test of some classical hypotheses – with application to sequential clinical trials. *Journal of the American Statistical Association* **61**, 577–594.
Cotton, S.C., Sharp, L. et al. (2006). Trial of management of borderline and other low-grade abnormal smears (TOMBOLA): Trial design. *Contemporary Clinical Trials* **27**(5), 449–471.
DeMets, D., Furberg, C. et al. (2006). *Data Monitoring in Clinical Trials: A Case Studies Approach.* Springer, New York.
Donner, A., Brown, K. (1990). A methodological review of non-therapeutic intervention trials employing cluster randomization. *International Journal of Epidemiology* **19**(4), 795–800.
Donner, A., Klar, N. (2000). *Design and Analysis of Cluster Randomization Trials in Health Research.* Arnold, London.
Donner, A., Klar, N. (2004). Methods for statistical analysis of binary data in split-cluster designs. *Biometrics* **60**(4), 919–925.
Elfring, G.L., Schultz, J.R. et al. (1973). Group sequential designs for clinical trials. *Biometrics* **29**(3), 471–477.
Ellenberg, S.S. (2001). Independent monitoring committees: Rationale, operations, and controversies. *Statistics in Medicine* **20**, 2573–2583.
Ellenberg, S.S., Fleming, T. et al. (2006). *Data Monitoring Committees in Clinical Trials: A Practical Perspective.* Wiley, London.
Emerson, S. (1996). Statistical packages for group sequential methods. *The American Statistician* **50**, 183–192.
Emerson, S., Fleming, T. (1990). Parameter estimation following group sequential hypothesis testing. *Biometrika* **77**, 875–892.
Fayers, P.M., Ashby, D. et al. (1997). Tutorial in biostatistics: Bayesian data monitoring in clinical trials. *Statistics in Medicine* **16**, 1413–1430.
Fleming, T., DeMets, D. (1993). Monitoring of clinical trials: Issues and recommendations. *Controlled Clinical Trials* **14**(3), 183–197.
Fleming, T.R., Green, S. (1984). Considerations for monitoring and evaluating treatment effect in clinical trials. *Controlled Clinical Trials* **5**, 55–66.

Fleming, T.R., Watelet, L.F. (1989). Approaches to monitoring clinical trials. *Journal of the National Cancer Institute* **81**, 188–193.

Freedman, L., Spiegelhalter, D. et al. (1994). The what, why, and how of Bayesian clinical trials monitoring. *Statistics in Medicine* **13**, 1371–1383.

Friedman, L., Demets, D., et al. (2003). Data and safety monitoring in the Beta-Blocker Heart Attach Trial: Early experience in formal monitoring methods.

Frustaci, S., Gherlinzoni, F. et al. (2001). Adjuvant chemotherapy for adult soft tissue sarcomas of the extremities and girdles: Results of the Italian randomized cooperative trial. *Journal of Clinical Oncology* **19**, 1238–1247.

Furberg, C., Friedwald, W. (Eds.) (1978). Effects of chronic administration of beta-blockade on long-term survival following myocardial infarction. *Beta-Adrenergic Blockade: A New Era in Cardio-vascular Medicine*. Excerpta Medica, Amsterdam.

Gausche, M., Lewis, R.J. et al. (2000). Effect of out-of-hospital pediatric endotracheal intubation on survival and neurological outcome. *The Journal of the American Medical Association* **283**(6), 783–790.

Geller, N.L., Pocock, S.J. et al. (1987). Interim analyses in randomized clinical trials: Ramifications and guidelines for practitioners. *Biometrics* **43**(1), 213–223.

Halperin, M., Lan, K. et al. (1982). An aid to data monitoring in long-term clinical trials. *Controlled Clinical Trials* **3**, 311–323.

Jennison, D., Turnbull, B. (1983). Confidence interval for a bionomial parameter following a mul-tistage test with application to MIL-STD 105D and medical trials. *Technometrics* **25**, 49–63.

Jennison, C., Turnbull, B. (1984). Repeated confidence intervals for group sequential clinical trials. *Controlled Clinical Trials* **5**, 33–45.

Jennison, C., Turnbull, B. (1985). Repeated confidence intervals for the median survival time. *Biometrika* **72**, 619–625.

Jennison, C., Turnbull, B. (1989). Interim Analyses: The repeated confidence interval approach (with discussion). *Journal of Royal Statistical Society. Series B* **51**, 305–361.

Jennison, C., Turnbull, B.W. (1997). Group sequential analysis incorporating covariate information. *Journal of the American Statistical Association* **92**, 1330–1341.

Jennison, C., Turnbull, B.W. (2000). *Group Sequential Methods with Application to Clinical Trials*. Chapman & Hall.

Jennison, C., Turnbull, B.W. et al. (2005). Meta-analyses and adaptive group sequential designs in the clinical development process. *Journal of Biopharmaceutical Statistics* **15**(4), 537–558.

Jones, D., Newman, C. et al. (1982). The design of a sequential clinical trial for the comparison of two lung cancer treatments. *Statistics in Medicine* **1**(1), 73–82.

Kaplan, E., Meier, P. (1958). Nonparametric estimation from incomplete observations. *Journal of American Statistical Association* **53**, 457–481.

Kelly, K., Crowley, J. et al. (2001). Randomized phase III trial of paclitaxel plus carboplatin versus vinorelbine plus cisplatin in the treatment of patients with advanced non–small-cell lung cancer: A southwest oncology group trial. *Journal of Clinical Oncology* **19**, 3210–3218.

Kim, K., DeMets, D. (1992). Sample size determination for group sequential clinical trials with immediate response. *Statistics in Medicine* **11**(10), 1391–1399.

Kittelson, J., Emerson, S. (1999). A unifying family of group sequential test designs. *Biometrics* **55**, 874–882.

Kpozehouen, A., Alioum, A. et al. (2005). Use of a Bayesian approach to decide when to stop a therapeutic trial: The case of a chemoprophylaxis trial in human immunodeficiency virus infection. *American Journal of Epidemiology*, **161**(6), 595–603, (see comment).

Kuehn, B. (2006). Industry, FDA warm to "Adaptive" trials. *The Journal of the American Medical Association* **296**(16), 1955–1971.

Lan, K., DeMets, D.L. (1989). Group sequential procedures: Calendar versus information time. *Statistics in Medicine* **8**, 1191–1198.

Lan, K., Demets, D. (1983). Discrete sequential boundaries for clinical trials. *Biometrika* **70**, 659–663.

Lan, K., Simon, R. et al. (1982). Stochastically curtailed tests in long-term clinical trials. *Communications in Statistics C* **1**, 207–219.

Lan, K., Wittes, J. (1988). The B-value: A tool for monitoring data. *Biometrics* **44**, 579–585.

Lan, K., Zucker, D. (1993). Sequential monitoring of clinical trials: The role of information and Brownian motion. *Statistics in Medicine* **12**, 753–765.

Lee, J., Demets, D. (1991). Sequential comparison of changes with repeated measurement data. *Journal of American Statistical Association* **86**, 757–762.

Mantel, N. (1966). Evaluation of survival data and two new rank order statistics arising in its consideration. *Cancer Chemotherapy Reports* **50**, 163–170.

Mazumdar, M. (2004). Group sequential design for comparative diagnostic accuracy studies: Implications and guidelines for practitioners. *Medical Decision Making: An International Journal of the Society for Medical Decision Making* **24**(5), 525–533.

Mazumdar, M., Liu, A. (2003). Group sequential design for comparative diagnostic accuracy studies. *Statistics in Medicine* **22**(5), 727–739.

McPherson, K. (1974). Statistics: The problem of examining accumulating data more than once. *New England Journal of Medicine* **290**, 501–502.

Motzer, R., Nichols, C. et al. (2007). Phase III randomized trial of conventional-dose chemotherapy with or without high-dose chemotherapy and autologous hematopoietic stem-cell rescue as first-line treatment for patients with poor-prognosis metastatic germ cell tumors. *Journal of Clinical Oncology* **25**(3), 247–256.

Murray, D.M. (1998). *Design and Analysis of Group-randomized Trials*. Oxford University Press, New York.

Nicholls, S.J., Sipahi, I. et al. (2006). Intravascular ultrasound assessment of novel antiatherosclerotic therapies: Rationale and design of the Acyl-CoA:Cholesterol Acyltransferase Intravascular Atherosclerosis Treatment Evaluation (ACTIVATE) Study. *American Heart Journal* **152**(1), 67–74.

O'Brien, P., Fleming, T. (1979). A multiple testing procedure for clinical trials. *Biometrics* **35**, 549–556.

Pampallona, S., Tsiatis, A. (1994). Group sequential designs for one-sided and two-sided hypothesis testing with provision for early stopping in favor of null hypothesis. *Journal of Statistical Planning and Inference* **42**, 19–35.

Parmar, M., Spiegelhalter, D. et al. (1994). The CHART trials: Bayesian design and monitoring in practice. *Statistics in Medicine* **13**, 1297–1312.

Pepe, M., Anderson, G. (1992). Two-stage experimental designs: Early stopping with a negative result. *Applied Statistics* **41**(1), 181–190.

Pocock, S.J. (1977). Group sequential methods in the design and analysis of clinical trials. *Biometrika* **64**, 191–199.

Proschan, M., Lan, K. et al. (2006). *Statistical Monitoring of Clinical Trials: A Unified Approach*. Springer.

Reboussin, D., Lan, K. et al. (1992). Group Sequential Testing of Longitudinal Data. Tech Report No. 72, Department of Biostatistics, University of Wisconsin.

Reboussin, D.M., DeMets, D.L. et al. (2000). Computations for group sequential boundaries using the Lan–DeMets spending function method. *Controlled Clinical Trials* **21**(3), 190–207.

Sacco, R.L., DeRosa, J.T. et al. (2001). Glycine antagonist in neuroprotection for patients with acute stroke: GAIN Americas – a randomized controlled trial. *The Journal of the American Medical Association* **285**(13), 1719–1728.

Scharfstein, D., Tsiatis, A. et al. (1997). Semiparametric efficiency and its implication on the design and analysis of group-sequential studies. *Journal of the American Statistical Association* **92**, 1342–1350.

Schoenfeld, D.A. (2001). A simple algorithm for designing group sequential clinical trials. *Biometrics* **57**(3), 972–974.

Sebille, V., Bellissant, E. (2003). Sequential methods and group sequential designs for comparative clinical trials. *Fundamental and Clinical Pharmacology* **17**(5), 505–516.

Spiegelhalter, D., Freedman, L. et al. (1994). Bayesian approaches to clinical trials (with discussion). *Journal of Royal Statistics Society Association* **157**, 357–416.

Spiegelhalter, D., Freedman, L. et al. (1986). Monitoring clinical trials: Conditional or predictive power? *Controlled Clinical Trials* **7**, 8–17.

Tsiatis, A., Boucher, H. et al. (1995). Sequential methods for parametric survival models. *Biometrics* **82**, 165–173.

Tsiatis, A., Rosner, G. et al. (1984). Exact confidence intervals following a group sequential test. *Biometrics* **40**, 797–803.

Tsiatis, A.A., Mehta, C.R. (2003). On the inefficiency of the adaptive design for monitoring clinical trials. *Biometrika* **90**(2), 367–378.

URL: http://cancertrials.nci.nih.gov Policy of the National Cancer Institute for Data and Safety Monitoring of Clinical Trials.

Wald, A. (1947). *Sequential Analysis*. Wiley, New York.

Wang, S.K., Tsiatis, A.A. et al. (1987). Approximately optimal one-parameter boundaries for group sequential trials. *Biometrics* **43**(1), 193–199.

Wang, Y., Leung, D. (1997). Bias reduction via resampling for estimation following sequential tests. *Sequential Analysis* **16**, 298–340.

Wassmer, G. (2006). Planning and analyzing adaptive group sequential survival trials. *Biometrical Journal* **48**(4), 714–729.

Wassmer, G., Vandemeulebroecke, M. (2006). A brief review on software developments for group sequential and adaptive designs. *Biometrical Journal* **48**(4), 732–737.

Whitehead, J. (1986). On the bias of maximum likelihood estimation following a sequential test. *Biometrika* **73**, 573–581.

Whitehead, J. (1997). *The Design and Analysis of Sequential Clinical Trials*. Wiley, Chichester.

Zou, G.Y., Donner, A. et al. (2005). Group sequential methods for cluster randomization trials with binary outcomes. *Clinical Trials* **2**(6), 479–487.

Handbook of Statistics, Vol. 27
ISSN: 0169-7161
© 2007 Elsevier B.V. All rights reserved
DOI: 10.1016/S0169-7161(07)27025-7

Estimation of Marginal Regression Models with Multiple Source Predictors

Heather J. Litman, Nicholas J. Horton, Bernardo Hernández and Nan M. Laird

Abstract

Researchers frequently use multiple informants to predict a single outcome and compare the marginal relationships of each informant with response; a common application is diagnostic testing where the goal is to determine which diagnostic test best predicts disease. We review generalized estimating equations (GEE) for marginal regression models using continuous multiple source predictors with a continuous outcome and introduce a new maximum likelihood (ML) approach. ML and GEE yield the same regression coefficient estimates when (1) allowing different regression coefficients for each informant report, (2) assuming equal variance for the two multiple informant reports and constraining the marginal regression coefficients to be equal and (3) including non-multiple informant covariates with cases 1 or 2. With the ML technique, likelihood ratio tests (LRTs) can be formed to easily compare regression models and a broader array of models can be fit. Using asymptotic relative efficiency (ARE), we show that a constrained model assuming equal variance is more efficient than an unconstrained model. We apply the methods to a study investigating the effect of vigorous exercise on body mass index (BMI) with measures of exercise collected on two informants: children and their mothers.

1. Introduction

Multiple informant data refer to information obtained from different individuals or sources used to measure a single construct. We use the term multiple informant data to describe data obtained from either multiple sources or multiple measures on a commensurate scale. Typically, researchers are interested in the relationship of each multiple informant predictor with response (Horton et al., 1999; Horton and Fitzmaurice, 2004). For example, Field et al. (2003) conducted a study to estimate the marginal correlation of different measures of body mass index (BMI) with a gold standard measurement of percentage body fat; the aim of the study is to find the best measure of BMI. Pepe et al. (1999) compared results from different informants to predict adult obesity from childhood obesity. We consider a validation study by Hernández et al. (1999) used to design a larger study of the relationship between physical activity/inactivity and obesity in children. Physical activity and inactivity in the validation study are reported by multiple informants: children and their mothers, but feasibility issues dictate that only children's responses will be used in the main study. Our goal is to compare the relationship of child's report of physical activity and BMI with the relationship of mother's report of physical activity and BMI in the context of study design. In some settings, if both informants yield similar results, it may be useful to obtain a more efficient and robust estimate of the effect by fitting a model with common slopes. For instance, Horton et al. (2001) predict mortality in a 16-year follow-up period of Stirling County Study subjects from multiple informants (self and physician report) about psychiatric disorders; their final model has a constrained estimate of the association between diagnosis and overall mortality (controlling for age and gender).

For simplicity, we define the response as Y and the two reports of physical activity measured by informants as X_1 and X_2, though extensions to more than two informants can be accommodated. In general, multiple informants can be used either as outcomes or as predictors in a standard regression model. Multiple informant outcomes have been considered by Fitzmaurice et al. (1995, 1996), Kuo et al. (2000) and Goldwasser and Fitzmaurice (2001). As described above, we instead consider the case where the multiple informants are predictors.

Over the years, researchers have developed many 'ad hoc' techniques to analyze multiple informants as predictors. One analysis method is to pool reports from the multiple informants (Offord et al., 1996). However, this method does not take into account the potential differences between the informants. Investigators also proposed models predicting $E(Y|X_1, X_2)$ where all multiple informants are in the model simultaneously (Horton and Fitzmaurice, 2004). In this case, the regression coefficient for a given multiple informant covariate is conditional on all other multiple informants in the model. However, as in the Field et al. (2003) study, the objective is not to best predict percentage body fat using all multiple informants, but rather to find the single measure of BMI that best predicts body fat. Thus, rather than fitting a model with all the multiple informants where we obtain a regression coefficient for each covariate that is conditional on the others in the model, we model the univariate relationship between percentage body fat and one BMI measure by predicting $E(Y|X_1)$ and also model the relationship between percentage body fat and another BMI measure by predicting $E(Y|X_2)$ (Horton and Fitzmaurice, 2004). Performing separate analyses such as this (Gould et al., 1996) has been done, but because measures from the different informants are not independent of one another, separate analyses are not amenable to comparing coefficients from the two models and it is not clear how to interpret a combined analysis.

Pepe et al. (1999) and Horton et al. (1999) independently developed a nonstandard application of generalized estimating equations (GEE) (Liang and Zeger, 1986; Zeger and Liang, 1986) in regression analyses with multiple informants as predictors. The technique provides marginal estimates of the multiple informants while appropriately controlling for the outcomes being the same. Using GEE requires fewer assumptions than maximum likelihood (ML); in particular, it only assumes that the model for the mean is correctly specified. We review this approach in Section 2.

This paper describes a ML approach for analysis of multiple informants as predictors and introduces constrained models that can increase efficiency. For simplicity, only the complete-data case is considered here, although additional research has been performed considering missingness (Litman et al., 2007). ML has been previously used for analysis of multiple informants as covariates when the responses and multiple informants are discrete (O'Brien et al., 2006). This research showed no loss of efficiency associated with using GEE compared with ML when there are no shared parameters. With a common parameter for the association between outcome and two multiple informant predictors, efficiency loss is modest with the minimum asymptotic relative efficiency (ARE) over a range of conditional parameter values being approximately 0.90 (O'Brien et al., 2006). Our paper instead considers a continuous outcome and continuous predictors. For simplicity, we consider a model from the Hernández et al. (1999) dataset with one univariate response and one predictor measured by two informants. Section 3 describes our new ML technique. Simulations to compare GEE and ML variance estimates are presented in Section 4 and efficiency of a constrained model is discussed in Section 5. Application of ML to the Hernández et al. (1999) study is presented in Section 6.

2. Review of the generalized estimating equations approach

We briefly review the method introduced by Horton et al. (1999) and Pepe et al. (1999) that was originally presented for a binary response using a logit link function, but here we assume a linear model. We define an outcome $\mathbf{Y}$ and K multiple source predictors $\mathbf{X}_1, \ldots, \mathbf{X}_k$. The GEE approach models the marginal associations between $\mathbf{Y}$ and $\mathbf{X}_k$, defined as $E(\mathbf{Y}|\mathbf{X}_k)$ for $k = 1, \ldots, K$. In the simplest case with no covariates and distinct parameters for each informant, the model fit is

$$E(\mathbf{Y}|\mathbf{X}_k) = \alpha_k + \beta_k \mathbf{X}_k \quad \text{for } k = 1, \ldots, K, \tag{1}$$

where α_k and β_k are parameters in the kth regression. Defining

$$\tilde{\mathbf{Y}} = \begin{pmatrix} Y_i \\ Y_i \\ \vdots \\ Y_i \end{pmatrix}_{(K \times 1)} \qquad \mathbf{X}_i = \begin{pmatrix} 1 & X_{i1} & 0 & 0 & \cdots & 0 & 0 \\ 0 & 0 & 1 & X_{i2} & \cdots & 0 & 0 \\ \vdots & & & & & & \\ 0 & 0 & 0 & 0 & \cdots & 1 & X_{iK} \end{pmatrix}_{(K \times 2K)} \qquad \beta = \begin{pmatrix} \alpha_1 \\ \beta_1 \\ \alpha_2 \\ \beta_2 \\ \vdots \\ \alpha_K \\ \beta_K \end{pmatrix}_{(2K \times 1)},$$

the GEE equations assuming an identity link, constant variance and a working independence correlation matrix simplify to the ordinary least squares (OLS) equations:

$$\sum_{i=1}^{n} \mathbf{X}_i^T(\tilde{\mathbf{Y}}_i - \mathbf{X}_i\beta) = 0. \tag{2}$$

Note that each vector of responses, $\tilde{\mathbf{Y}}_i$, consists of the same response K times (Pepe et al., 1999). Also, the data records from each subject are treated as independent clusters. We assume an independence working correlation matrix as have previous papers developing GEE (Horton et al., 1999; Pepe et al., 1999); we show later that the use of this matrix is optimal under the likelihood model. Solving Eq. (2), we find that $\hat{\beta} = \Sigma_{i=1}^{n}(\mathbf{X}_i^T\mathbf{X}_i)^{-1}\mathbf{X}_i^T\tilde{\mathbf{Y}}_i$ where $\hat{\alpha}_k$ and $\hat{\beta}_k$ are the intercept and slope estimates from a univariate regression model with response $\mathbf{Y}$ and a single predictor $\mathbf{X}_k$. A strength of the GEE approach is that it provides a joint variance–covariance matrix for the $2K$ univariate parameter estimates (Pepe et al., 1999).

Estimates of var($\hat{\beta}$) can be derived using empirical or model-based variance formulas. The empirical or 'sandwich' variance estimator has traditionally been used because it allows the variance of the response to depend on the design matrix while taking the correlation of the residuals into account (Huber, 1967). Using the empirical variance formula and assuming working independence,

$$\widehat{\mathrm{var}}(\hat{\beta}) = \left(\sum_{i=1}^{n}\mathbf{X}_i^T\mathbf{X}_i\right)^{-1}\left(\sum_{i=1}^{n}\mathbf{X}_i^T(\tilde{\mathbf{Y}}_i - \mathbf{X}_i\hat{\beta})(\tilde{\mathbf{Y}}_i - \mathbf{X}_i\hat{\beta})^T\mathbf{X}_i\right)$$
$$\times \left(\sum_{i=1}^{n}\mathbf{X}_i^T\mathbf{X}_i\right)^{-1}. \tag{3}$$

Since the 'sandwich' variance makes no modeling assumptions, it provides a robust expression appropriate for many applications. Because ML assumes var($\mathbf{Y}_i$) does not depend on $\mathbf{X}_i$, to facilitate comparison of ML to GEE, we use a version of the model-based variance for the GEE estimator:

$$\widehat{\mathrm{var}}(\hat{\beta}) = \left(\sum_{i=1}^{n}\mathbf{X}_i^T\mathbf{X}_i\right)^{-1}\left(\sum_{i=1}^{n}\mathbf{X}_i^T\hat{\Sigma}\mathbf{X}_i\right)\left(\sum_{i=1}^{n}\mathbf{X}_i^T\mathbf{X}_i\right)^{-1}, \tag{4}$$

where

$$\hat{\Sigma} = \frac{\sum_{i=1}^{n}(\tilde{\mathbf{Y}}_i - \mathbf{X}_i\hat{\beta})(\tilde{\mathbf{Y}}_i - \mathbf{X}_i\hat{\beta})^T}{n}. \tag{5}$$

We define the diagonal elements of $\hat{\Sigma}$ as $\hat{\Sigma}_{11}, \ldots, \hat{\Sigma}_{KK}$ (estimated variances) and the off-diagonal elements as $\hat{\Sigma}_{12}, \ldots, \hat{\Sigma}_{(K-1)K}$ (estimated covariances). The variance in Eq. (4) is model-based since it assumes the same $\hat{\Sigma}$ for each individual and $\hat{\Sigma}$ does not depend on the design matrix. Using Eq. (4) and because $\Sigma_{i=1}^{n}\mathbf{X}_i^T\mathbf{X}_i$

is block diagonal, the estimated variance–covariance matrix for the slopes can be expressed as

$$
\widehat{\text{var}}
\begin{pmatrix}
\hat{\beta}_1 \\
\hat{\beta}_2 \\
\vdots \\
\hat{\beta}_K
\end{pmatrix}
=
\begin{pmatrix}
\dfrac{\hat{\Sigma}_{11}}{\text{SS}_{X_1^2}} & \cdots & \dfrac{\text{SS}_{X_1,X_K}\hat{\Sigma}_{1K}}{\text{SS}_{X_1^2}\text{SS}_{X_K^2}} \\
\vdots & & \\
\dfrac{\text{SS}_{X_1,X_K}\hat{\Sigma}_{1K}}{\text{SS}_{X_1^2}\text{SS}_{X_K^2}} & \cdots & \dfrac{\hat{\Sigma}_{KK}}{\text{SS}_{X_K^2}}
\end{pmatrix},
\tag{6}
$$

where

$$
\text{SS}_{X_k^2} = \sum_{i=1}^{n}(X_{ik} - \bar{X}_k)^2,
$$

and

$$
\text{SS}_{X_k X_l} = \sum_{i=1}^{n}(X_{ik} - \bar{X}_k)(X_{il} - \bar{X}_l).
$$

We also consider a constrained model with $\beta_1 = \beta_2 = \ldots = \beta_K = \beta_C$ defined as

$$
E(\mathbf{Y}|\mathbf{X}_k) = \alpha_k + \beta_C \mathbf{X}_k \qquad \text{for } k = 1,\ldots,K,
\tag{7}
$$

where $\tilde{\mathbf{Y}}_i$ remain the same as in the unconstrained model,

$$
\mathbf{X}_i =
\begin{pmatrix}
1 & 0 & \cdots & 0 & X_{i1} \\
0 & 1 & \cdots & 0 & X_{i2} \\
\vdots & & & & \\
0 & 0 & \cdots & 1 & X_{iK}
\end{pmatrix}
\quad \text{and } \beta = (\alpha_1, \alpha_2, \ldots, \alpha_K, \beta_C)^T.
$$

The same general expression for $\hat{\beta}$ holds and it is again straightforward to show that

$$
\hat{\beta} = \left(\bar{Y} - \hat{\beta}_C \bar{X}_1, \ldots, \bar{Y} - \hat{\beta}_C \bar{X}_K, \right.
$$

$$
\left. \frac{\sum_{i=1}^{n}(X_{i1} - \bar{X}_1)(Y_i - \bar{Y}) + \cdots + \sum_{i=1}^{n}(X_{iK} - \bar{X}_K)(Y_i - \bar{Y})}{\sum_{i=1}^{n}(X_{i1} - \bar{X}_1)^2 + \cdots + \sum_{i=1}^{n}(X_{iK} - \bar{X}_K)^2} \right)^T,
$$

and from Eq. (4),

$$
\widehat{\text{var}}(\hat{\beta}_C) = \frac{\text{SS}_{X_1^2}\hat{\Sigma}_{11} + \cdots + \text{SS}_{X_K^2}\hat{\Sigma}_{KK} + \sum_{i>j}\text{SS}_{X_i,X_j}\hat{\Sigma}_{ij}}{(\text{SS}_{X_1^2} + \cdots + \text{SS}_{X_K^2})^2}.
\tag{8}
$$

We also extend the model to incorporate a vector of continuous or discrete covariates $\mathbf{Z}$ not measured by multiple informants. We predict $E(\mathbf{Y}|\mathbf{X}_k,\mathbf{Z})$ using the following model:

$$
E(\mathbf{Y}|\mathbf{X}_k, \mathbf{Z}) = \alpha_k + \beta_k \mathbf{X}_k + \gamma_k \mathbf{Z} \quad \text{for } k = 1,\ldots,K.
\tag{9}
$$

This model is a simplification of a more general one that includes an interaction between each $\mathbf{X}_k$ and $\mathbf{Z}$. Our simplified model makes the standard regression assumption that the variance–covariance matrix of $(\mathbf{Y}, \mathbf{X}_1, \mathbf{X}_2, \ldots, \mathbf{X}_K)$ is conditioned on $\mathbf{Z}$, but does not depend explicitly on $\mathbf{Z}$, e.g., is not a function of $\mathbf{Z}$. To implement the GEE approach we modify $\mathbf{X}_i$ and β as

$$
\mathbf{X}_i = \begin{pmatrix}
1 & X_{i1} & Z_i & 0 & 0 & 0 & \cdots & 0 & 0 & 0 \\
0 & 0 & 0 & 1 & X_{i2} & Z_i & \cdots & 0 & 0 & 0 \\
\vdots & & & & & & & & & \\
0 & 0 & 0 & 0 & 0 & 0 & \cdots & 1 & X_{iK} & Z_i
\end{pmatrix}
$$

$$
\beta = (\alpha_1, \beta_1, \gamma_1, \alpha_2, \beta_2, \gamma_2, \ldots, \alpha_K, \beta_K, \gamma_K)^T.
$$

Similar to the case without covariates, $\hat{\alpha}_k$, $\hat{\beta}_k$ and $\hat{\gamma}_k$ are estimates from a univariate regression model with response $\mathbf{Y}$, multiple informant $\mathbf{X}_k$ and covariates $\mathbf{Z}$. Using Eq. (4), we can obtain variances as in the case without covariates.

3. Maximum likelihood estimation

To use ML we assume a joint multivariate distribution for the outcome and multiple informants. For simplicity, we consider only two predictors here but the model extends straightforwardly. For each of n observations, let $\mathbf{Q}_i = (Y_i, X_{1i}, X_{2i})^T$ and thus

$$
\mathbf{Q}_i \sim MVN \left(\begin{pmatrix} \mu_Y \\ \mu_{X_1} \\ \mu_{X_2} \end{pmatrix}, \begin{pmatrix} \sigma_Y^2 & \sigma_{X_1,Y} & \sigma_{X_2,Y} \\ \sigma_{X_1,Y} & \sigma_{X_1}^2 & \sigma_{X_1,X_2} \\ \sigma_{X_2,Y} & \sigma_{X_1,X_2} & \sigma_{X_2}^2 \end{pmatrix} \right).
$$

From this distribution, we find estimates for $\theta = (\mu_Y, \mu_{X_1}, \mu_{X_2}, \sigma_Y^2, \sigma_{X_1,Y}, \sigma_{X_2,Y}, \sigma_{X_1,X_2}, \sigma_{X_1}^2, \sigma_{X_2}^2)^T$. However, we are interested in the regression parameter estimates from Eq. (1) with $K = 2$. Thus, we make a transformation from the original parameters, θ, to the parameters of interest $\tau = (\alpha_1, \beta_1, \alpha_2, \beta_2, V_{11}, V_{22}, V_{12})^T$. To make the transformation full rank, we include two parameters, μ_Y and σ_Y^2, from θ into τ. Using conditional mean formulas for the multivariate normal distribution, we find $E(\mathbf{Y}|\mathbf{X}_i) = \mu_Y + \sigma_{X_i,Y}(\mathbf{X}_i - \mu_{X_i})/\sigma_{X_i}^2$, where $i = 1, 2$. We define $\alpha_i = \mu_Y - \beta_i \mu_{X_i}$ and $\beta_i = \sigma_{X_i,Y}/\sigma_{X_i}^2$, where $i = 1, 2$ and thus Eq. (1) follows. We also define V_{11}, V_{22} and V_{12} in terms of θ by utilizing conditional variance formulas for the multivariate normal distribution, e.g., $V_{11} = \mathrm{var}(\mathbf{Y}|\mathbf{X}_1)$, $V_{22} = \mathrm{var}(\mathbf{Y}|\mathbf{X}_2)$ and $V_{12} = \mathrm{cov}(\mathbf{Y}|\mathbf{X}_1, \mathbf{Y}|\mathbf{X}_2)$.

From standard ML theory, $\hat{\theta}$ are sample means, variances and covariances with n in the denominators of the variances and covariances; we then make the full rank transformation to obtain $\hat{\tau}$ and find that the ML estimates of β are identical to the estimates found by GEE. Furthermore, using the multivariate normal model, we find $\mathrm{var}(\hat{\beta}) = \mathbf{J}\mathrm{var}(\hat{\theta})\mathbf{J}^{T}$, where $\mathbf{J}$ is the 9×9 Jacobian matrix for the transformation from θ to τ. Thus, asymptotically

$$\mathrm{var}\begin{pmatrix} \sqrt{n}\hat{\beta}_1 \\ \sqrt{n}\hat{\beta}_2 \end{pmatrix} \rightarrow \begin{pmatrix} \dfrac{\sigma_Y^2(1 - \rho_{X_1,Y}^2)}{\sigma_{X_1}^2} & \dfrac{\sigma_Y^2(1 - A)\sigma_{X_1,X_2}}{\sigma_{X_1}^2 \sigma_{X_2}^2} \\ \dfrac{\sigma_Y^2(1 - A)\sigma_{X_1,X_2}}{\sigma_{X_1}^2 \sigma_{X_2}^2} & \dfrac{\sigma_Y^2(1 - \rho_{X_2,Y}^2)}{\sigma_{X_2}^2} \end{pmatrix}, \tag{10}$$

where

$$A = 2(\rho_{X_1,Y}^2 + \rho_{X_2,Y}^2 - \rho_{X_1,Y}\rho_{X_2,Y}\rho_{X_1,X_2}) - \frac{\rho_{X_1,Y}\rho_{X_2,Y}}{\rho_{X_1,X_2}}.$$

If we estimate the asymptotic ML variance using the ML estimates of $\sigma_{X_1,Y}$, $\sigma_{X_2,Y}$, σ_{X_1,X_2}, the estimated variances of GEE and ML are the same; the estimated covariances given by GEE and ML are not identical but are quite similar in practice (results not presented).

We also consider the constrained model where $\beta_1 = \beta_2 = \beta_C$; one approach is to define

$$\sigma_{X_1,Y} = \beta_C \sigma_{X_1}^2, \sigma_{X_2,Y} = \beta_C \sigma_{X_2}^2 \tag{11}$$

and all other variance–covariance terms remain as in the unconstrained model. ML estimation assuming Eq. (11), where β_C is the common slope and no assumption is made regarding equality of the multiple informant variances, does not lead to closed form solutions. We find no obvious way to set up GEE to reproduce the model assuming Eq. (11). However, if we constrain the slopes to be equal and also assume equal multiple informant variances, we can derive the same estimates as obtained by fitting Eq. (7) using GEE when assuming

$$\sigma_{X_1,Y} = \sigma_{X_2,Y} = \sigma_{X,Y}, \sigma_{X_1}^2 = \sigma_{X_2}^2 = \sigma_X^2. \tag{12}$$

The model assuming Eq. (12) implies that $\beta_1 = \beta_2 = \beta_C$ when assuming the variances for the two covariates are equal and also implies equal correlation of each informant with the response. Similar to the unconstrained case, we define $\theta = (\mu_Y, \mu_{X_1}, \mu_{X_2}, \sigma_Y^2, \sigma_{X,Y}, \sigma_{X_1,X_2}, \sigma_X^2)^T$ and $\tau = (\alpha_1, \alpha_2, \beta_C, V_{11C}, V_{12C})^T$. Equation (7) follows directly with $\alpha_k = \mu_Y - \beta_C\mu_{X_k}$ for $k = 1, 2$ and $\beta_C = \sigma_{X,Y}/\sigma_X^2$. The ML estimates of θ under the constrained model are the same as in the unconstrained case except with $\hat{\sigma}_{X,Y} = (\Sigma_{i=1}^n(X_{i1} - \bar{X}_1)(Y_i - \bar{Y}) + \Sigma_{i=1}^n(X_{i2} - \bar{X}_2)(Y_i - \bar{Y}))/2n$ and $\hat{\sigma}_X^2 = (\Sigma_{i=1}^n(X_{i1} - \bar{X}_1)^2 + \Sigma_{i=1}^n(X_{i2} - \bar{X}_2)^2)/2n$; furthermore, we find that $\hat{\beta}_C$ is the same for GEE and ML. An expression for $\mathrm{var}(\hat{\beta}_C)$ is derived; asymptotically

$$\mathrm{var}(\sqrt{n}\hat{\beta}_C) \rightarrow \left(\frac{\sigma_Y^2(1 + \rho_{X_1,X_2})(1 - \rho_{Y|X_1,X_2}^{(C)2})}{2\sigma_X^2}\right), \tag{13}$$

where

$$\rho^{(C)^2}_{Y|X_1,X_2} = \frac{2\rho^2_{X,Y}}{1+\rho_{X_1,X_2}}.$$

Next we incorporate a vector of covariates $\mathbf{Z}$ not measured by multiple informants using the model in Eq. (9) and find the same estimates as derived by the GEE approach. We assume that

$$\mathbf{Q}_i \sim MVN\left(\begin{pmatrix}\mu_0+\mu_1\mathbf{Z}\\ \delta_0+\delta_1\mathbf{Z}\\ v_0+v_1\mathbf{Z}\end{pmatrix}, \begin{pmatrix}\sigma^2_{Y|Z} & \sigma_{X_1,Y|Z} & \sigma_{X_2,Y|Z}\\ \sigma_{X_1,Y|Z} & \sigma^2_{X_1|Z} & \sigma_{X_1,X_2|Z}\\ \sigma_{X_2,Y|Z} & \sigma_{X_1,X_2|Z} & \sigma^2_{X_2|Z}\end{pmatrix}\right),$$

and make no distributional assumptions on $\mathbf{Z}$. As done previously, we obtain mean expressions for $\mathbf{Y}$ given $(\mathbf{X}_1, \mathbf{Z})$ and $\mathbf{Y}$ given $(\mathbf{X}_2, \mathbf{Z})$ and relate these to Eq. (9). Using the results of standard multivariate normal regression theory, estimates for θ are obtained from three separate regressions. In summary, (μ_0, μ_1) are regression coefficients from fitting $E(\mathbf{Y}|\mathbf{Z})$, (δ_0, δ_1) are from $E(\mathbf{X}_1|\mathbf{Z})$ and (v_0, v_1) are from $E(\mathbf{X}_2|\mathbf{Z})$. After obtaining these estimates, we make a transformation to τ; the vector consists of the regression coefficients from Eq. (9) (β), variance–covariance terms that condition on $\mathbf{Z}$ and values from θ that ensure a full rank transformation. We find that estimates of β obtained from ML are the same as those from GEE. We calculate var($\hat{\beta}$) using the same technique as without covariates.

In this section, we have found that ML and GEE give the same estimates under an unconstrained model, assuming a constrained model with equal variances and with inclusion of covariates not measured by multiple informants. To obtain ML estimates, we have assumed multivariate normality. However, in the situations where the ML and GEE estimates are identical, ML is clearly robust to the distributional assumptions on the multiple informants.

4. Simulations

We performed 10,000 simulations to compare the empirical GEE, model-based GEE and ML variances. We generate our first dataset from the trivariate normal distribution with response $\mathbf{Y}$ and multiple informants $\mathbf{X}_1$ and $\mathbf{X}_2$ for $i = 1, \ldots, 500$. For the subsequent 9999 draws, we generate each of the 500 $\mathbf{Y}$ values from a normal distribution with mean $E(\mathbf{Y}|\mathbf{X}_1,\mathbf{X}_2)$ and variance var($\mathbf{Y}|\mathbf{X}_1,\mathbf{X}_2$); thus $\mathbf{X}_1$ and $\mathbf{X}_2$ are fixed since each iteration has the same set of 500 $\mathbf{X}_1, \mathbf{X}_2$ values. We consider four scenarios assuming different unconstrained parameters; the first case we present, $\sigma_{X_1,Y} = -0.142$, $\sigma_{X_2,Y} = -0.156$ and $\sigma_{X_1,X_2} = 0.333$, are values from the illustration described in Section 6. Table 1 gives the slope variances from the simulations using Eqs (3) and (6) for the empirical GEE and model-based GEE variances, respectively. We calculate the ML variance

Table 1
Variance simulation results – unconstrained model

$\mathrm{var}(\hat{\beta}_1)$

$\sigma_{X_1,Y}$	$\sigma_{X_2,Y}$	σ_{X_1,X_2} [a]	Empirical	Model-Based	ML	Simulation
-0.142	-0.156	0.333	0.00229	0.00229	0.00229	0.00231
0.300	0.600	0.600	0.00327	0.00324	0.00324	0.00270
0.800	0.500	0.000	0.00459	0.00459	0.00459	0.00415
0.000	0.000	0.333	0.00171	0.00172	0.00172	0.00173

$\mathrm{cov}(\hat{\beta}_1, \hat{\beta}_2)$

$\sigma_{X_1,Y}$	$\sigma_{X_2,Y}$	σ_{X_1,X_2} [a]	Empirical	Model-Based	ML	Simulation
-0.142	-0.156	0.333	0.00062	0.00061	0.00061	0.00061
0.300	0.600	0.600	0.00156	0.00161	0.00158	0.00162
0.800	0.500	0.000	0.00111	0.00032	0.00032	0.00028
0.000	0.000	0.333	0.00074	0.00074	0.00074	0.00078

[a] $\sigma_Y^2 = \sigma_{X_1}^2 = \sigma_{X_2}^2 = 1$.

using

$$\widehat{\text{var}}\begin{pmatrix} \sqrt{n}\hat{\beta}_1 \\ \sqrt{n}\hat{\beta}_2 \end{pmatrix} = \begin{pmatrix} \dfrac{\hat{\sigma}_Y^2(1 - \hat{\rho}_{X_1,Y}^2)}{\hat{\sigma}_{X_1}^2} & \dfrac{\hat{\sigma}_Y^2(1 - \hat{\rho}_{Y|X_1,X_2}^2)\hat{\sigma}_{X_1,X_2}}{\hat{\sigma}_{X_1}^2 \hat{\sigma}_{X_2}^2} \\ \dfrac{\hat{\sigma}_Y^2(1 - \hat{\rho}_{Y|X_1,X_2}^2)\hat{\sigma}_{X_1,X_2}}{\hat{\sigma}_{X_1}^2 \hat{\sigma}_{X_2}^2} & \dfrac{\hat{\sigma}_Y^2(1 - \hat{\rho}_{X_2,Y}^2)}{\hat{\sigma}_{X_2}^2} \end{pmatrix},$$

(14)

where

$$\hat{\rho}_{Y|X_1,X_2}^2 = \frac{\hat{\sigma}_{X_2}^2 \hat{\sigma}_{X_1,Y}^2 - 2\hat{\sigma}_{X_1,Y}\hat{\sigma}_{X_1,X_2} + \hat{\sigma}_{X_1}^2 \hat{\sigma}_{X_2,Y}^2}{(\hat{\sigma}_{X_1}^2 \hat{\sigma}_{X_2}^2 - \hat{\sigma}_{X_1,X_2}^2)\hat{\sigma}_Y^2}.$$

We omit $\text{var}(\hat{\beta}_2)$ since its results are similar to $\text{var}(\hat{\beta}_1)$; we also present the covariance between the slopes, $\text{cov}(\hat{\beta}_1, \hat{\beta}_2)$.

We compare the variance using each of the three methods (empirical GEE and model-based GEE and ML) to the variance of the simulations (reported in the column of Table 1 entitled Simulation) calculated as

$$\text{var}(\hat{\beta}_1) = \frac{\sum_{i=1}^{m}(\hat{\beta}_{1i} - \overline{\hat{\beta}_1})^2}{m},$$

(15)

where m is the number of simulations and $\overline{\hat{\beta}_1}$ is the average of the $\hat{\beta}_{1i}^{(1)}$ values over all simulations. We compare the covariance using a similar technique. Nonparametric 95% confidence intervals (not reported) for the empirical, model-based and ML variances illustrate that the estimated variances are similar and closely approximate the simulated variances in most cases. In general, we find that the empirical estimates are more variable than their model-based and ML counterparts. The largest difference occurred when $\sigma_{X_1,Y} = 0.8$, $\sigma_{X_2,Y} = 0.5$ and $\sigma_{X_1,X_2} = 0$, for example, the empirical covariance appears inconsistent with the simulated covariance, but its confidence interval (0.00054, 0.00174) nearly includes the simulated value. All other empirical values fell within the nonparametric confidence intervals, and hence were trivial differences. Table 2 presents results when assuming a constrained model with equal variances (Eq. (12)) under three scenarios assuming different constrained parameters. As in the unconstrained case, the estimated variances from the GEE and ML

Table 2
Variance simulation results – constrained model

$\sigma_{X_1,Y}$	$\sigma_{X_2,Y}$	σ_{X_1,X_2} [a]	var($\hat{\beta}_C$)			
			Empirical	Model-Based	ML	Simulation
−0.149	−0.149	0.333	0.00125	0.00125	0.00124	0.00123
0.400	0.400	0.600	0.00206	0.00204	0.00201	0.00198
0.500	0.500	0.000	0.00217	0.00194	0.00169	0.00173

[a] $\sigma_Y^2 = \sigma_{X_1}^2 = \sigma_{X_2}^2 = 1$.

techniques are similar and both are consistent with the true variance estimates for the constrained case.

5. Efficiency calculations

We now discuss when using a constrained model leads to efficiency gains by comparing the variances of the slope estimates under the unconstrained model and the constrained model assumed in Eq. (12) using ARE, defined as the ratio of two asymptotic variances. Specifically, ARE is the ratio of $\text{var}(\hat{\beta}_1)$ to $\text{var}(\hat{\beta}_C)$ assuming $\beta_1 = \beta_2 = \beta_C$ since $\text{var}(\hat{\beta}_1) = \text{var}(\hat{\beta}_2)$ under the constrained model. If the ARE is greater than 1, then the estimated slope variance of the constrained model is more efficient than the estimated slope of the unconstrained model; this leads to increased power for detecting associations between multiple informants and response.

Using the asymptotic ML variances derived in Section 3 and assuming $\sigma_{X_1,Y} = \sigma_{X_2,Y} = \sigma_{X,Y}$ and $\sigma_{X_1}^2 = \sigma_{X_2}^2 = \sigma_X^2$, we calculate

$$\text{ARE} = \frac{2(1 - \rho_{X,Y}^2)}{(1 + \rho_{X_1,X_2})(1 - \rho_{Y|X_1,X_2}^2)}.$$

Because $\rho_{Y|X_1,X_2}^2 \geq \rho_{X,Y}^2 \geq 0$ and $-1 \leq \rho_{X_1,X_2} \leq 1$ it follows that $\text{ARE} \geq 1$ for all values of ρ_{X_1,X_2}, $\rho_{X,Y}^2$ and $\rho_{Y|X_1,X_2}^2$. Therefore, the slope estimate under the constrained model is always as efficient or more efficient than the unconstrained estimate when the constrained model holds. We consider ARE at particular values of ρ_{X_1,X_2}; for instance, with $\rho_{X_1,X_2} = 0$, ARE increases as the difference between $\rho_{Y|X_1,X_2}^2$ and $\rho_{X,Y}^2$ increases (Fig. 1). As ρ_{X_1,X_2} increases, the general

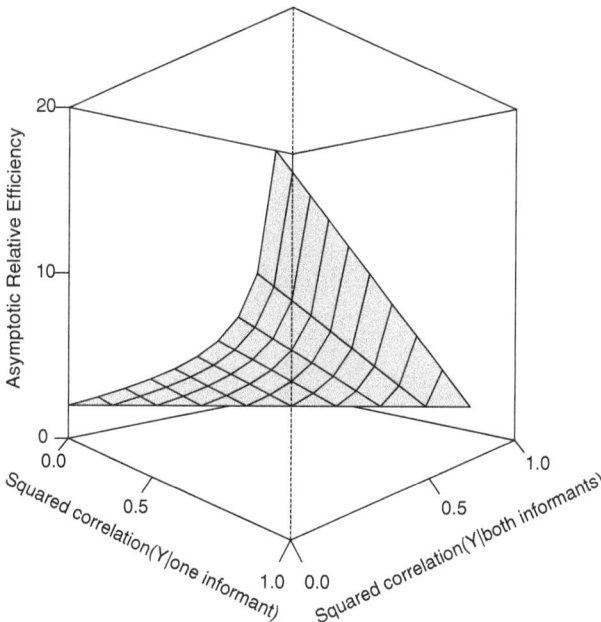

Fig. 1. Asymptotic relative efficiency ($\rho_{X_1,X_2} = 0$).

shape of the ARE function remains the same but both the minimum and maximum ARE values decrease. In summary, if the slopes are similar, fitting a constrained model offers efficiency in the slope estimate over fitting an unconstrained model.

6. Illustration

In 1996, a study investigating the association between physical activity/inactivity and obesity was performed in two towns of Mexico City (Hernández et al., 1999, 2000, Hernández, 1998). Our goal is to compare the marginal relationship between BMI (**Y**) and vigorous exercise as reported by the child (**X$_1$**) and the relationship between BMI and vigorous exercise reported by the child's mother (**X$_2$**). We also fit a constrained model for increased efficiency. Although we could control for many covariates concerning the child (age, grade, gender, school, socioeconomic status, whether or not the child was sick on the evaluation day, nutritional status and whether or not the child was obese), for illustration we include only child's grade level in school. Grade is dichotomized with elementary school children of grades 5 and 6 in one category compared with secondary school children of grades 1 and 2. Complete information is available for 82 observations.

The raw summary measures for BMI and vigorous exercise are given in Table 3. Because the vigorous exercise measurements are highly skewed and the multiple informant variances are not equal, we convert the measurements to normal scores and then mean center and standardize these in order to compare the covariance of BMI and each covariate on the same scale. Grade is also mean centered and standardized for simplicity. Table 4 provides a summary of the estimates derived from GEE or ML and their standard errors (empirical GEE, model-based GEE/ML) for models of BMI and vigorous exercise fit using R (2004).

The marginal relationship between BMI and child's report of vigorous exercise, $\hat{\beta}_1$, and the marginal relationship between BMI and mother's report, $\hat{\beta}_2$, are not statistically significantly different; furthermore, both measures have a

Table 3
Estimated means and variance–covariance matrix for vigorous exercise

Variable	Estimated Mean
BMI (**Y**)	21.382
Vigorous exercise reported by child (**X$_1$**)	0.986
Vigorous exercise reported by mother (**X$_2$**)	0.786

Σ

	Y	**X$_1$**	**X$_2$**
Y	12.108	−0.374	−0.413
X$_1$	−0.374	0.897	0.150
X$_2$	−0.413	0.150	0.455

Table 4
Parameter estimates and standard errors for models using vigorous exercise to predict BMI

$\hat{\beta}_1$	Emp/ML[a] $\widehat{se}(\hat{\beta}_1)$	$\hat{\beta}_2$	Emp/ML[a] $\widehat{se}(\hat{\beta}_2)$	$\hat{\gamma}_1$	Emp/ML[a] $\widehat{se}(\hat{\gamma}_1)$	$\hat{\gamma}_2$	Emp/ML[a] $\widehat{se}(\hat{\gamma}_2)$
-0.511	0.341/0.380	-0.561	0.345/0.379				
-0.536[b]	0.249/0.308[b]						
-0.377	0.360/0.381	-0.514	0.353/0.372	-0.673	0.401/0.381	-0.714	0.369/0.372
-0.447[b]	0.264/0.305[b]			-0.659	0.384/0.378	-0.718	0.373/0.371

[a] Empirical GEE standard error/ML standard error.
[b] Constrained slope estimate.

Table 5
−2 log likelihood values

Model	−2 log(Likelihood)
Unconstrained model	437.856
Constrained model	437.869
Unconstrained model with covariate	431.437
Constrained model with covariate	431.572

negative relationship with BMI and neither are statistically significant predictors of BMI. Thus, we fit a constrained model to gain efficiency (although physical activity is still not statistically significantly related to BMI); the constrained slope coefficient is −0.536, indicating that for every one unit increase in vigorous exercise a child receives, BMI decreases by over one half of a unit. In addition, fitting a constrained slope is more efficient than fitting two separate slopes ($\widehat{ARE} = 1.51$); the estimated variance of the constrained slope is approximately 50% smaller than when fitting an unconstrained model and provides more power to assess the association between vigorous exercise and BMI. We report −2 log (likelihood) values to compare models by constructing likelihood ratio tests (LRTs) in Table 5; according to a one degree of freedom LRT, fitting a constrained model as compared with the unconstrained model is appropriate. We also include grade in the models; according to a two degree of freedom LRT, adding grade is reasonable (p-value = 0.04). We also find that fitting a model where we constrain the slope to be equal in the presence of grade is appropriate according to a one degree of freedom LRT. Therefore, the relationship between vigorous exercise and BMI is similar regardless of respondent. Fitting a constrained model is simpler and more efficient; adding the covariate increases the predictive power. With regard to design issues, using either mother or child responses should yield similar results. Including both would increase power, although may not be feasible.

7. Conclusion

In this paper, we review a nonstandard application of GEE (Horton et al., 1999, Pepe et al., 1999) and introduce a novel ML method for modeling marginal regression models with multiple source predictors. ML and GEE yield the same estimates of the regression coefficients in the following situations: (1) unconstrained model, (2) constrained model with the multiple informants having equal variances (assuming Eq. (12)) and (3) including covariates not measured by multiple informants (assuming covariates have possibly different slopes). The model-based GEE and ML variances are similar; in practice, the covariances are as well. Our work also demonstrates that, at least in simple cases, the working correlation matrix recommended by Pepe et al. (1999) is optimal. The GEE empirical variance yields similar variance and covariance estimates as the model-based GEE and ML estimates, but the GEE empirical variance quantities are more variable than the former.

Throughout this paper, our goal has been to estimate the marginal relationship of each multiple informant covariate with response; we have presented two approaches to do so. Alternative techniques include use of latent variable or measurement error models; in both cases, the problem could be construed as each of the multiple informants being an imprecise surrogate for the true value (Horton and Fitzmaurice, 2004). However, when comparing diagnostic tests in practice researchers are interested in the actual reports and how they compare.

The ML technique can be extended to include more than two sets of multiple informants. For example, the Hernández et al. (1999) study had additional multiple informant measures including video viewing, moderate exercise and video-game playing. To implement ML in this setting, two equations with sets of regression slope coefficients for each additional multiple informant measure are necessary. This provides estimates of each multiple informant measure conditional on the other multiple informant measures in the model. If we take the case of two sets of multiple informants with $\mathbf{X}_{ij}$, where $i =$ set, $j =$ multiple informant, instead of using $E(\mathbf{Y}|\mathbf{X}_1)$ and $E(\mathbf{Y}|\mathbf{X}_2)$ to find the transformation from θ to τ, $E(\mathbf{Y}|\mathbf{X}_{11},\mathbf{X}_{21})$ and $\mathrm{E}(\mathbf{Y}|\mathbf{X}_{12},\mathbf{X}_{22})$ is used. Aside from the proliferation of parameters, solutions should extend from the existing methods.

Another extension is dealing with one construct measured with more than two multiple informants $(K>2)$. In this situation, K separate regression equations are fit rather than 2. This may lead to estimation of a large number of parameters and a Jacobian matrix for the transformation from θ to τ of high dimension; e.g., with $K = 3$, θ consists of 14 parameters. The models can also be extended to include a vector of covariates not measured by multiple informants. Rather than predicting $\mathbf{Y}$, $\mathbf{X}_1$, $\mathbf{X}_2$ from $\mathbf{Z}$ using an intercept and a slope, the model would be a multiple linear regression with an intercept and K slopes. Using a potentially cumbersome transformation from θ to τ, the $2(K+1)$ regression parameters are found as previously described. While extending the ML technique leads to additional parameters, ML can accommodate constrained models where the slope parameters are equal. In addition to providing efficiency gains, constraining coefficients also helps maintain parsimonious models.

Considering the advantages and disadvantages of using GEE and ML for analysis of multiple informants as predictors, GEE is more flexible than ML since it does not require a model for the multiple informants nor does it need normality of the multiple informants or the dependent variable. However, because ML and GEE yield the same solutions in most situations, ML does not require the multivariate normality assumption to be valid. In fact, the vigorous activity multiple informant measurements in the Hernández et al. (1999) dataset were skewed to the left; although we standardized this data, an analysis without standardization reveals that ML is still equivalent to GEE, thus confirming the robustness of ML to deviations from normality. A drawback of the GEE approach is that the independence working correlation structure must be assumed for the model to be valid (Pepe and Anderson, 1994). However, we have shown that the use of the independence working correlation matrix is optimal for certain models when assuming normality where the GEE and ML approaches yield identical estimates and standard errors.

An advantage of ML is the ability to fit a broader range of models than what can be fit using GEE; for example, ML can fit a model when a constrained effect is desired but the variance differs across levels of X_1 and X_2 (e.g. with large amounts of missing data on the multiple informants). Another positive aspect of the ML approach is that likelihood-based tests can be constructed to easily compare models; this is particularly helpful when considering many models. Perhaps the biggest advantage ML can offer is an efficiency gain compared with GEE when considering data with missingness (Litman et al., 2007).

Acknowledgement

We are grateful for the support provided by the National Institute of Mental Health (NIMH) grant number MH54693 and National Institute of Health (NIH) grant number T32-MH017119.

References

Field, A.E., Laird, N.M., Steinberg, E., Fallon, E., Semega-Janneh, M., Yanovski, J.A. (2003). Which metric of relative weight best captures body fatness in children? *Obesity Research* **11**, 1345–1352.

Fitzmaurice, G.M., Laird, N.M., Zahner, G.E.P. (1996). Multivariate logistic models for incomplete binary responses. *Journal of the American Statistical Association* **91**(433), 99–108.

Fitzmaurice, G.M., Laird, N.M., Zahner, G.E.P., Daskalakis, C. (1995). Bivariate logistic regression analysis of child psychopathology ratings using multiple informants. *American Journal of Epidemiology* **142**(11), 1194–1203.

Goldwasser, M.A., Fitzmaurice, G.M. (2001). Multivariate linear regression of childhood psychopathology using multiple informant data. *International Journal of Methods in Psychiatric Research* **20**, 1–11.

Gould, M.S., Fisher, P., Parides, M., Flory, M., Shaffer, D. (1996). Psychosocial risk factors of child and adolescent completed suicide. *Archives of General Psychiatry* **53**, 1155–1162.

Hernández, B. (1998). *Diet, physical activity and obesity in Mexican children*. PhD thesis. Harvard School of Public Health, Boston, MA, USA.

Hernández, B., Gortmaker, S.L., Colditz, G.A., Peterson, K.E., Laird, N.M., Parra-Cabrera, S. (1999). Association of obesity with physical activity, television programs and other forms of video viewing among children in Mexico City. *International Journal of Obesity* **23**, 845–854.

Hernández, B., Gortmaker, S.L., Laird, N.M., Colditz, G.A., Parra-Cabrera, S., Peterson, K.E. (2000). Validity and reproducibility of a physical activity and inactivity questionnaire for Mexico City's schoolchildren. *Salud Publica de Mexico* **42**(4), 315–323.

Horton, N.J., Fitzmaurice, G.M. (2004). Tutorial in biostatistics: Regression analysis of multiple source and multiple informant data from complex survey samples. *Statistics in Medicine* **23**(18), 2911–2933.

Horton, N.J., Laird, N.M., Murphy, J.M., Monson, R.R., Sobol, A.M., Leighton, A.H. (2001). Multiple informants: Mortality associated with psychiatric disorders in the Stirling County Study. *American Journal of Epidemiology* **154**(7), 649–656.

Horton, N.J., Laird, N.M., Zahner, G.E.P. (1999). Use of multiple informant data as a predictor in psychiatric epidemiology. *International Journal of Methods in Psychiatric Research* **8**, 6–18.

Huber, P.J. (1967). The behaviour of maximum likelihood estimators under non-standard conditions. In: LeCam, L.M., Neyman, J. (Eds.),**Vol. 1** *Proceedings of the Fifth Berkeley Symposium on Mathematical Statistics and Probability*. University of California Press, pp. 221–233.

Kuo, M., Mohler, B., Raudenbush, S.L., Earls, F.J. (2000). Assessing exposure to violence using multiple informants: Application of hierarchical linear models. *Journal of Child Psychology and Psychiatry and Allied Disciplines* **41**, 1049–1056.

Liang, K., Zeger, S.L. (1986). Longitudinal data analysis using generalized linear models. *Biometrika* **73**(1), 13–22.

Litman, H.J., Horton, N.J., Hernández, B., Laird, N.M. (2007). Incorporating missingness for estimation of marginal regression models with multiple source predictors. *Statistics in Medicine* **26**, 1055–1068.

O'Brien, L.M., Fitzmaurice, G.M., Horton, N.J. (2006). Maximum likelihood estimation of marginal pairwise associations with multiple source predictors. *Biometrical Journal* **48**(5), 860–875.

Offord, D.R., Boyle, M.H., Racine, Y., Szatmari, P., Fleming, J.E., Sanford, M., Lipman, E.L. (1996). Integrating assessment data from multiple informants. *Journal of the American Academy of Child and Adolescent Psychiatry* **35**(8), 1078–1085.

Pepe, M.S., Anderson, G.L. (1994). A cautionary note on inference for marginal regression models with longitudinal data and general correlated response data. *Communications in Statistics* **23**(4), 939–951.

Pepe, M.S., Whitaker, R.C., Seidel, K. (1999). Estimating and comparing univariate associations with application to the prediction of adult obesity. *Statistics in Medicine* **18**, 163–173.

R Development Core Team (2004). *R: A language and environment for statistical computing.* R Foundation for Statistical Computing, Vienna, Austria.

Zeger, S.L., Liang, K. (1986). Longitudinal data analysis for discrete and continuous outcomes. *Biometrics* **42**, 121–130.

Handbook of Statistics, Vol. 27
ISSN: 0169-7161
DOI: 10.1016/S0169-7161(07)27027-0

11

The Bayesian Approach to Experimental Data Analysis

Bruno Lecoutre

Abstract

This chapter introduces the conceptual basis of the objective Bayesian approach to experimental data analysis and reviews some of its methodological improvements. The presentation is essentially non-technical and, within this perspective, restricted to relatively simple situations of inference about proportions. Bayesian computations and softwares are also briefly reviewed and some further topics are introduced.

> It is their straightforward, natural approach to inference that makes them [Bayesian methods] so attractive.
>
> (Schmitt, 1969, preface)

Preamble: and if you were a Bayesian without knowing it?

In a popular statistical textbook that claims the goal of "understanding statistics," Pagano (1990, p. 288) describes a 95% confidence interval as

> an interval such that the probability is 0.95 that the interval contains the population value.

If you agree with this statement, or if you feel that it is not the correct interpretation but that it is desirable, you should ask yourselves: "and if I was a Bayesian without knowing it?"

The *correct* frequentist interpretation of a 95% confidence interval involves a long-run repetition of the same experiment: in the long run 95% of computed confidence intervals will contain the "true value" of the parameter; each interval in isolation has either a 0 or 100% probability of containing it. Unfortunately, treating the data as random *even after observation* is so strange that this "correct" interpretation does not make sense for most users. Actually, virtually all users interpret frequentist confidence intervals in terms of "a *fixed* interval having a 95% chance of including the true value of interest."

In the same way, many statistical users misinterpret the p-values of null hypothesis significance tests as "inverse" probabilities: $1 - p$ is "the probability that the alternative hypothesis is true." Even experienced users and experts in statistics (Neyman himself) are not immune from *conceptual* confusions.

> In these conditions [a p-value of $1/15$], the odds of 14 to 1 that this loss was caused by seeding [of clouds] do not appear negligible to us. (Battan et al., 1969)

After many attempts to rectify these (Bayesian) interpretations of frequentist procedures, I completely agree with Freeman (1993, p. 1446) that in these attempts "we are fighting a losing battle."

> It would not be scientifically sound to justify a procedure by frequentist arguments and to interpret it in Bayesian terms. (Rouanet, 2000b, p. 54)

We then naturally have to ask ourselves whether the "Bayesian choice" will not, sooner or later, be unavoidable (Lecoutre et al., 2001).

1. Introduction

Efron (1998, p. 106) wrote

> A widely accepted objective Bayes theory, which fiducial inference was intended to be, would be of immense theoretical and practical importance. A successful objective Bayes theory would have to provide good frequentist properties in familiar situations, for instance, reasonable coverage probabilities for whatever replaces confidence intervals.

I suggest that such a theory is by no means a speculative viewpoint but, on the contrary, is perfectly feasible (see especially, Berger, 2004). It is better suited to the needs of users than frequentist approach and provides scientists with relevant answers to essential questions raised by experimental data analysis.

1.1. What is Bayesian inference for experimental data analysis?

One of the most important objective of controlled clinical trials is to impact on public health, so that their results need to be accepted by a large community of scientists and physicians. For this purpose, null hypothesis significance testing (NHST) has been long conventionally required in most scientific publications for analyzing experimental data. This publication practice dichotomizes each experimental result (significant vs. non-significant) according to the NHST outcome.

But scientists cannot in this way find all the answers to the precise questions posed in experimental investigations, especially in terms of effect size evaluation.

> But the primary aim of a scientific experiment is not to precipitate decisions, but to make an appropriate adjustment in the degree to which one accepts, or believes, the hypothesis or hypotheses being tested. (Rozeboom, 1960)

By their insistence on the decision-theoretic elements of the Bayesian approach, many authors have obscured the contribution of Bayesian inference to experimental data analysis and scientific reporting. Within this context, many Bayesians place emphasis on a *subjective* perspective. This can be the reasons why until now scientists have been reluctant to use Bayesian inferential procedures in practice for analyzing their data. It is not surprising that the most common (and easy) criticism of the Bayesian approach by frequentists is the need for prior probabilities. Without dismissing the merits of the decision-theoretic viewpoint, it must be recognized that there is another approach that is just as Bayesian, which was developed by Jeffreys in 1930s (Jeffreys, 1961/1939). Following the lead of Laplace (1986/1825), this approach aimed at assigning the prior probability when nothing was known about the value of the parameter. In practice, these *non-informative* prior probabilities are vague distributions that, a priori, do not favor any particular value. Consequently, they let the data "speak for themselves" (Box and Tiao, 1973, p. 2). In this form, the Bayesian paradigm provides, if not objective methods, at least *reference* methods appropriate for situations involving scientific reporting. This approach of Bayesian inference is now recognized as a standard.

> A common misconception is that Bayesian analysis is a subjective theory; this is neither true historically nor in practice. The first Bayesians, Bayes (see Bayes (1763)) and Laplace (see Laplace (1812)) performed Bayesian analysis using a constant prior distribution for unknown parameters ... (Berger, 2004, p. 3)

1.2. Routine Bayesian methods for experimental data analysis

For more than 30 years now, with other colleagues in France we have worked in order to develop routine Bayesian methods for the most familiar situations encountered in experimental data analysis. These methods can be learned and used as easily, if not more, as the t, F or χ^2 tests. We argued that they offer promising new ways in statistical methodology (Rouanet et al., 2000).

We have especially developed methods based on non-informative priors. In order to promote them, it seemed important to us to give them a more explicit name than "standard," "non-informative" or "reference." Recently, Berger (2004) proposed the name *objective Bayesian analysis*.

> The statistics profession, in general, hurts itself by not using attractive names for its methodologies, and we should start systematically accepting the 'objective Bayes' name before it is co-opted by others. (Berger, 2004, p. 3)

With the same incentive, we argued for the name *fiducial Bayesian* (Lecoutre, 2000; Lecoutre et al., 2001). This deliberately provocative name pays tribute to Fisher's work on scientific inference for research workers (Fisher, 1990/1925). It indicates their specificity and their aim to let the statistical analysis express *what the data have to say* independently of any outside information.

An objective (or fiducial) Bayesian analysis has a privileged status in order to gain public use statements. However, this does not preclude using other Bayesian techniques when appropriate.

1.3. The aim of this chapter

The aim of this chapter is to introduce the conceptual basis of objective Bayesian analysis and to illustrate some of its methodological improvements. The presentation will be essentially non-technical and, within this perspective, restricted to simple situations of inference about proportions. A similar presentation for inferences about means in the analysis of variance framework is available elsewhere (Lecoutre, 2006a).

The chapter is divided into four sections. (1) I briefly discuss the frequentist and Bayesian approaches to statistical inference and show the difficulties of the frequentist conception. I conclude that the Bayesian approach is highly desirable, if not unavoidable. (2) Its feasibility is illustrated in detail from a simple illustrative example of inference about a proportion in a clinical trial; basic Bayesian procedures are contrasted with usual frequentist techniques and their advantages are outlined. (3) Other examples of inferences about proportions serve me to show that these basic Bayesian procedures can be straightforward extended to deal with more complex situations. (4) The concluding remarks summarize the main advantages of the Bayesian methodology for experimental data analysis. Bayesian computations and softwares are also briefly reviewed. At last, some further topics are introduced.

The reader interested in more advanced aspects of Bayesian inference, with an emphasis on modeling and computation, is especially referred to the Volume 25 of this series (Dey and Rao, 2005).

2. Frequentist and Bayesian inference

2.1. Two conceptions of probabilities

Nowadays, probability has at least two main definitions (Jaynes, 2003). (1) Probability is the long-run frequency of occurrence of an event, either in a sequence of repeated trials or in an ensemble of "identically" prepared systems. This is the "frequentist" conception of probability, which seems to make probability an observable ("objective") property, existing in the nature independently of us, that should be based on empirical frequencies. (2) Probability is a measure of the degree of belief (or confidence) in the occurrence of an event or in a proposition. This is the "Bayesian" conception of probability.

This dualistic conception was already present in Bernoulli (1713), who clearly recognized the distinction between probability ("degree of certainty") and frequency, deriving the relationship between probability of occurrence in a single trial and frequency of occurrence in a large number of independent trials.

Assigning a frequentist probability to a single-case event is often not obvious, since it requires imagining a reference set of events or a series of repeated experiments in order to get empirical frequencies. Unfortunately, such sets are seldom available for assignment of probabilities in real problems. By contrast, the Bayesian definition is more general: it is not conceptually problematic to assign a probability to a unique event (Savage, 1954; de Finetti, 1974).

> It is beyond any reasonable doubt that for most people, probabilities about single events do make sense even though this sense may be naive and fall short from numerical accuracy. (Rouanet, 2000a, p. 26)

The Bayesian definition fits the meaning of the term probability in everyday language, and so the Bayesian probability theory appears to be much more closely related to how people intuitively reason in the presence of uncertainty.

2.2. Two approaches to statistical inference

The frequentist approach to statistical inference is self-proclaimed *objective* contrary to the Bayesian conception that should be necessary *subjective*. However, the Bayesian definition can clearly serve to describe "objective knowledge," in particular based on symmetry arguments or on frequency data. So Bayesian statistical inference is no less objective than frequentist inference. It is even the contrary in many contexts.

Statistical inference is typically concerned with both known quantities – the observed data – and unknown quantities – the parameters and the data that have not been observed. In the frequentist inference, all probabilities are conditional on parameters that are assumed known. This leads in particular to

- significance tests, where the parameter value of at least one parameter is fixed by hypothesis;
- confidence intervals.

In the Bayesian inference, parameters can also be probabilized. This results in distributions of probabilities that express our uncertainty:

- before observations (they do not depend on data): *prior* probabilities;
- after observations (conditional on data): *posterior* (or *revised*) probabilities;
- about future data: *predictive* probabilities.

As a simple illustration let us consider a finite population of size 20 with a dichotomous variable success/failure and a proportion φ (the *unknown parameter*) of success. A sample of size 5 has been observed, hence these *known data:*

$$0 \quad 0 \quad 0 \quad 1 \quad 0 \qquad f = 1/5$$

The inductive reasoning is fundamentally a generalization from a known quantity (here the data $f = 1/5$) to an unknown quantity (here the parameter φ).

2.3. The frequentist approach: from unknown to known

In the frequentist framework, we have no probabilities and consequently no possible inference. The situation must be reversed, but we have no more probabilities ... unless we fix a parameter value. Let us assume, for instance, $\varphi = 0.75$.

Then we get sampling probabilities $\Pr(f|\varphi = 0.75)$ – that is frequencies – involving *imaginary repetitions* of the observations. They can be obtained by simulating repeated drawing of samples of 5 marbles (without replacement) from a box that contains 15 black and 5 white marbles. Alternatively, they can be (exactly) computed from a hypergeometric distribution. These sampling probabilities serve to define a null hypothesis significance test. If the null hypothesis is true ($\varphi = 0.75$), one find in 99.5% of the repetitions a value $f > 1/5$ (the proportion of black marbles in the sample), greater than the observation in hand: the null hypothesis $\varphi = 0.75$ is rejected ("significant test": $p = 0.005$). Note that I do not enter here in the one-sided/two-sided test discussion, which is irrelevant for my purpose.

However, this conclusion is based on the probability of the samples *that have not been observed*, what Jeffreys (1961, Section 7.2) ironically expressed in the following terms:

> If P is small, that means that there have been unexpectedly large departures from prediction. But why should these be stated in terms of P? The latter gives the probability of departures, measured in a particular way, equal to or greater than the observed set, and the contribution from the actual value is nearly always negligible. What the use of P implies, therefore, is that a hypothesis that may be true may be rejected because it has not predicted observable results that have not occurred. This seems a remarkable procedure.

As another example of null hypothesis, let us assume $\varphi = 0.50$. In this case, if the null hypothesis is true ($\varphi = 0.50$), one find in 84.8% of the repetitions a value $f > 1/5$, greater than the observation: the null hypothesis $\varphi = 0.50$ is not rejected by the data in hand. Obviously, *this does not prove that $\varphi = 0.50$!*

Now a frequentist confidence interval can be constructed as the set of possible parameter values that are not rejected by the data. Given the data in hand we get the following 95% confidence interval: [0.05, 0.60]. How to interpret the confidence 95%? The frequentist interpretation is based on the universal statement:

> whatever the fixed value of the parameter is, in 95% (at least) of the repetitions the interval that should be computed includes this value.

But this interpretation is very strange since *it does not involve the data in hand*! It is at least unrealistic, as outlined by Fisher (1990/1973, p. 71):

> Objection has sometimes been made that the method of calculating Confidence Limits by setting an assigned value such as 1% on the frequency of observing 3 or less (or at the other end of observing 3 or more) is unrealistic in treating the values less than 3, which have not been observed, in exactly the same manner as the value 3, which is the one that has been observed. This feature is indeed not very defensible save as an approximation.

2.4. The Bayesian approach: from known to unknown

> As long as we are uncertain about values of parameters, we will fall into the
> Bayesian camp. (Iversen, 2000)

Let us return to the inductive reasoning, starting from the known data, and adopting a Bayesian viewpoint. We can now use, in addition to sampling probabilities, probabilities that express our uncertainty about all possible values of the parameter. In the Bayesian inference, we consider, not the frequentist probabilities of imaginary samples but the frequentist probabilities of *the observed data* $\Pr(f = 1/5|\varphi)$ for all possible values of the parameter. This is the *likelihood* function that is denoted by

$$\ell(\varphi|\text{data}).$$

We assume prior probabilities $\Pr(\varphi)$ before observations. Then, by a simple product, we get the joint probabilities of the parameter values and the data:

$$\Pr\left(\varphi \text{ and } f = \frac{1}{5}\right) = \Pr\left(f = \frac{1}{5}\middle|\varphi\right) \times \Pr(\varphi) = \ell(\varphi|\text{data}) \times \Pr(\varphi).$$

The sum of the joint probabilities gives the marginal predictive probability of the data, before observation:

$$\Pr\left(f = \frac{1}{5}\right) = \sum_{\varphi} \Pr\left(\varphi \text{ and } f = \frac{1}{5}\right).$$

The result is very intuitive since the predictive probability is a weighted average of the likelihood function, the weights being the prior probabilities.

Finally, we compute the posterior probabilities after observation, by application of the definition of conditional probabilities. The posterior distribution (given by Bayes' theorem) is simply the normalized product of the prior and the likelihood:

$$\Pr\left(\varphi\middle|f = \frac{1}{5}\right) \propto \ell(\varphi|\text{data}) \times \Pr(\varphi) = \frac{\Pr(\varphi \text{ and } f = 1/5)}{\Pr(f = 1/5)}.$$

2.5. The desirability of the Bayesian alternative

We can conclude with Berry (1997):

> Bayesian statistics is difficult in the sense that thinking is difficult.

In fact, it is the frequentist approach that involves considerable difficulties due to the mysterious and unrealistic use of the sampling distribution for justifying null hypothesis significance tests and confidence intervals. As a consequence, even experts in statistics are not immune from *conceptual* confusions about frequentist confidence intervals.

For instance, in a methodological paper, Rosnow and Rosenthal (1996, p. 336) take the example of an observed difference between two means $d = +0.266$. They consider the interval [0, +0.532] whose bounds are the "null hypothesis" (0) and what they call the "counternull value" ($2d = +0.532$), computed as the symmetrical value of 0 with regard to d. They interpret this specific interval [0, +0.532] as "a 77% confidence interval" ($0.77 = 1 - 2 \times 0.115$, where 0.115 is the one-sided p-value for the usual t-test). If we repeat the experience, the counternull value and the p-value will be different, and, in a long-run repetition, the proportion of null–counternull intervals that contain the true value of the difference δ will not be 77%. Clearly, 0.77 is here a *data-dependent* probability, which needs a Bayesian approach to be correctly interpreted. Such difficulties are not encountered with the Bayesian inference: the posterior distribution, being conditional on data, only involves the sampling probability of the data *in hand*, via the likelihood function $\ell(\varphi|\text{data})$ that writes the sampling distribution in the *natural order:* "from unknown to known."

Moreover, since most people use "inverse probability" statements to interpret NHST and confidence intervals, the Bayesian definition of probability, conditional probabilities and Bayes' formula are already – at least implicitly – involved in the use of frequentist methods. Which is simply required by the Bayesian approach is a very natural shift of emphasis about these concepts, showing that they can be used consistently and appropriately in statistical analysis. This makes this approach highly desirable, if not unavoidable.

With the Bayesian inference, intuitive justifications and interpretations of procedures can be given. Moreover, an empirical understanding of probability concepts is gained by applying Bayesian procedures, especially with the help of computer programs.

2.6. Training strategy

The reality of the current use of statistical inference in experimental research cannot be ignored. On the one hand, experimental publications are full of significance tests and students and researchers are (and will be again in the future) constantly confronted to their use. My opinion is that NHST is an inadequate method for experimental data analysis (which has been denounced by the most eminent and most experienced scientists), not because it is an incorrect normative model, just because it does not address the questions that scientific research requires (Lecoutre et al., 2003; Lecoutre, 2006a, 2006b). However, NHST is such an integral part of experimental teaching and scientists' behavior that its misuses and abuses should not be discontinued by flinging it out of the window.

On the one hand, confidence intervals could quickly become a compulsory norm in experimental publications. On the other hand, for many reasons due to their frequentist conception, confidence intervals can hardly be viewed as the ultimate method. In practice, two probabilities can be routinely associated with a specific interval estimate computed from a particular sample.

- The first probability is "the proportion of repeated intervals that contain the parameter." It is usually termed the coverage probability.
- The second probability is the Bayesian "posterior probability that this interval contains the parameter," assuming a non-informative prior distribution.

In the frequentist approach, it is forbidden to use the second probability. On the contrary, in the Bayesian approach, the two probabilities are valid. Moreover, an objective Bayes interval is often "a great frequentist procedure" (Berger, 2004).

As a consequence, it is a challenge for statistical instructors to introduce Bayesian inference without discarding either NHST or the "official guidelines" that tend to supplant it by confidence intervals. I argue that the sole effective strategy is *a smooth transition towards the Bayesian paradigm* (Lecoutre et al., 2001).

The suggested training strategy is to introduce Bayesian methods as follows: (1) to present natural *Bayesian interpretations* of NHST outcomes to call attention about their shortcomings. (2) To create as a result of this the need for *a change of emphasis in the presentation and interpretation* of results. (3) Finally, to equip users with a real possibility of *thinking sensibly about statistical inference* problems and behaving in a more reasonable manner.

3. An illustrative example

My first example of application will concern the inference about a proportion in a clinical trial (Lecoutre et al., 1995). The patients under study were post-myocardial infarction patients, treated with a low-molecular-weight heparin as a prophylaxis of an intra-cardial left ventricular thrombosis. Because of the limited knowledge available on drug potential efficacy, the trial aimed at abandoning further development as early as possible if the drug was likely to be not effective, and at estimating its efficacy if it turned out to be promising. It was considered that 0.85 was the success rate (no thrombosis) above which the drug would be attractive, and that 0.70 was the success rate below which the drug would be of no interest.

The trial was initially designed within the traditional Neyman–Pearson framework. Considering the null hypothesis H_0: $\varphi = 0.70$, the investigators planned a one-sided fixed sample Binomial test with specified respective Type I and Type II error probabilities $\alpha = 0.05$ and $\beta = 0.20$, hence a power $1-\beta = 0.80$ at the alternative H_a: $\varphi = 0.85$ (the hypothesis that they wish to accept!). The associated sample size was $n = 59$, for which the Binomial test rejects H_0 at level 0.05 if the observed number of success a is greater than 47. Indeed, for a sample of size n, the probability of observing a successes is given by the Binomial distribution

$$a|\varphi \sim \text{Bin}(\varphi, n),$$

$$\Pr(a|\varphi) = \binom{n}{a} \varphi^a (1 - \varphi)^{n-a},$$

hence the likelihood function

$$\ell(\varphi|\text{data}) \sim \varphi^a (1 - \varphi)^{n-a}.$$

For $n = 59$ (which can be found by successive iterations), we get:

$$\Pr(a > 47|H_0 : \varphi = 0.70) = 0.035 < 0.05 \ (\alpha)$$
$$\Pr(a > 47|H_a : \varphi = 0.85) = 0.834 > 0.80 \ (1 - \beta).$$

Note that, due to the discreteness of the distribution, the actual Type I error rate and the actual power differ from α and $1 - \beta$.

Since it would be preferable to stop the experiment as early as possible if the drug was likely to be ineffective, the investigators planned an interim analysis after 20 patients have been included. Since the traditional Neyman–Pearson framework requires specification of all possibilities in advance, they designed a stochastically curtailed test. Stochastic curtailment suggests that an experiment be stopped at an interim stage when the available information determines the outcome of the experiment with high probability under either H_0 or H_a. The notations are summarized in Table 1.

3.1. Stochastically curtailed testing and conditional power

Stochastically curtailed testing uses the "conditional power" at interim analysis, which is defined as the probability, given φ and the available data, that the test rejects H_0 at the planned termination. At interim analysis, termination occurs to reject H_0 if the conditional power at the null hypothesis value is high, say greater than 0.80. In our example, even if after 20 observations 20 successes have been observed, we do not stop the trial.

Similarly, early termination may be allowed to accept H_0 if the conditional power at the alternative hypothesis value is weak, say smaller than 0.20. For instance, if 12 successes have been observed after 20 observations this rule suggests stopping and accepting the null hypothesis. A criticism addressed to this procedure is that there seems little point in considering a prediction that is based on hypotheses that may be no longer fairly plausible given the available data. In fact, the procedure ignores the knowledge about the parameter accumulated by the time of the interim analysis.

3.2. An hybrid solution: the predictive power

Many authors have advocated calculating the "predictive power," averaging conditional power over values of the parameter in a Bayesian calculation. We are led to a Bayesian approach, but still with a frequentist test in mind. Formally, the prediction uses the posterior distribution of φ given a prior and the data available

Table 1
Summary of the notations for the inference about a proportion

	Number of Successes	Number of Errors	Sample Size
Current data at interim stage	a_1	$n_1 - a_1$	$n_1 = 20$
Future data	a_2	$n_2 - a_2$	$n_1 = 39$
Complete data	$a = a_1 + a_2$	$n - a$	$n = 59$

at the interim analysis. For the inference about a proportion, the calculations are particularly simple if we choose a conjugate Beta prior distribution

$$\varphi \sim \text{Beta}(a_0, b_0),$$

with density

$$p(\varphi) = \frac{1}{\text{B}(a_0, b_0)} \varphi^{a_0 - 1} (1 - \varphi)^{b_0 - 1}.$$

The advantage is that the posterior is also a Beta distribution (hence the name conjugate), with density

$$p(\varphi|\text{data}) \propto \ell(\varphi|\text{data}) \times p(\varphi) \propto \varphi^{a_0 + a - 1}(1 - \varphi)^{b_0 + b - 1}.$$

The prior weights a_0 and b_0 are added to the observed counts a_1 and b_1, so that at the interim analysis

$$\varphi|\text{data} \sim \varphi|a_1 \sim \text{Beta}(a_1 + a_0, b_1 + b_0).$$

The predictive distribution, which is a mixture of Binomial distributions, is naturally called a Beta–Binomial distribution

$$a_2|a_1 \sim \text{Beta} - \text{Bin}(a_1 + a_0, b_1 + b_0; n_2).$$

A vague or *non-informative* prior is generally considered. It is typically defined by small weights a_0 and b_0, included between 0 and 1. Here, I have retained a Beta prior with parameters 0 and 1

$$\varphi \sim \text{Beta}(0, 1).$$

This choice is consistent with the test procedure. I shall address this issue in greater detail later on.

In the example above with $n_1 = 20$ and $a_1 = 20$, the predictive probability of rejecting H_0 at the planned termination ($n = 59$) explicitly takes into account the available data (no failure has been observed). It is with no surprise largely greater than the probability conditional on the null hypothesis value

$$\Pr(a > 47|a_1 = 20) = \Pr(a_2 > 27|a_1 = 20) = 0.997 > 0.80,$$

hence the decision to stop and reject H_0.

This predictive probability is a weighted average of the probabilities conditional to φ, the weights being given by the posterior distribution

$$\Pr(a > 47|a_1 = 20 \text{ and } \varphi) = \Pr(a_2 > 27|a_1 = 20 \text{ and } \varphi),$$

some examples of which being

φ	$\longmapsto$	$\Pr(a > 47|a_1 = 20 \text{ and } \varphi)$
1		1
0.95		0.9999997
0.85		0.990
0.70		0.482

Since the predictive power approach is a hybrid one, it is most unsatisfactory. In particular, it does not give us direct Bayesian information about φ. The trouble is that a decision (to accept H_0 or to accept H_a) is taken at the final analysis (or eventually at an interim analysis), even if the observed proportion falls in the no-decision region [0.70, 0.85], in which case *nothing has been proved.*

What the investigators need is to evaluate at any stage of the experiment the probability of some specified regions of interest and the ability of a future sample to support and corroborate findings already obtained. The Bayesian analysis addresses these issues.

3.3. The Bayesian solution

Bayesian methodology enables the probabilities of the pre-specified regions of interest to be obtained. Such statements give straight answers to the question of effect sizes and have no frequentist counterpart. Consider the following example of Bayesian interim analysis, with 10 observed successes ($n_1 = 20$ and $a_1 = 10$).

3.3.1. Evaluating the probability of specified regions

Let us assume the Jeffreys prior Beta(1/2, 1/2) – hence the posterior Beta(10.5, 10.5) shown in Fig. 1 – that will give the privileged non-informative solution (I shall also address this issue later on).

In this case it is very likely that the drug is ineffective ($\varphi < 0.70$), as indicated by the following statements

$$\Pr(\varphi < 0.70|a_1 = 10) = 0.971$$
$$\Pr(0.70 < \varphi < 0.85|a_1 = 10) = 0.029 \quad \Pr(\varphi > 0.85|a_1 = 10) = 0.0001.$$

Note that in this case, the Bayesian inference about φ at the interim analysis does not explicitly integrate the stopping rule (which is nevertheless taken into account in the predictive probability). In the frequentist framework, the interim inferences are usually modified according to the stopping rule. This issue – that could appear as an area of disagreement between the frequentist and Bayesian approaches – will be considered later on. Resorting to computers solves the technical problems involved in the use of Bayesian distributions. This gives the users an attractive and intuitive way of understanding the impact of sample sizes,

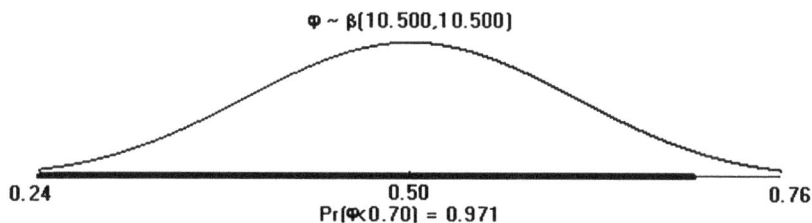

$\varphi \sim \beta(10.500, 10.500)$

| 0.24 | 0.50 | 0.76 |

Pr(φ<0.70) = 0.971

Fig. 1. Example of interim analysis ($n_1 = 20$ and $a_1 = 10$). Density of the posterior distribution Beta(10.5, 10.5) associated with the prior Beta(1/2, 1/2).

320   B. Lecoutre

data and prior distributions. The posterior distribution can be investigated by means of visual display.

3.3.2. Evaluating the ability of a future sample to corroborate the available results

As a summary to help in the decision whether to continue or to terminate the trial, it is useful to assess the predictive probability of confirming the conclusion of ineffectiveness. If a guarantee of at least 0.95 for the final conclusion is wanted, that is $\Pr(\varphi<0.70|a)>0.95$, the total number of successes a must be less than 36 out of 59. Since $a_1 = 10$ successes have been obtained, we must compute the predictive probability of observing $0\leq a_2\leq25$ successes in the future data. Here, given the current data, there is about 87% chance that the conclusion of ineffectiveness will be confirmed. Table 2 gives a summary of the analyses for the previous example and for another example more favorable to the new drug.

3.3.3. Determining the sample size

Predictive procedures are also useful tools to help in the choice of the sample size. Suppose that in order to plan a trial to demonstrate the effectiveness of the drug, we have realized a pilot study: for instance, with $n_0 = 10$ patients, we have observed zero failure. In this case, the posterior probability from the pilot experiment (starting with the Jeffreys prior) is used as prior distribution. Here, for this prior, $\Pr(\varphi>0.85) = 0.932$. If the preliminary data of the pilot study are integrated in the analysis ("full Bayesian" approach), the procedure is exactly the same as that of the interim analysis. However, in most experimental devices, the preliminary data are not included, and the analysis is conducted using a non-informative prior, here Beta(1/2, 1/2).

The procedure remains analogous: we compute the predictive probability that in the future sample of size n (not in the whole data), the conclusion of

Table 2
Summary of the Bayesian interim analyses

Prior Distribution Beta(1/2, 1/2)	
Example 1: $n_1 = 20$ and $a_1 = 10$	
Inference about φ	Predictive probability ($n = 59$)
Posterior probability	Conclusion with guarantee ≥ 0.95
$\Pr(\varphi<0.70|a_1 = 10)$	$\varphi<0.70$
0.971	0.873 ($a<36$)
$\Pr(\varphi<0.85|a_1 = 10)$	$\varphi<0.85$
0.9999	0.9998 ($a<46$)
Example 2: $n_1 = 20$ and $a_1 = 18$	
Inference about φ	Predictive probability ($n = 59$)
Posterior probability	Conclusion with guarantee ≥ 0.95
$\Pr(\varphi<0.70|a_1 = 10)$	$\varphi >0.70$
0.982	0.939 ($a>46$)
$\Pr(\varphi<0.85|a_1 = 10)$	$\varphi>0.85$
0.717	0.301 ($a>54$)

effectiveness ($\varphi > 0.85$) will be reached with a given guarantee γ. Hence, for instance, the following predictive probabilities for $\gamma = 0.95$

$$n = 20 \mapsto 0.582 \ (a > 19) \quad n = 30 \mapsto 0.696 \ (a > 28)$$
$$n = 40 \mapsto 0.744 \ (a > 37) \quad n = 50 \mapsto 0.770 \ (a > 46)$$
$$n = 60 \mapsto 0.787 \ (a > 55) \quad n = 70 \mapsto 0.696 \ (a > 64)$$
$$n = 71 \mapsto 0.795 \ (a > 65) \quad n = 72 \mapsto 0.829 \ (a > 65).$$

Values within parentheses indicate those values of a that satisfy the condition

$$\Pr(\varphi > 0.85 | a) \geq 0.95.$$

Based on the preliminary data, there are 80% chances to demonstrate effectiveness with a sample size about 70. Note that it is not surprising that the probabilities can be non-increasing: this results in the discreteness of the variable (it is the same for power).

3.4. A comment about the choice of the prior distribution: Bayesian procedures are no more arbitrary than frequentist ones

Many potential users of Bayesian methods continue to think that they are too subjective to be scientifically acceptable. However, frequentist methods are full of more or less ad hoc conventions. Thus, the p-value is traditionally based on the samples that are "more extreme" than the observed data (under the null hypothesis). But, for discrete data, it depends on whether the observed data are included or not in the critical region. So, for the usual Binomial one-tailed test for the null hypothesis, $\varphi = \varphi_0$ against the alternative $\varphi > \varphi_0$, this test is *conservative*, but if the observed data are excluded, it becomes *liberal*. A typical solution to overcome this problem consists in considering a mid-p-value, but it has only ad hoc justifications.

In our example, suppose that 47 successes are observed at the final analysis ($n = 59$ and $a = 47$), that is the value above which the Binomial test rejects $H_0 : \varphi = 0.70$. The p-value can then be computed according to the three following possibilities:

(1) $p_{\text{inc}} = \Pr(a \geq 47 | H_0 : \varphi = 0.70) = 0.066$ ["including" solution]
  $\Rightarrow H_0$ is not rejected at level $\alpha = 0.05$ (conservative test)
(2) $p_{\text{exc}} = \Pr(a > 47 | H_0 : \varphi = 0.70) = 0.035$ ["excluding" solution]
  $\Rightarrow H_0$ is rejected at level $\alpha = 0.05$ (liberal test)
(3) $p_{\text{mid}} = 1/2(p_{\text{inc}} + p_{\text{exc}}) = 0.051$ [mid-p-value]

Obviously, in this case the choice of a non-informative prior distribution cannot avoid conventions. But the particular choice of such a prior is an exact counterpart of the arbitrariness involved within the frequentist approach. For Binomial sampling, different non-informative priors have been proposed (for a discussion, see, e.g., Lee, 2004, pp. 79–81). In fact, there exist two extreme non-informative priors that are, respectively, the most unfavorable and the most favorable priors with respect to the null hypothesis. They are respectively the

Beta distribution of parameters 1 and 0 and the Beta distribution of parameters 0 and 1. These priors lead to the Bayesian interpretation of the Binomial test: the observed significance levels of the inclusive and exclusive conventions are exactly the posterior Bayesian probabilities that φ is greater than φ_0, respectively, associated with these two extreme priors. Note that these two priors constitute an a priori "ignorance zone" (Bernard, 1996), which is related to the notion of imprecise probability (see Walley, 1996).

(1) $\Pr(\varphi < 0.70 | a = 47) = 0.066 = p_{\text{inc}}$
    for the prior $\varphi \sim \text{Beta}(0, 1)$ (the most favorable to H_0)
    hence the posterior $\varphi | a \sim \text{Beta}(47, 13)$
(2) $\Pr(\varphi < 0.70 | a = 47) = 0.035 = p_{\text{exc}}$
    for the prior $\varphi \sim \text{Beta}(1, 0)$ (the most unfavorable to H_0)
    hence the posterior $\varphi | a \sim \text{Beta}(48, 12)$
(3) $\Pr(\varphi < 0.70 | a = 47) = 0.049 \approx p_{\text{mid}}$
    for the prior $\varphi \sim \text{Beta}(1/2, 1/2)$
    hence the posterior $\varphi | a \sim \text{Beta}(47.5, 12.5)$

Then the usual criticism of frequentists towards the divergence of Bayesians with respect to the choice of a non-informative prior can be easily reversed. Furthermore, the Jeffreys prior, which is very naturally the intermediate Beta distribution of parameters 1/2 and 1/2, gives a posterior probability, fully justified, close to the observed mid-p-value. The Bayesian response should not be to underestimate the impact of the choice of a particular non-informative prior, as it is often done,

> In fact, the [different non informative priors] do not differ enough to make much difference with even a fairly small amount of data. (Lee, 2004, p. 81)

but on the contrary to assume it.

3.5. Bayesian credible intervals and frequentist coverage probabilities

In other situations, where there is no particular value of interest for the proportion, we may consider an interval (or more generally a region) estimate for φ. In the Bayesian framework, such an interval is usually termed a *credible interval* (or *credibility interval*), which explicitly accounts for the difference in interpretation with the frequentist confidence interval.

3.5.1. Equal-tails intervals
Table 3 gives 95% equal-tails credible intervals for the following two examples, assuming different non-informative priors.

The prior Beta(1, 0), which gives the largest limits, has the following frequentist properties: the proportion of samples for which the upper limit is less than φ is smaller than $\alpha/2$ and the proportion of samples for which the lower limit is more than φ is larger than $\alpha/2$. The prior Beta(0, 1), which gives the smallest

Table 3
Example of 95% credible intervals assuming different non-informative priors

Beta(0, 1)	Beta(1, 1)	Beta(1/2, 1/2)	Beta(0, 0)	Beta(1, 0)
$n_1 = 20$, $a_1 = 19$				
[0.7513, 0.9877]	[0.7618, 0.9883]	[0.7892, 0.9946]	[0.8235, 0.9987]	[0.8316, 0.9987]
$n_1 = 59$, $a_1 = 32$				
[0.4075, 0.6570]	[0.4161, 0.6633]	[0.4158, 0.6649]	[0.4240, 0.6728]	[0.4240, 0.6728]

limits, has the reverse properties. Consequently, simultaneously considering the limits of these two intervals protects the user both from erroneous acceptation and rejection of hypotheses about φ. This is undoubtedly an objective Bayesian analysis. If a single limit is wanted for summarizing and reporting results, these properties lead to retain the *intermediate* symmetrical prior Beta(1/2, 1/2) (which is the Jeffreys prior). Actually, the Jeffreys credible interval has remarkable frequentist properties. Its coverage probability is very close to the nominal level, even for small-size samples, and it can be favorably compared to most frequentist intervals (Brown et al., 2001; Agresti and Min, 2005).

> We revisit the problem of interval estimation of a Binomial proportion ... We begin by showing that the chaotic coverage properties of the Wald interval are far more persistent than is appreciated ... We recommend the Wilson interval or the equal-tailed Jeffreys prior interval for small n. (Brown et al., 2001, p. 101)

Note that similar results are obtained for *negative*-Binomial (or *Pascal*) sampling, in which we observe the number of patients n until a *fixed number of successes a* is obtained. In this case, the observed significance levels of the inclusive and exclusive conventions are exactly the posterior Bayesian probabilities associated with the two respective priors Beta(0, 0) and Beta(0, 1). This suggests privileging the intermediate Beta distribution of parameters 0 and 1/2, which is precisely the Jeffreys prior. This result concerns an important issue related to the "likelihood principle." I shall address it in greater detail further on.

3.5.2. Highest posterior density intervals
A frequently recommended alternative approach is to consider the *highest posterior density* (HPD) credible interval. For such an interval, which can be in fact an union of disjoint intervals (if the distribution is not unimodal), every point included has higher probability density than every point excluded. The aim is to get the shortest possible interval. However, except for a symmetric distribution, each of the two one-sided probabilities is different from $\alpha/2$. This property is generally undesirable in experimental data analysis, since more questions are "one-sided" as in the present example.

Moreover, such an interval is not invariant under transformation (except for a linear transformation), which can be considered with Agresti and Min (2005,

p. 3) as "a fatal disadvantage." So, for the data $n = 59$, $a = 32$ and the prior Beta(1/2, 1/2), we get the HPD intervals

$$[0.4167, 0.6658] \text{ for } \varphi \text{ and } [0.7481, 2.1594] \text{ for } \frac{\varphi}{1 - \varphi},$$

with the one-sided probabilities

$$\Pr(\varphi < 0.4167) = 0.026 \text{ and } \Pr\left(\frac{\varphi}{1 - \varphi} < 0.7481\right) = 0.039,$$

$$\Pr(\varphi < 0.6658) = 0.024 \text{ and } \Pr\left(\frac{\varphi}{1 - \varphi} < 2.1594\right) = 0.011.$$

It must be emphasized, from this example, that the posterior distribution of $\varphi/(1-\varphi)$ is easily obtained: it is a Fisher–Snedecor F distribution. We find the 95% equal-tails interval [0.712, 1.984].

3.6. The contribution of informative priors

When an objective Bayesian analysis suggests a given conclusion, various prior distributions expressing results from other experiments or subjective opinions from specific, well-informed individuals ("experts"), whether *skeptical* or *convinced* (*enthusiastic*), can be investigated to assess the robustness of conclusions (see, in particular, Spiegelhalter et al., 1994).

The elicitation of a prior distribution from the opinions of "experts" in the field can be useful in some studies, but it must be emphasized that this needs appropriate techniques (see for an example in clinical trials Tan et al., 2003) and should be used with caution. The following examples are provided to understand how the Bayesian inference combines information, and are not intended to correspond to a realistic situation (in the current situation, no good prior information was available). I leave the reader the task to appreciate the potential contribution of these methods.

3.6.1. Skeptical and convinced priors

Consider again the example of data $n = 59$, $a = 32$, for which the objective Bayesian procedure concludes to inefficiency ($\varphi < 0.70$). For the purpose of illustration, let us assume the two priors, a priori, respectively, very skeptical and very convinced about the drug:

$$\varphi \sim \text{Beta}(20, 80) \quad \text{with mean } 0.200 \quad \text{for which } \Pr(\varphi < 0.70) \approx 1,$$
$$\varphi \sim \text{Beta}(98, 2) \quad \text{with mean } 0.980 \quad \text{for which } \Pr(\varphi > 0.85) = 0.999998.$$

The respective posteriors are

$$\varphi \sim \text{Beta}(52, 107) \quad \text{with mean } 0.327 \quad \text{for which } \Pr(\varphi < 0.70) \approx 1,$$
$$\varphi \sim \text{Beta}(130, 29) \quad \text{with mean } 0.818 \quad \text{for which } \Pr(\varphi > 0.85) = 0.143.$$

Of course the first prior reinforces the conclusion of inefficiency. Figure 2 shows this prior density (thick line) and the posterior (medium line), which can be

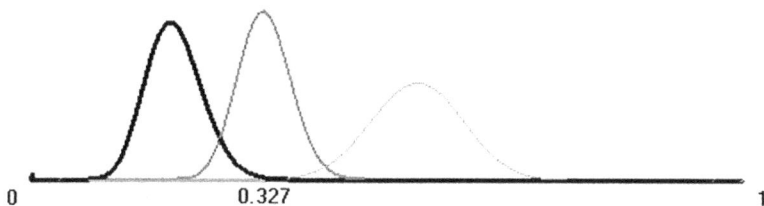

Fig. 2. Example of skeptical prior for the data $n = 59$ and $a = 32$. Densities of the prior Beta(20, 80) (thick line) and of the posterior distributions associated with this prior (medium line) and with the prior Beta(1/2, 1/2) (thin line).

compared to the objective posterior for the prior Beta(1/2, 1/2) (thin line). However, for the planned sample size, this prior opinion does not have any chance of being infirmed by the data. Even if 59 successes and 0 error had been observed, one would have $\Pr(\varphi < 0.70) | a = 59) = 0.99999995$.

The second prior allows a clearly less unfavorable conclusion. However, the efficiency of the drug cannot be asserted:

$$\Pr(\varphi > 0.70 | a = 32) = 0.997 \quad \text{but} \quad \Pr(\varphi > 0.85 | a = 32) = 0.143.$$

It is enlightening to examine the impact of the prior Beta(a_0, b_0) on the posterior mean. Letting $n_0 = a_0 + b_0$, the ratios $n_0/(n_0 + n)$ and $n/(n_0 + n)$ represent the relative weights of the prior and of the data. The posterior mean can be written

$$\frac{a_0 + a}{n_0 + n} = \frac{n_0}{n_0 + n}\frac{a_0}{n_0} + \frac{n}{n_0 + n}\frac{a}{n},$$

and is consequently equal to

prior relative weight $\times$ prior mean $+$ data relative weight $\times$ observed mean.

The posterior means are as follows:

$$100/159 \times 0.200 + 59/159 \times 0.542 = 0.327 \text{ for the prior } \varphi \sim \text{Beta}(20, 80),$$

$$100/159 \times 0.980 + 59/159 \times 0.542 = 0.818 \text{ for the prior } \varphi \sim \text{Beta}(98, 2).$$

3.6.2. Mixtures of Beta densities

A technique that remains simple to manage is to use a prior with a density defined as a mixture of prior densities of Beta distributions. The posterior is again such a mixture. This prior has two main interests, on the one hand to approximate any arbitrary complex prior that otherwise would need numerical integration methods, and on the other hand to combine several pieces of information (or different opinions). As an illustration, let us consider for the same data a mixture of the two previous distributions with equal weights, that is

$$\varphi \sim \frac{1}{2}\text{Beta}(20, 80) \oplus \frac{1}{2}\text{Beta}(98, 2),$$

where ⊕ refers to a mixture of densities, that is symbolically written

$$p(\varphi) = \frac{1}{2}p(\text{Beta}(20, 80)) + \frac{1}{2}p(\text{Beta}(98, 2)).$$

Note that this distribution must not be confounded with the distribution of the linear combination of two variables with independent Beta distributions (that would have a much more complex density).

Figure 3 shows the prior density (thick line), which is bimodal, the corresponding posterior (medium line) and the Jeffreys posterior (thin line). In fact, in this case, the data $n = 59$, $a = 32$ allow us, in some sense, to discriminate between the two distributions of the mixture, as the posterior distribution is

$$0.999999903\text{Beta}(52, 107) \oplus 0.000000097\text{Beta}(130, 29),$$

so that it is virtually confounded with the distribution Beta(52, 107) associated with the prior Beta(20, 80).

It is enlightening to note that the weight associated with each Beta distribution of the posterior mixture is proportional to the product of the prior weight times the predictive probability of the data associated with the corresponding Beta prior.

If the number of patients is multiplied by 10, with the same proportion of successes ($n = 590$, $a = 320$), the posterior density, shown in Fig. 4, is virtually confounded with the posterior Beta(340, 350) associated with the prior Beta(20, 80). Of course, it is closer to the Jeffreys solution.

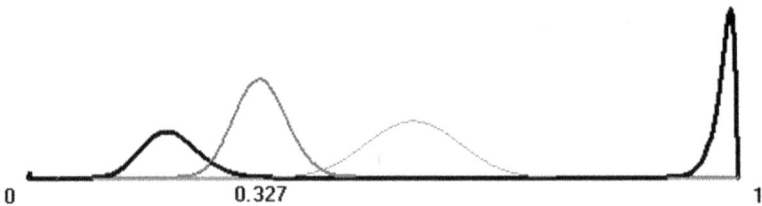

Fig. 3. Example of mixture prior for the data $n = 59$ and $a = 32$. Densities of the bimodal prior (1/2)Beta(20, 80)⊕(1/2)Beta(98, 2) (thick line) and of the posterior distributions associated with this prior (medium line) and with the prior Beta(1/2, 1/2) (thin line).

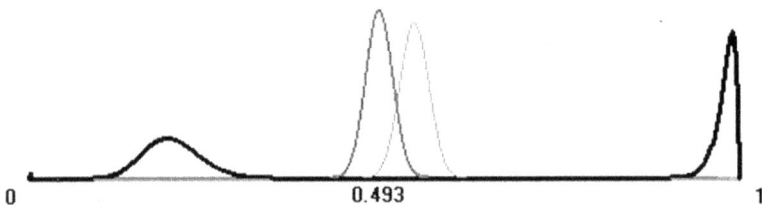

Fig. 4. Example of mixture prior for the data $n = 590$ and $a = 320$. Densities of the bimodal prior (1/2)Beta(20, 80)⊕(1/2)Beta(98, 2) (thick line) and of the posterior distributions associated with this prior (medium line) and with the prior Beta(1/2, 1/2) (thin line).

3.7. The Bayes factor

In order to complete the presentation of the Bayesian tools, I shall present the *Bayes factor*. Consider again the example of data $n = 59$, $a = 32$, with the convinced prior $\varphi \sim \text{Beta}(98, 2)$ and the corresponding a priori probabilities $\Pr(\varphi > 0.85) = 0.99999810$ (that will be denoted π_a), and consequently $\Pr(\varphi < 0.85) = 0.00000190$ (π_0). The notations π_0 and π_a are usual, since the Bayes factor is generally presented as a Bayesian approach to classical hypothesis testing; in this framework, π_0 and π_a are the respective prior probabilities of the null H_0 and alternative H_a hypotheses.

It is then quite natural to consider:

• the ratio of these two prior probabilities, hence

$$\frac{\pi_0}{\pi_a} = \frac{\Pr(\varphi < 0.85)}{\Pr(\varphi > 0.85)} = 0.0000019,$$

which here is of course very small,
• and their posterior ratio, hence

$$\frac{p_0}{p_a} = \frac{\Pr(\varphi < 0.85 | a = 32)}{\Pr(\varphi > 0.85 | a = 32)} = \frac{0.8570}{0.1430} = 5.99,$$

which is now distinctly larger than 1.

The Bayes factor (associated with the observation a) is then defined as the ratio of these two ratios

$$B(a) = \frac{p_0/p_a}{\pi_0/\pi_a} = \frac{p_0 \pi_a}{p_a \pi_0} = 3154986,$$

which evaluates the modification of the relative likelihood of the null hypothesis due to the observation. However, the Bayes factor is only an incomplete summary, which cannot replace the information given by the posterior probabilities.

The Bayes factor applies in the same way to non-complementary hypotheses H_0 and H_a, for instance, here $\varphi < 0.70$ and $\varphi > 0.85$. However, in this case the interpretation is again more problematic, since the "no-decision" region $0.70 < \varphi < 0.85$ is ignored.

In the particular case of two simple hypotheses H_0: $\varphi = \varphi_0$ and H_a: $\varphi = \varphi_a$, the Bayes factor is simply the classical *likelihood ratio*

$$B(a) = \frac{p(\varphi_0 | a) p(\varphi_a)}{p(\varphi_a | a) p(\varphi_0)} = \frac{p(a | \varphi_0)}{p(a | \varphi_a)},$$

since $p(\varphi_0 | a) \propto p(a | \varphi_0) p(\varphi_0)$ and $p(\varphi_a | a) \propto p(a | \varphi_a) p(\varphi_a)$.

Note again that when H_0 and H_a are complementary hypotheses (hence $p_a = 1 - p_0$), as in the example above, their posterior probabilities can be computed from the prior probabilities ($\pi_a = 1-\pi_0$) and the Bayes ratio. Indeed, it can be easily verified that

$$\frac{1}{p_0} = 1 + \frac{1 - \pi_0}{\pi_0} \frac{1}{B(a)}.$$

4. Other examples of inferences about proportions

4.1. Comparison of two independent proportions

Conceptually, all the Bayesian procedures for a proportion can be easily extended to two Binomial independent samples, assuming two independent priors (see Lecoutre et al., 1995). In order to illustrate the conceptual simplicity and the flexibility of Bayesian inference, I give in the subsequent subsection an application of these procedures for a different sampling model.

4.2. Comparison of two proportions for the play-the-winner rule

From ethical point of view, adaptative designs can be desirable. In such designs subjects are assumed to arrive sequentially and they are assigned to a treatment with a probability that is updated as a function of the previous events. The intent is to favor the "most effective treatment" given available information. The *play-the-winner* allocation rule is designed for two treatments t^1 and t^2 with a dichotomous (e.g., success/failure) outcome (Zelen, 1969). It involves an "all-or-none" process: if subject $k-1$ is assigned to treatment t (t^1 or t^2) and if the outcome is a success (with probability φ_t), subject k is assigned to the same treatment; if, on the contrary, the outcome is a failure (with probability $1-\varphi_t$), subject k is assigned to the other treatment.

For simplicity, it is assumed here that the outcome of subject $k-1$ is known when subject k is included.

For a fixed number n of subjects, the sequel of treatment allocations ($t_1, t_2,\ldots,$ $t_k, t_{k+1}, \ldots, t_{n+1}$) contains all the information in the data. Indeed, $t_k = t_{k+1}$ implies that a success to t_k has been observed and $t_k \neq t_{k+1}$ implies that a failure to t_k has been observed. Moreover, the likelihood function is simply

$$\ell(\varphi_1, \varphi_2)|(t_1,\ldots,t_{n+1}) = \frac{1}{2}\varphi_1^{n_{11}}(1 - \varphi_1)^{n_{10}}\varphi_2^{n_{21}}(1 - \varphi_2)^{n_{20}},$$

where n_{ij} is the number of pairs (t_k, t_{k+1}) equal to (t^i, t^j), so that n_{11} and n_{21} are the respective numbers of success to treatments t^1 and t^2, and n_{10} and n_{20} are the numbers of failure (1/2 is the probability of t_1).

Since Bayesian methods only involve the likelihood function, they are immediately available. Moreover, since the likelihood function is identical (up to a multiplicative constant) with the likelihood function associated with the comparison of two independent binomial proportions, the same Bayesian procedures apply here, even if the sampling probabilities are very different. On the contrary, with the frequentist approach, specific procedures must be developed. Due to the complexity of the sampling distribution, only asymptotic solutions are easily available. Of course, except for large samples, they are not satisfactory.

4.2.1. Numerical example

Let us consider for illustration the results of a trial with $n = 150$ subjects. The observed rates of success are, respectively, 74 out of 94 attributions for treatment t^1 and 35 out of 56 attributions for treatment t^2. Note that, from the definition of the rule, the numbers of failures (here 20 and 21) can differ at most by 1. A joint probability statement is, in a way, the best summary of the posterior distribution. For instance, if we assume the Jeffreys prior, that is two independent Beta(1/2, 1/2) distributions for φ_1 and φ_2, the marginal posteriors Beta(74.5, 20.5) and Beta (35.5, 21.5) are again independent, so that a joint probability statement can be immediately obtained. We get, for instance,

$$\Pr(\varphi_1 > 0.697 \text{ and } \varphi_2 < 0.743 | \text{data}) = 0.95$$

which is deduced from $\Pr(\varphi_1 > 0.697) = \Pr(\varphi_2 > 0.743) = \sqrt{0.95} = 0.9747$, obtained as in the case of the inference about a single proportion.

It is, in a way, the best summary of the posterior distribution. However, a statement that deals with the comparison of the two treatments directly would be preferable. So we have a probability 0.984 that $\varphi_2 > \varphi_1$. Furthermore, the distribution of any derived parameter of interest can be easily obtained from the joint posterior distribution using numerical methods. We find the 95% equal-tails credible intervals:

$$[+0.013, +0.312] \text{ for } \varphi_1 - \varphi_2 [1.02, 1.62] \text{ for } \frac{\varphi_1}{\varphi_2} [1.07, 4.64] \text{ for } \frac{\varphi_1/(1-\varphi_1)}{\varphi_2/(1-\varphi_2)}.$$

For the Jeffreys prior, Bayesian methods have fairly good frequentist coverage properties for interval estimates (Lecoutre and ElQasyr, 2005).

4.2.2. The reference prior approach

For multidimensional parameter problems, the *reference prior* approach introduced by Bernardo (1979) (see also Berger and Bernardo, 1992) can constitute a successful refinement of the Jeffreys prior. This approach presupposes that we are interested in a particular derived parameter θ. It aims at finding the optimal objective prior, given that θ is the parameter of interest and the resulting prior is consequently dependent on this parameter. An objection can be raised against this approach in the context of experimental data analysis. Even when a particular parameter is privileged to summarize the findings, we are also interested in other parameters, so that joint prior and posterior distributions are generally wanted.

4.3. A generalization with three proportions: medical diagnosis

Berger (2004, p. 5) considered the following situation (Mossman and Berger, 2001; see also in a different context Zaykin et al., 2004).

Within a population for which $\varphi_0 = \mathrm{Pr}(\text{Disease } D)$, a diagnostic test results in either a Positive ($+$) or Negative ($-$) reading. Let $\varphi_1 = \mathrm{Pr}(+|\text{patient has } D)$ and ($\varphi_2 = \mathrm{Pr}(+|\text{patient does not have } D)$. [the authors notations p_i have been changed to φ_i]

By Bayes' theorem, one get the probability θ that the patient has the disease given a positive diagnostic test

$$\theta = \mathrm{Pr}(D|+) = \frac{\mathrm{Pr}(+|D)\mathrm{Pr}(D)}{\mathrm{Pr}(+|D)\mathrm{Pr}(D) + \mathrm{Pr}(+|-D)\mathrm{Pr}(-D)} = \frac{\varphi_1\varphi_0}{\varphi_1\varphi_0 + \varphi_2(1-\varphi_0)}.$$

It is assumed that for $i = 0, 1, 2$ there are available (independent) data a_i, having Binomial distributions

$$a_i|\varphi_i \sim \mathrm{Bin}(\varphi_i, n_i),$$

hence a straightforward generalization of the inference about two independent proportions. Note that, conditionally to φ_0, the situation is that of inference about the ratio of two independent Binomial proportions, since for instance

$$\mathrm{Pr}(\theta < u|\varphi_0) = \mathrm{Pr}\left(\frac{\varphi_2}{\varphi_1} > \frac{1-\varphi_0}{\varphi_0}\frac{1-u}{u}\right).$$

The marginal probability is a mixture of these conditional probabilities.

It results "a simple and easy to use procedure, routinely usable on a host of applications," which, from a frequentist perspective "has better performance [...] than any of the classically derived confidence intervals" (Berger, 2004, pp. 6–7).

Another situation that involves a different sampling model but leads to the same structure is presented in greater detail hereafter.

4.4. Logical models in a contingency table

Let us consider a group of n patients, with two sets of binary attributes, respectively, $V = \{v1, v0\}$ and $W = \{w1, w0\}$. To fix ideas, let us suppose that W is cardiac mortality (yes/no) and that V is myocardial infarction (yes/no). Let us consider the following example of logical model (Lecoutre and Charron, 2000).

An absolute (or logical) *implication* $v1 \Rightarrow w1$ (for instance) exists if all the patient having the modality v_1 also have the modality $w1$, whereas the converse is not necessarily true.

However, the hypothesis of an absolute implication (here "myocardial infarction implies cardiac mortality") is of little practical interest, since a single observation of the event ($v1$, $w0$) is sufficient to falsify it.

Consequently, we have to consider the weaker hypothesis "$v1$ implies in most cases $w0$" ($v1 \hookrightarrow w1$).

The issue is to evaluate the departure from the logical model "the cell $(v1, w0)$ should be empty." A departure index $\eta_{v1 \hookrightarrow w1}$ can be defined from the cell proportions

	$W1$	$w0$	
$v1$	φ_{11}	φ_{10}	$\varphi_{1.}$
$v0$	φ_{01}	φ_{00}	$\varphi_{0.}$
	$\varphi_{.1}$	$\varphi_{.0}$	1

as

$$\eta_{v1 \hookrightarrow w1} = 1 - \frac{\varphi_{10}}{\varphi_{1.}\varphi_{.0}} \quad (-\infty < \eta_{v1 \hookrightarrow w1} < +1).$$

This index has been actually considered in various frameworks, with different approaches. It can be viewed as a measure of *predictive efficiency* of the model when predicting the outcome of W given $v1$.

- The prediction is perfect (there is an absolute implication) when $\eta_{v1 \hookrightarrow w1} = +1$.
- The closer to 1 $\eta_{v1 \hookrightarrow w1}$ is, the more efficient the prediction.
- In case of independence, $\eta_{v1 \hookrightarrow w1} = 0$.
- A null or negative value means that the model is a prediction failure.

Consequently, in order to investigate the predictive efficiency of the model, we have to demonstrate that $\eta_{v1 \hookrightarrow w1}$ has a value close to $+1$. Of course, one can define in the same way the indexes $\eta_{v1 \hookrightarrow w0}$, $\eta_{w1 \hookrightarrow v1}$, and $\eta_{w0 \hookrightarrow v0}$ One can, again, characterize the *equivalence* between two modalities. An absolute equivalence between $v1$ and $w1$ (for instance) exists if $\eta_{v1 \hookrightarrow w1} = +1$ and $\eta_{v0 \hookrightarrow w0} = +1$ (the two cells $[v1, w0]$ and $[v0, w1]$ are empty). Consequently, the minimum of these two indexes is an index of departure from equivalence.

Let us assume a multinomial sampling model, hence for a sample of size n, the probability of observing the cell counts n_{ij}

$$\Pr(n_{11}, n_{10}, n_{01}, n_{00} | \varphi_{11}, \varphi_{10}, \varphi_{01}, \varphi_{00}) = \frac{n!}{n_{11}!n_{10}!n_{01}!n_{00}!} \varphi_{11}^{n_{11}} \varphi_{10}^{n_{10}} \varphi_{01}^{n_{01}} \varphi_{00}^{n_{00}}.$$

4.5. Frequentist solutions

Asymptotic procedures (see, e.g., Fleiss, 1981) are clearly inappropriate for small samples. Alternative procedures based on Fisher's conditional test (Copas and Loeber, 1990; Lecoutre and Charron, 2000) have been proposed. This test involves the sampling distribution of n_{11} (for instance). A classical result is that this distribution, given fixed observed margins, only depends on the cross product $\rho = \varphi_{11}\varphi_{00}/\varphi_{10}\varphi_{01}$ (Cox, 1970, p. 4). The null hypothesis $\rho = \rho_0$ can be tested against the alternative $\rho < \rho_0$ (or against $\rho > \rho_0$), by using the probability that n_{11} exceeds the observed value in the appropriate direction.

Consequently, the procedure is analogous to the Binomial test considered for the inference about a proportion. We can define in the same way an "including" solution and an "excluding" solution.

In the particular case $\rho_0 = 0$, this test is the Fisher's randomization test of the null hypothesis $\rho = 1$ (i.e., $\eta_{v1 \hookrightarrow w1} = 0$) against $\rho < 1$ ($\eta_{v1 \hookrightarrow w1} < 0$).

By inverting this conditional test, confidence intervals can be computed for the cross product ρ. An interval for $\eta_{v1 \hookrightarrow w1}$ is then deduced by replacing ρ by its confidence limits in the following expression that gives $\eta_{v1 \hookrightarrow w1}$ as a function of ρ

$$\eta_{v1 \hookrightarrow w1} = \frac{1 + (\rho - 1)(\varphi_{1.} + \varphi_{.1} - \varphi_{1.}\varphi_{.1}) - [(1 + (\varphi_{1.} + \varphi_{.1})(\rho - 1))^2 - 4\varphi_{1.}\varphi_{.1}\rho(\rho - 1)]^{1/2}}{2(\rho - 1)\varphi_{.1}(1 - \varphi_{1.})}.$$

Unfortunately, these limits depend on the true margin values $\varphi_{.1}$ and $\varphi_{1.}$. The most common procedure consists in simply replacing these *nuisance parameters* by their estimates $f_{.1}$ and $f_{1.}$. It is much more performing than asymptotic solutions, but is unsatisfactory for extreme parameter values. More efficient principles for dealing with nuisance parameters exist (for instance, Toecher, 1950; Rice, 1988). However, one comes up against a problem that is eternal within the frequentist inference, and that is of course entirely avoided in the Bayesian approach. In any case, Bayesian inference copes with the problem of nuisance parameters. Moreover, it explicitly handles the problems of discreteness and unobserved events (null counts) by way of the prior distribution.

4.6. The Bayesian solution

The Bayesian solution is a direct generalization of the Binomial case. Let us assume a joint (conjugate) *Dirichlet* prior distribution, which is a multidimensional extension of the Beta distribution

$$(\varphi_{11}, \varphi_{10}, \varphi_{01}, \varphi_{00}) \sim \text{Dirichlet}(v_{11}, v_{10}, v_{01}, v_{00}).$$

The posterior distribution is also a Dirichlet in which the prior weights are simply added to the observed cell counts.

$$(\varphi_{11}, \varphi_{10}, \varphi_{01}, \varphi_{00})|\text{data} \sim \text{Dirichlet}(n_{11} + v_{11}, n_{10} + v_{10}, n_{01} + v_{01}, n_{00} + v_{00}).$$

From the basic properties of the Dirichlet distribution (see, e.g., Bernardo and Smith, 1994, p. 135), the marginal posterior distribution for the derived parameter η_{11} can be characterized as a function of three independent Beta distributions

$$X = \varphi_{10}|\text{data} \sim \text{Beta}(n_{10} + v_{10}, n_{11} + v_{11} + n_{01} + v_{01} + n_{00} + v_{00}),$$

$$Y = \frac{\varphi_{00}}{1 - \varphi_{10}} = \frac{\varphi_{00}}{1 - X}|\text{data} \sim \text{Beta}(n_{00} + v_{00}, n_{11} + v_{11} + n_{01} + v_{01}),$$

$$Z = \frac{\varphi_{11}}{1 - \varphi_{10} - \varphi_{00}} = \frac{\varphi_{11}}{(1 - Y)(1 - X)}|\text{data} \sim \text{Beta}(n_{11} + v_{11}, n_{01} + v_{01}),$$

since

$$\eta_{v1 \hookrightarrow w1} = 1 - \frac{X}{(X + Z(1 - Y)(1 - X))(X + Y(1 - X))}$$

This leads to straightforward numerical methods.

4.7. Numerical example: mortality study

4.7.1. Non-treated patients

The data in Table 4 were obtained for 340 high-risk patients who received no medical treatment. Let us consider the implication "Myocardial infarction $\hookrightarrow$ Cardiac mortality within 2 years."

The observed values of the index are

- for the implication "Infarction $\hookrightarrow$ Decease" (cell [yes,no] empty): $H_{v1 \hookrightarrow w1} = 0.12$,
- for the implication "Decease $\hookrightarrow$ Infarction" (cell [no,yes] empty): $H_{v1 \hookrightarrow w1} = 0.37$.

The marginal proportions of decease are (fortunately!) rather small – respectively, 0.22 after infarction and 0.07 without infarction – so that the count 72 in the cell [yes,no] is proportionally large. Consequently, relatively small values of the index are here "clinically significant." Assuming the Jeffreys prior Dirichlet $(1/2, 1/2, 1/2, 1/2)$, we get the posterior

$$\Phi = (\varphi_{11}, \varphi_{10}, \varphi_{01}, \varphi_{00}) | \text{data} \sim \text{Dirichlet}(20.5, 72.5, 17.5, 231.5).$$

from which we derive the marginal posteriors. Figure 5 shows the decreasing distribution function of the posterior of $\eta_{v1 \hookrightarrow w1}$ and its associated 90% credible interval.

From the two credible intervals,

- "Infarction $\hookrightarrow$ Decease": $\Pr(+0.06 < \eta_{v1 \hookrightarrow w1} < +0.19) = 0.90$
- "Decease $\hookrightarrow$ Infarction": $\Pr(+0.20 < \eta_{w1 \hookrightarrow v1} < +0.54) = 0.90$.

Table 4
Mortality data for 340 high-risk patients who received no medical treatment

		Decease			
		Yes	No		
Myocardial infarction	Yes	20	72	92	[20/92 = 0.22]
	No	17	231	248	[17/248 = 0.07]
		37	303	340	

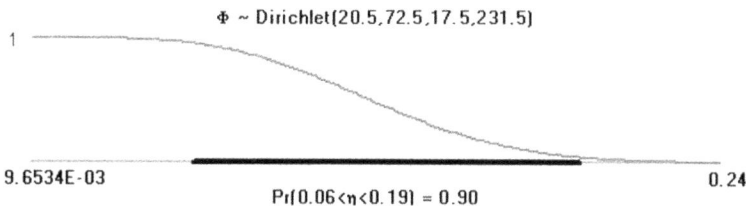

Fig. 5. Implication "Infarction $\hookrightarrow$ Decease" (non-treated patients). Decreasing distribution function for $\eta_{v1 \hookrightarrow w1}$ [$\Pr(\eta_{v1 \hookrightarrow w1} < x)$] associated with the prior Dirichlet$(1/2, 1/2, 1/2, 1/2)$.

Table 5
Mortality data for 357 high-risk patients who received a preventive treatment

| | | Decease | | | |
		Yes	No		
Myocardial infarction	Yes	1	78	79	$[1/79 = 0.01]$
	No	13	265	278	$[13/278 = 0.05]$
		14	343	357	

we can assert an implication of limited importance. In fact, it appears that decease is a better prognostic factor for infarction than the reverse.

4.7.2. Treated patients
Other data reported in Table 5 were obtained for 357 high-risk patients who received a preventive treatment.

Here, it is, of course, expected that the treatment would reduce the number of deceases after infarction. Ideally, if there was no cardiac decease among the treated patients after infarction (cell [yes,yes] empty), there would be an absolute implication "Infarction $\Rightarrow$ No decease." We get the following results for this implication:

"Infarction $\hookrightarrow$ No decease" : $H_{v1 \hookrightarrow w0} = +0.68$ and $\Pr(-0.10 < \eta_{v1 \hookrightarrow w0} < +0.94) = 0.90$.

Here, in spite of a distinctly higher observed value, it cannot be concluded to the existence of an implication. The width of the credible interval shows a poor precision. This is a consequence of the very small observed proportions of decease. Of course, it cannot be concluded that there is no implication or that the implication is small. This illustrate the abuse of interpreting the non-significant result of usual "tests of independence" (chi-square for instance) in favor of the null hypothesis.

4.8. Non-informative priors and interpretation of the observed level of Fisher's permutation tests

The Bayesian interpretation of the permutation test (conditional to margins) generalizes the interpretation of the Binomial test. For the usual one-sided test (including solution), the null hypothesis H_0: $\eta_{v1 \hookrightarrow w0} = 0$ is not rejected ($p_{inc} = 0.145$). It is well known that this test is conservative, but if we consider the excluding solution, we get a definitely smaller p-value $p_{exc} = 0.028$. This results from the poor experimental accuracy. As in the case of a single proportion, there exist two extreme non-informative priors, Dirichlet(1, 0, 0, 1) and Dirichlet(0, 1, 1, 0) that constitute the ignorance zone. They give an enlightening interpretation of these two p-values, together with an objective Bayesian analysis.

(1) $\Pr(\eta_{v1 \hookrightarrow w0} < 0) = 0.145 = p_{inc}$
    for the prior Dirichlet(1, 0, 0, 1) (the most favorable to H_0)
    hence the posterior Dirichlet(2, 78, 13, 266)

(2) $\Pr(\eta_{v1 \hookrightarrow w0} < 0) = 0.028 = p_{\text{exc}}$
   for the prior Dirichlet(0, 1, 1, 0) (the most unfavorable to H_0)
   hence the posterior Dirichlet(1, 79, 14, 265)
(3) $\Pr(\eta_{v1 \hookrightarrow w0} < 0) = 0.072 \approx (p_{\text{inc}} + p_{\text{exc}})/2 = 0.086$
   for the prior Dirichlet(1/2, 1/2, 1/2, 1/2)
   hence the posterior Dirichlet(1.5, 78.5, 13.5, 265.5)

4.8.1. The choice of a non-informative prior

As for a single proportion, the choice of a non-informative prior is no more arbitrary or subjective than the conventions of frequentist procedures. Moreover, simulation studies of frequentist coverage probabilities favorably compare Bayesian credible intervals with conditional confidence intervals (Lecoutre and Charron, 2000). For each lower and upper limits of the $1-\alpha$ credible interval, the frequentist error rates associated with the two *extreme* priors always include $\alpha/2$. Moreover, if a single limit is wanted for summarizing and reporting results, the symmetrical *intermediate* prior Dirichlet(1/2, 1/2, 1/2, 1/2) has fairly good coverage properties, including the cases of moderate sample sizes and small parameter values. Of course the differences between the different priors in the ignorance zone is less for small or medium values of $\eta_{v1 \hookrightarrow w1}$ and vanishes as the sample size increases.

4.9. Further analyses

There is no difficulty in extending the Bayesian procedures to any situation involving the multinomial sampling model, for instance, the comparison of two proportions based on paired data. Here, in particular, the distribution of the minimum of the two indexes for asserting equivalence is easily obtained by simulation. Moreover, the procedures can be extended to compare the indexes associated with two independent groups (for instance, here treated and non-treated patients).

   Of course, in all these situations, informative priors and predictive probabilities can be used in the same way as for a single proportion.

   Note again that binary and polychotomous response data can also be analyzed by Bayesian regression methods. Relevant references are Albert and Chib (1993) and Congdon (2005).

5. Concluding remarks and some further topics

Time's up to come to a positive agreement for procedures of experimental data analysis that bypass the common misuses of NHST. This agreement should fills up its role of "an aid to judgment," which "should not be confused with automatic acceptance tests, or 'decision functions'" (Fisher, 1990/1925, p. 128). Undoubtedly, there is an increasing acceptance that Bayesian inference can be ideally suited for this purpose. It fulfills the requirements of scientists: objective procedures (including traditional p-values), procedures about effect sizes (beyond p-values) and procedures for designing and monitoring experiments. Then, why scientists, and in particular experimental investigators, really appear to want a different kind of inference but seem reluctant to use Bayesian inferential procedures in practice? In a very lucid paper, Winkler (1974, p. 129) answered that "this state of affairs appears to be due to a combination of factors including philosophical conviction, tradition, statistical training, lack of 'availability', computational difficulties, reporting difficulties, and perceived resistance by journal editors." He concluded that if we leave to one side the choice of philosophical approach, none of the mentioned arguments are entirely convincing. Although Winkler's paper was written more than 30 years ago, it appears as if it had been written today.

> We [statisticians] will all be Bayesians in 2020, and then we can be a united profession. (Lindley, in Smith, 1995, p. 317)

In fact the times we are living in at the moment appear to be crucial. On the one hand, an important practical obstacle is that the standard statistical packages that are nowadays extensively used do not include Bayesian methods. On the other hand, one of the decisive factors could be the recent "draft guidance document" of the US Food and Drug Administration (FDA, 2006). This document reviews "the least burdensome way of addressing the relevant issues related to the use of Bayesian statistics in medical device clinical trials." It opens the possibility for experimental investigators to really be Bayesian in practice.

5.1. Some advantages of Bayesian inference

5.1.1. A better understanding of frequentist procedures

> Students [exposed to a Bayesian approach] come to understand the frequentist concepts of confidence intervals and P values better than do students exposed only to a frequentist approach. (Berry, 1997)

To take another illustration, let us consider the basic situation of the inference about the difference δ between two normal means. It is especially illustrative of how the Bayesian procedures combine descriptive statistics and significance tests.

Let us denote by d (assuming $d \neq 0$) the observed difference and by t the value of the Student's test statistic. Assuming the usual non-informative prior, the posterior for δ is a generalized (or scaled) t distribution (with the same degrees of freedom as the t-test), centered on d and with scale factor the ratio $e = d/t$ (see, e.g., Lecoutre, 2006a).

From this *technical* link with the t statistic, it results *conceptual* links. The one-sided p-value of the t-test is exactly the posterior Bayesian probability that the difference δ has the opposite sign of the observed difference. Given the data, if for instance $d > 0$, there is a p posterior probability of a negative difference and a $1-p$ complementary probability of a positive difference. In the Bayesian framework these statements are *statistically correct*. Another important feature is the interpretation of the usual confidence interval in natural terms. It becomes correct to say that "there is a 95% [for instance] probability of δ being included between the fixed bounds of the interval" (conditionally on the data).

In this way, Bayesian methods allow users to overcome usual difficulties encountered with the frequentist approach. In particular, using the Bayesian interpretations of significance tests and confidence intervals in the language of probabilities about unknown parameters is quite natural for the users. In return, the common misuses and abuses of NHST are more clearly understood. In particular, users of Bayesian methods become quickly alerted that non-significant results cannot be interpreted as "proof of no effect."

5.1.2. Combining information from several sources

An analysis of experimental data should always include an objective Bayesian analysis in order to express *what the data have to say* independently of any outside information. However, informative Bayesian priors also have an important role to play in experimental investigations. They may help refining inference and investigating the sensitivity of conclusions to the choice of the prior. With regard to scientists' need for objectivity, it could be argued with Dickey (1986, p. 135) that

> an objective scientific report is a report of the whole prior-to-posterior mapping of a relevant range of prior probability distributions, keyed to meaningful uncertainty interpretations.

Informative Bayesian techniques are ideally suited for *combining information* from the data in hand and from other studies, and therefore planning a series of experiments. More or less realistic and convincing uses have been proposed (for a discussion of how to introduce these techniques in medical trials, see, e.g., Irony and Pennello, 2001). Ideally, when "good prior information is available," it could (should) be used to reach the same conclusion that an "objective Bayesian analysis," but with a smaller sample size. Of course, they should integrate a real knowledge based on data rather than expert opinions, which are generally controversial. However, in my opinion, the use of these techniques must be more extensively explored before appreciating their precise contribution to experimental data analysis.

5.1.3. The predictive probabilities: a very appealing tool

> An essential aspect of the process of evaluating design strategies is the ability to calculate predictive probabilities of potential results. (Berry, 1991, p. 81)

A major strength of the Bayesian paradigm is the ease with which one can make predictions about future observations. The predictive idea is central in experimental investigations, as "the essence of science is replication: a scientist should always be concerned about what would happen if he or another scientist were to repeat his experiment" (Guttman, 1983). Bayesian predictive procedures give users a very appealing method to answer essential questions such as: "how big should be the experiment to have a reasonable chance of demonstrating a given conclusion?" "given the current data, what is the chance that the final result will be in some sense conclusive, or on the contrary inconclusive?" These questions are unconditional in that they require consideration of all possible values of parameters. Whereas traditional frequentist practice does not address these questions, predictive probabilities give them direct and natural answer.

In particular, from a pilot study, the predictive probabilities on credible limits give a useful summary to help in the choice of the sample size of an experiment (for parallels between Bayesian and frequentist methods, see Inoue et al., 2005).

The predictive approach is a very appealing method (Baum et al., 1989) to aid the decision to stop an experiment at an interim stage. On the one hand, if the predictive probability that it will be successful appears poor, it can be used as a rule to abandon the experiment for futility. On the other hand, if the predictive probability is sufficiently high, this suggests to early stop the experiment and conclude success.

Predictive probabilities are also a valuable tool for missing data imputation. Note that interim analyses are a kind of such imputation. The case of censored survival data is particularly illustrative. At the time of interim analysis, available data are divided into three categories: (1) included patients for whom the event of interest has been observed, (2) included patients definitely censored and (3) included patients under current observation for whom the maximum observation period has not ended. Consequently, the missing data to be predicted are respectively related to these last patients for which we have partial information and to the new patients planned to be included for which we have no direct information. The Bayesian approach gives us straightforward and effective ways to deal with this situation (Lecoutre et al., 2002).

It can again be outlined that the predictive distributions are also a useful tool for constructing a subjective prior, as it is often easier to express an opinion relative to expected data.

5.2. Bayesian computations and statistical packages

There is currently increasingly widespread application of Bayesian inference for experimental data analysis. However, an obstacle to the routine use of objective Bayesian methods is the lack of user-friendly general purpose software that would be a counterpart to the standard frequentist software. This obstacle may be expected to be removed in the future. Some packages have been designed to learn elementary Bayesian inference: see, for example, First Bayes (O'Hagan, 1996) and a package of Minitab macros (Albert, 1996). With a more ambitious perspective, we have developed a statistical software for Bayesian analysis of variance (Lecoutre and Poitevineau, 1992; Lecoutre, 1996). It incorporates both traditional frequentist practices (significance tests, confidence intervals) and routine Bayesian procedures (non-informative and conjugate priors). These procedures are applicable to general experimental designs (in particular, repeated measures designs), balanced or not balanced, with univariate or multivariate data, and covariables. This software also includes the basic Bayesian procedures for inference about proportions presented in this chapter.

At a more advanced level, the privileged tool for the Bayesian analysis of complex models is a method called Markov Chain Monte Carlo (MCMC). The principle of MCMC techniques (Gilks et al., 1996; Gamerman, 1997) is to simulate, and consequently approximate, the posterior and predictive distributions (when they cannot be determined analytically). This can be done for virtually any Bayesian analysis. WinBUGS (a part of the BUGS project) is an any general purpose flexible and efficient Bayesian software. It "aims to make practical MCMC methods available to applied statisticians" and largely contributes to the increasing use of Bayesian methods. It can be freely downloaded from the web site: http://www.mrc-bsu.cam.ac.uk/bugs/welcome.shtml. However, it can hardly be recommended to beginners unless they are highly motivated.

Very recently, Bayesian analysis has been added in some procedures of the SAS/STAT software. In addition to the full functionality of the original ones, the new procedures produce Bayesian modeling and inference capability in generalized linear models, accelerated life failure models, Cox regression models, and piecewise constant baseline hazard models (SAS Institute Inc., 2006).

5.3. Some further topics

I do not intend to give here an exhaustive selection of topics, but rather to simply outline some areas of research that seems to me particularly important for the methodological development of objective Bayesian analysis for experimental data.

5.3.1. The interplay of frequentist and Bayesian inference

Bayarri and Berger (2004) gave an interesting view of the interplay of frequentist and Bayesian inference. They argued that the traditional frequentist argument, involving "repetitions of the same problem with different data" is not what is done in practice. Consequently, it is "a joint frequentist–Bayesian principle" that is practically relevant: a given procedure (for instance, a 95% confidence interval for a normal mean) is in practice used "on a series of different problems involving a series of different normal means with a corresponding series of data" (p. 60). More generally, they reviewed current issues in the Bayesian–frequentist synthesis from a methodological perspective. It seems a reasonable conclusion to hope a methodological unification, but not a philosophical unification.

> Philosophical unification of the Bayesian and frequentist positions is not likely, nor desirable, since each illuminates a different aspect of statistical inference. We can hope, however, that we will eventually have a general methodological unification, with both Bayesians and frequentists agreeing on a body of standard statistical procedures for general use. (Bayarri and Berger, 2004, p. 78)

In this perspective, an active area of research aims at finding "probability matching priors" for which the posterior probabilities of certain specified sets are equal (at least approximately) to their coverage probabilities: see Fraser et al. (2003) and Sweeting (2005).

5.3.2. Exchangeability and hierarchical models

Roughly speaking, random events are *exchangeable* "if we attribute the same probability to an assertion about any given number of them" (de Finetti, 1972, p. 213). This is a key notion in statistical inference. For instance, future patients must be assumed to be exchangeable with the patients who have already been observed in order to make predictive probabilities reasonable. In the same way, similar experiments must be assumed to be exchangeable for a coherent integration of the information.

The notion of exchangeability is very important and useful in the Bayesian framework. Using multilevel prior specifications, it allows a flexible modeling of related experimental devices by means of *hierarchical models* (Bernardo, 1996).

> If a sequence of observations is judged to be exchangeable, then any subset of them must be regarded as a random sample from some model, and there exist a prior distribution on the parameter of such model, hence requiring a Bayesian approach. (Bernardo, 1996, p. 5)

Hierarchical models are important to make full use of the data from a multicenter experiment. They are also particularly suitable for meta-analysis in which we have data from a number of relevant studies that may be exchangeable on some levels but not on others (Dumouchel, 1990). In all cases, the problem can be decomposed into a series of simpler conditional models, using the hierarchical Bayesian methodology (Good, 1980).

5.3.3. The stopping rule principle: a need to rethink

Experimental designs often involve interim looks at the data for the purpose of possibly stopping the experiment before its planned termination. Most experimental investigators feel that the possibility of early stopping cannot be ignored, since it may induce a bias on the inference that must be explicitly corrected. Consequently, they regret the fact that the Bayesian methods, unlike the frequentist practice, generally ignore this specificity of the design. Bayarri and Berger (2004) considered this desideratum as an area of current disagreement between the frequentist and Bayesian approaches. This is due to the compliance of most Bayesians with the *likelihood principle* (a consequence of Bayes' theorem), which implies the *stopping rule principle* in interim analysis:

> Once the data have been obtained, the reasons for stopping experimentation should have no bearing on the evidence reported about unknown model parameters. (Bayarri and Berger, 2004, p. 81)

Would the fact that "people resist an idea so patently right" (Savage, 1954) be fatal to the claim that "they are Bayesian without knowing it?" This is not so sure, experimental investigators could well be right! They feel that the experimental design (incorporating the stopping rule) is prior to the sampling information and that *the information on the design is one part of the evidence*. It is precisely the point of view developed by de Cristofaro (1996, 2004, 2006), who persuasively argued that the correct version of Bayes' formula must integrate the parameter θ, the design d, the initial evidence (prior to designing) e_0, and the statistical information i. Consequently, it must be written in the following form:

$$p(\theta|i, e_0, d) \propto (\theta|e_0, d)p(i|\theta, e_0, d).$$

It becomes evident that the *prior depends on d*. With this formulation, both the likelihood principle and the stopping rule principle are no longer automatic consequences. It is not true that, under the same likelihood, the inference about θ is the same, irrespective of d. Note that the role of the sampling model in the derivation of the Jeffreys prior in Bernoulli sampling for the Binomial and the *Pascal* models was previously discussed by Box and Tiao (1973, pp. 45–46), who stated that the Jeffreys priors are different as the two sampling models are also different. In both cases, the resulting posterior distribution have remarkable frequentist properties (i.e., coverage probabilities of credible intervals).

This result can be extended to general stopping rules (Bunouf, 2006). The basic principle is that the design information, which is ignored in the likelihood function, *can be recovered in the Fisher's information*. Within this framework, we can get a coherent and fully justified Bayesian answer to the issue of sequential analysis, which furthermore satisfy the experimental investigators desideratum (Bunouf and Lecoutre, 2006).

References

Agresti, A., Min, Y. (2005). Frequentist performance of Bayesian confidence intervals for comparing proportions in 2×2 contingency tables. *Biometrics* **61**, 515–523.

Albert, J. (1996). *Bayesian Computation Using Minitab*. Wadsworth Publishing Company, Belmont.

Albert, J., Chib, S. (1993). Bayesian analysis of binary and polychotomous response data. *Journal of the American Statistical Association* **88**, 669–679.

Battan, L.J., Neyman, J., Scott, E.L., Smith, J.A. (1969). Whitetop experiment. *Science* **165**, 618.

Baum, M., Houghton, J., Abrams, K.R. (1989). Early stopping rules: clinical perspectives and ethical considerations. *Statistics in Medicine* **13**, 1459–1469.

Bayarri, M.J., Berger, J.O. (2004). The interplay of Bayesian and frequentist analysis. *Statistical Science* **19**, 58–80.

Berger, J. (2004). The case for objective Bayesian analysis. *Bayesian Analysis* **1**, 1–17.

Berger, J.O., Bernardo, J.M. (1992). On the development of reference priors (with discussion). In: Bernardo, J.M., Berger, J.O., Dawid, A.P., Smith, A.F.M. (Eds.), *Bayesian Statistics 4. Proceedings of the Fourth Valencia International Meeting*. Oxford University Press, Oxford, pp. 35–60.

Bernard, J.-M. (1996). Bayesian interpretation of frequentist procedures for a Bernoulli process. *The American Statistician* **50**, 7–13.

Bernardo, J.M. (1979). Reference posterior distributions for Bayesian inference (with discussion). *Journal of the Royal Statistical Society, Series B, Methodological* **41**, 113–147.

Bernardo, J.M. (1996). The concept of exchangeability and its applications. *Far East Journal of Mathematical Sciences* **4**, 111–121.

Bernardo, J., Smith, A.F.M. (1994). *Bayesian Theory*. Wiley, New York.

Bernoulli, J. (1713). *Ars Conjectandi* (English translation by Bing Sung as Technical report No. 2 of the Department of Statistics of Harvard University, February 12, 1966), Basel, Switzerland.

Berry, D.A. (1991). Experimental design for drug development: a Bayesian approach. *Journal of Biopharmaceutical Statistics* **1**, 81–101.

Berry, D.A. (1997). Teaching elementary Bayesian statistics with real applications in science. *The American Statistician* **51**, 241–246.

Box, G.E.P., Tiao, G.C. (1973). *Bayesian Inference in Statistical Analysis*. Addison Wesley, Reading, MA.

Brown, L.D., Cai, T., DasGupta, A. (2001). Interval estimation for a binomial proportion (with discussion). *Statistical Science* **16**, 101–133.

Bunouf, P. (2006). *Lois Bayesiennes a priori dans un Plan Binomial Sequentiel*. Unpublished Doctoral Thesis in Mathematics, Université de Rouen, France.

Bunouf, P., Lecoutre, B. (2006). Bayesian priors in sequential binomial design. *Comptes Rendus de L'Academie des Sciences Paris, Série I* **343**, 339–344.

Congdon, P. (2005). *Bayesian Models for Categorical Data*. Wiley, Chichester.

Copas, J.B., Loeber, R. (1990). Relative improvement over chance (RIOC) for 2×2 tables. *British Journal of Mathematical and Statistical Psychology* **43**, 293–307.

Cox, D.R. (1970). *The Analysis of Binary Data*. Methuen, London.

de Cristofaro, R. (1996). L'influence du plan d'echantillonnage dans inférence statistique. *Journal de la Société Statistique de Paris* **137**, 23–34.

de Cristofaro, R. (2004). On the foundations of likelihood principle. *Journal of Statistical Planning and Inference* **126**, 401–411.

de Cristofaro, R. (2006). Foundations of the 'objective Bayesian inference'. In: *First Symposium on Philosophy, History and Methodology of ERROR*. Virginia Tech., Blacksburg, VA.

de Finetti, B. (1972). *Probability, Induction and Statistics: The Art of Guessing*. Wiley, London.

de Finetti, B. (1974). *Theory of Probability* Vol. 1, Wiley, New York.

Dey, D., Rao, C.R. (eds.) (2005). Handbook of Statistics, 25, Bayesian Thinking, Modeling and Computation. Elsevier, North Holland.

Dickey, J.M. (1986). Discussion of Racine, A., Grieve, A. P., Fliihler, H. and Smith, A. F. M., Bayesian methods in practice: experiences in the pharmaceutical industry. *Applied Statistics* **35**, 93–150.

Dumouchel, W. (1990). Bayesian meta-analysis. In: Berry, D. (Ed.), *Statistical Methodology in Pharmaceutical Science*. Marcel-Dekker, New York, pp. 509–529.

Efron, B. (1998). R.A. Fisher in the 21st century [with discussion]. *Statistical Science* **13**, 95–122.

FDA. (2006). *Guidance for the Use of Bayesian Statistics in Medical Device, Draft Guidance for Industry and FDA Staff*. U.S. Department of Health and Human Services, Food and Drug Administration, Center for Devices and Radiological Health, Rockville MD.

Fisher, R.A. (1990/1925). *Statistical Methods for Research Workers* (Reprint, 14th ed., 1925, edited by J.H. Bennett). Oxford University Press, Oxford.

Fisher, R.A. (1990/1973). *Statistical Methods and Scientific Inference* (Reprint, 3rd ed., 1973, edited by J.H. Bennett). Oxford University Press, Oxford.

Fleiss, J.L. (1981). *Statistical Methods for Rates and Proportions*, 2nd ed. Wiley, New York.

Fraser, D.A.S., Reid, N., Wong, A., Yi, G.Y. (2003). Direct Bayes for interest parameters. In: Bernardo, J.M., Bayarri, M.J., Berger, J.O., Dawid, A.P., Heckerman, D., Smith, A.F.M., West, M. (Eds.), *Bayesian Statistics 7*. Oxford University Press, Oxford, pp. 529–534.

Freeman, P.R. (1993). The role of p-values in analysing trial results. *Statistics in Medicine* **12**, 1443–1452.

Gamerman, D. (1997). *Markov chain Monte Carlo: stochastic simulation for Bayesian inference*. Chapman & Hall, London.

Gilks, W.R., Richardson, S., Spiegelhalter, D.J. (1996). *Markov Chain Monte Carlo in Practice*. Chapman & Hall, London.

Good, I.J. (1980). Some history of the hierarchical Bayesian methodology. In: Bernardo, J.M., DeGroot, M.H., Lindley, D.V., Smith, A.F.M. (Eds.), *Bayesian Statistics*. Valencia University Press, Valencia, pp. 489–519.

Guttman, L. (1983). What is not what in statistics? *The Statistician* **26**, 81–107.

Inoue, L.Y.T., Berry, D.A., Parmigiani, G. (2005). Relationship between Bayesian and frequentist sample size determination. *The American Statistician* **59**, 79–87.

Irony, T.Z., Pennello, G.A. (2001). Choosing an appropriate prior for Bayesian medical device trials in the regulatory setting. In: *American Statistical Association 2001 Proceedings of the Biopharmaceutical Section*. American Statistical Association, Alexandria, VA.

Iversen, G.R. (2000). Why should we even teach statistics? A Bayesian perspective. In: *Proceedings of the IASE Round Table Conference on Training Researchers in the Use of Statistics*, The Institute of Statistical Mathematics, Tokyo, Japan.

Jaynes, E.T. (2003). In: Bretthorst, G.L. (Ed.), *Probability Theory: The Logic of Science*. Cambridge University Press, Cambridge.

Jeffreys, H. (1961). *Theory of Probability*, 3rd ed. Clarendon, Oxford (1st ed.: 1939).

Laplace, P.-S. (1986/1825). *Essai Philosophique sur les Probabilités* (Reprint, 5th ed., 1825). Christian Bourgois, Paris (English translation: *A Philosophical Essay on Probability*, 1952, Dover, New York).

Lecoutre, B. (1996). *Traitement statistique des donnees experimentales: des pratiques traditionnelles aux pratiques bayésiennes* [*Statistical Analysis of Experimental Data: From Traditional to Bayesian Procedures*]. DECISIA, Levallois-Perret, FR (with Windows Bayesian programs by B. Lecoutre and J. Poitevineau, freely available from the web site: http://www.univ-rouen.fr/LMRS/Persopage/Lecoutre/Eris).

Lecoutre, B. (2000). From significance tests to fiducial Bayesian inference. In: Rouanet, H., Bernard, J.-M., Bert, M.-C., Lecoutre, B., Lecoutre, M.-P., Le Roux, B. (Eds.), *New ways in statistical methodology: from significance tests to Bayesian inference (2nd ed.)*. Peter Lang, Bern, pp. 123–157.

Lecoutre, B. (2006a). Training students and researchers in Bayesian methods for experimental data analysis. *Journal of Data Science* **4**, 207–232.

Lecoutre, B. (2006b). And if you were a Bayesian without knowing it? In: Mohammad-Djafari, A. (Ed.), *26th Workshop on Bayesian Inference and Maximum Entropy Methods in Science and Engineering*. *AIP Conference Proceedings Vol. 872*, Melville, pp. 15–22.

Lecoutre, B., Charron, C. (2006b). Bayesian procedures for prediction analysis of implication hypotheses in 2 × 2 contingency tables. *Journal of Educational and Behavioral Statistics* **25**, 185–201.

Lecoutre, B., Derzko, G., Grouin, J.-M. (1995). Bayesian predictive approach for inference about proportions. *Statistics in Medicine* **14**, 1057–1063.

Lecoutre, B., ElQasyr, K. (2005). Play-the-winner rule in clinical trials: models for adaptive designs and Bayesian methods. In: Janssen, J., Lenca, P. (Eds.), *Applied Stochastic Models and Data Analysis Conference 2005 Proceedings, Part X. Health*. ENST Bretagne, Brest, France, pp. 1039–1050.

Lecoutre, B., Lecoutre, M.-P., Poitevineau, J. (2001). Uses, abuses and misuses of significance tests in the scientific community: won't the Bayesian choice be unavoidable? *International Statistical Review* **69**, 399–418.

Lecoutre, B., Mabika, B., Derzko, G. (2002). Assessment and monitoring in clinical trials when survival curves have distinct shapes in two groups: a Bayesian approach with Weibull modeling. *Statistics in Medicine* **21**, 663–674.

Lecoutre, B., Poitevineau, J. (1992). *PAC (Programme d Analyse des Comparaisons): Guide d'utilisation et manuel de reference*. CISIA-CERESTA, Montreuil, France.

Lecoutre, M.-P., Poitevineau, J., Lecoutre, B. (2003). Even statisticians are not immune to misinterpretations of null hypothesis significance tests. *International Journal of Psychology* **38**, 37–45.

Lee, P. (2004). *Bayesian Statistics: An Introduction*, 3rd ed. Oxford University Press, New York.

Mossman, D., Berger, J. (2001). Intervals for post-test probabilities: a comparison of five methods. *Medical Decision Making* **21**, 498–507.

O'Hagan, A. (1996). *First Bayes* [Teaching Package for Elementary Bayesian Statistics]. Retrieved January 10, 2007, from http://www.tonyohagan.co.uk/1b/.

Pagano, R.R. (1990). *Understanding Statistics in the Behavioral Sciences*, 3rd ed. West, St. Paul, MN.

Rice, W.R. (1988). A new probability model for determining exact *P* value for 2 × 2 contingency tables. *Biometrics* **44**, 1–22.

Rosnow, R.L., Rosenthal, R. (1996). Computing contrasts, effect sizes, and counternulls on other people's published data: general procedures for research consumers. *Psychological Methods* **1**, 331–340.

Rouanet, H. (2000a). Statistics for researchers. In: Rouanet, H., Bernard, J.-M., Bert, M.-C., Lecoutre, B., Lecoutre, M.-P., Le Roux, B. (Eds.), *New Ways in Statistical Methodology: From Significance Tests to Bayesian Inference (2nd ed.)*. Peter Lang, Bern, pp. 1–27.

Rouanet, H. (2000b). Statistical practice revisited. In: Rouanet, H., Bernard, J.-M., Bert, M.-C., Lecoutre, B., Lecoutre, M.-P., Le Roux, B. (Eds.), *New Ways in Statistical Methodology: From Significance Tests to Bayesian Inference (2nd ed.)*. Peter Lang, Bern, pp. 29–64.

Rouanet, H., Bernard, J.-M., Bert, M.-C., Lecoutre, B., Lecoutre, M.-P., Le Roux, B. (2000). *New Ways in Statistical Methodology: From Significance Tests to Bayesian Inference*, 2nd ed. Peter Lang, Bern.

Rozeboom, W.W. (1960). The fallacy of the null hypothesis significance test. *Psychological Bulletin* **57**, 416–428.

SAS Institute Inc. (2006). *Preliminary Capabilities for Bayesian Analysis in SAS/STAT® Software.* SAS Institute Inc, Cary, NC.

Savage, L. (1954). *The Foundations of Statistical Inference.* Wiley, New York.

Schmitt, S.A. (1969). *Measuring Uncertainty: An Elementary Introduction to Bayesian Statistics.* Addison Wesley, Reading, MA.

Smith, A. (1995). A conversation with Dennis Lindley. *Statistical Science* **10**, 305–319.

Spiegelhalter, D.J., Freedman, L.S., Parmar, M.K.B. (1994). Bayesian approaches to randomized trials. *Journal of the Royal Statistical Society, Series A* **157**, 357–416.

Sweeting, T.J. (2005). On the implementation of local probability matching priors for interest parameters. *Biometrika* **92**, 47–57.

Tan, S.B., Chung, Y.F.A., Tai, B.C., Cheung, Y.B., Machin, D. (2003). Elicitation of prior distributions for a phase III randomized controlled trial of adjuvant therapy with surgery for hepatocellular carcinoma. *Controlled Clinical Trials* **24**, 110–121.

Toecher, K.D. (1950). Extension of the Neyman–Pearson theory of tests to discontinuous variables. *Biometrika* **37**, 130–144.

Walley, P. (1996). Inferences from multinomial data: learning about a bag of marbles [with discussion]. *Journal of the Royal Statistical Society B* **58**, 3–57.

Winkler, R.L. (1974). Statistical analysis: theory versus practice. In: Stael Von Holstein, C.-A.S. (Ed.), *The Concept of Probability in Psychological Experiments.* D. Reidel, Dordrecht, pp. 127–140.

Zaykin, D.V., Meng, Z., Ghosh, S.K. (2004). Interval estimation of genetic susceptibility for retrospective case–control studies. *BMC Genetics* **5**(9), 1–11.

Zelen, M. (1969). Play the winner rule and the controlled clinical trial. *Journal of the American Statistical Association* **64**, 131–146.

Subject Index

www.ingramcontent.com/pod-product-compliance
Lightning Source LLC
Chambersburg PA
CBHW050454190326
41458CB00005B/1273

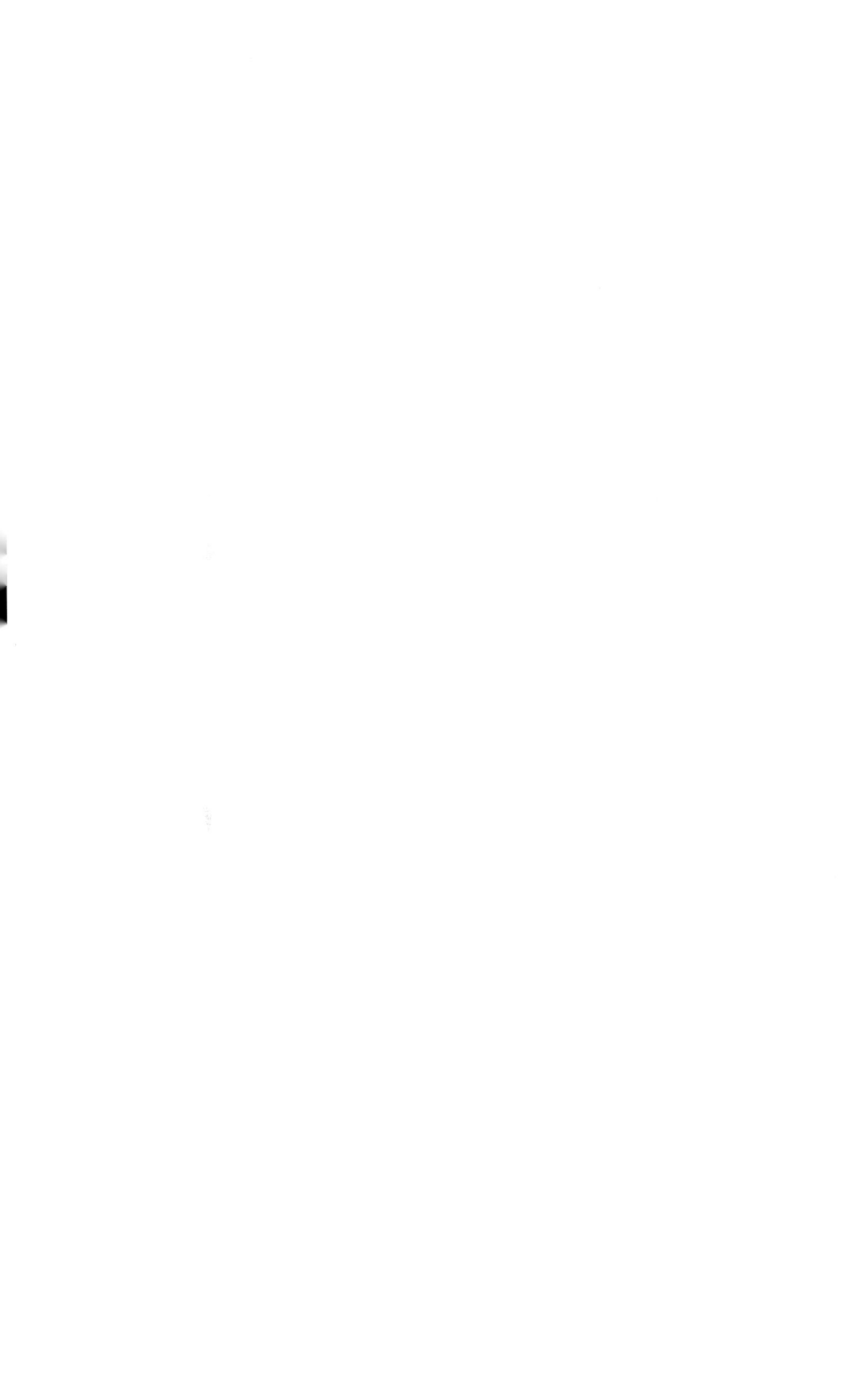